The Complete Keto Cookbook for Beginners

Easy Keto Diet Books with 600 Healthy Low-carb High-fat Recipes and 21 Days Meal Plan for Busy People to Burn Fat Fast

1000-Day Keto Recipe Book

Janet R. Smith

Copyright© 2020 By Janet R. Smith All Rights Reserved

The content contained within this book may not be reproduced, duplicated or transmitted without direct written permission from the author or the publisher.

Under no circumstances will any blame or legal responsibility be held against the publisher, or author, for any damages, reparation, or monetary loss due to the information contained within this book, either directly or indirectly.

Legal Notice:

This book is copyright protected. It is only for personal use. You cannot amend, distribute, sell, use, quote or paraphrase any part, or the content within this book, without the consent of the author or publisher.

Disclaimer Notice:

Please note the information contained within this document is for educational and entertainment purposes only. All effort has been executed to present accurate, up to date, reliable, complete information. No warranties of any kind are declared or implied. Readers acknowledge that the author is not engaged in the rendering of legal, financial, medical or professional advice. The content within this book has been derived from various sources. Please consult a licensed professional before attempting any techniques outlined in this book.

By reading this document, the reader agrees that under no circumstances is the author responsible for any losses, direct or indirect, that are incurred as a result of the use of the information contained within this document, including, but not limited to, errors, omissions, or inaccuracies.

Table of Content

Introduction 1

Chapter 1 The Basics of the Keto Diet 2

The Benefits of the Ketogenic Diet 3
How Keto Diet Works 4
8 Critical Tips for Entering Ketosis Quickly 5
Calculating and Tracking Your Macros 5
21-Day Meal Plan 8
Foods to Eat 10
Foods to Avoid 11
Tips for Successful and Happy Ketogenic Lifestyle 11
Some Effects You May Undergo During the Transition 13
Ketogenic Diet and Weight-Loss 13
5 Weight Loss Tips During the Keto Journey ... 14
Frequently Asked Questions 15

Chapter 2 Sauce and Dressing .. 18

1. Homemade Dijon Vinaigrette 18
2. Creamy Caesar Dressing 18
3. Tangy Avocado Crema 18
4. Avocado Mayonnaise 18
5. Chunky Lemony Blue Cheese 19
6. Bolognese Sauce 19
7. Cheesy Hot Crab Sauce 19
8. Spicy Enchilada Sauce 19
9. Basil Dressing 20
10. Fettuccine Alfredo 20
11. Bolognese Sauce 20
12. Sriracha Mayonnaise 20
13. Marinara Sauce 21
14. Hollandaise Sauce 21
15. Cheesy Spinach Basil Pesto 21
16. Basil Kale Pesto 22
17. Spanish Queso Sauce 22
18. Garlicky Mayonnaise 22
19. Tzatziki Sauce 22
20. Garlic Aioli Sauce 23
21. Asian Peanut Sauce 23
22. Oregano Balsamic Vinegar 23
Chapter 3 Egg and Dairy 25
23. Double Cheese Stuffed Bell Peppers 25
24. Mediterranean Aïoli 25
25. Egg Muffins 25
26. Herbed Cheese Balls 25
27. Cheesy Omelet and Vegetables 26
28. French Scrambled Eggs 26

29. Spicy Brown Mushroom Omelet 26
30. Scrambled Eggs and Baby Spinach 26
31. Egg, Scallion, Jalapeño Pepper Salad 27
32. Yogurt and Swiss Cheese Soup 27
33. Italian Bacon Omelet 27
34. Ham, Cheese and Egg Cups 27
35. Jalapeño Pepper Cream Cheese Omelet .. 28
36. Prosciutto and Egg Muffins 28
37. Greek Scrambled Eggs 28
38. Boiled Eggs with Lemony Avocado 29
39. Broccoli and Cauliflower Omelet 29
40. Paprika Egg Salad with Mayo 29
41. Old-Fashioned Greek Tirokroketes 29
42. Mediterranean Shakshuka 30
43. Crustless Cheesy Quiche Lorraine 30
44. Egg and Bacon Muffins with Kale 30
45. Goat Cheese Omelet 31
46. Bacon Frittata with Olives and Herbs 31
47. Cheesy Tomato Frittata 31
48. Fried Eggs with Canadian Bacon 31
49. Mangalore-Style Egg Curry 32
50. Two-Cheese Sausage Balls 32
51. Sausage Frittatas with Goat Cheese 32
52. Dilled Egg Salad with Dijon Mayo 32

Chapter 4 Pork 34

53. Pork and Beef Meatballs 34
54. Bacon and Pork Omelet 34
55. Mustard Pork Meatballs 34
56. Baked Cheesy Pork and Veggies 34
57. Cheesy Pork Nachos 35
58. Pork and Mashed Cauliflower Crust 35
59. Pork Chops and Bacon 35
60. Pork Steaks with Chimichurri Sauce 35
61. Balsamic Pork Loin Chops 36
62. Mediterranean Pork 36
63. Lemony Peanuts Pork Chops 36
64. Pork Shoulder and Sauerkraut Casserole .. 36
65. Pork Chops with Broccoli 37
66. Pork and Veggies Burgers 37
67. Golden Pork Burgers 37
68. Buttered Pork Chops 37
69. Creamy Pork Chops and Canadian Ham .. 38
70. Pork Chops with Blackberry Gravy 38
71. Lemony Pork Loin and Brussels Sprouts .. 38
72. Stewed Pork and Veggies 38
73. Pork Medallions with Rosemary 39
74. Lemony Pork Chops with Veggies 39
75. Pork with Raspberry Sauce 39
76. BBQ Grilled Pork Spare Ribs 39
77. Pork Steaks with Broccoli 40
78. Pork Lettuce Wraps 40

79. Pork Loin Chops 40
80. Lemony Pork Chops and Brussel Sprouts . 40
81. Tangy Pork Rib Roast 41
82. Pork Chops with Greek Salsa........................... 41
83. Tangy-Garlicky Pork Chops............................... 41
84. Pork and Butternut Squash Stew 42
85. Herbed Pork Chops with Cranberry Sauce . 42
86. Pork and Yellow Squash Traybake 42
87. Hearty Pork Stew Meat...................................... 43
88. Pork Meatballs in Pasta Sauce 43
89. Baked Pork Sausage and Bell Pepper 43
90. Pork Wraps with Veggies 44
91. Spicy Pork and Capers with Olives 44
92. Roasted Stuffed Pork Loin Steak 44
93. Parmesan Bacon-Stuffed Pork Roll 44
94. Tomato purée Pork Chops 45
95. Pork Kofte with Cauliflower Mash 45
96. Pork Pie 45
97. Homemade Pork Osso Bucco 45
98. Rosemary Lamb Chops 46
99. Lemony Pork Chops and Brussels Sprouts 46
100. Balsamic Pork Loin Chops 46
101. Pork Tenderloin with Lemon Chimichurri . 47
102. Herbed Pork Chops with Raspberry Sauce 47
103. Pork with Cranberry Sauce........................... 47
104. Garlicky Pork and Bell Peppers 48
105. Classic Carnitas... 48
106. Cranberry Pork Roast 48
107. Pork Patties with Caramelized Onion Rings 49
108. Lemony Pork Loin Roast 49

Chapter 5 Beef and Lamb 51

109. Skirt Steak with Green Beans 51
110. Zoodles with Beef Bolognese Sauce 51
111. Creole Beef Tripe Stew with Onions 51
112. King Size Beef Burgers 51
113. Ground Beef and Cauliflower Curry............. 52
114. Basil Feta Flank Steak Pinwheels 52
115. Creamy Reuben Soup with Sauerkraut 52
116. Beef and cauliflower rice Casserole 52
117. Beef Brisket with Red Wine 53
118. Grilled Ribeye Steaks with Green Beans ... 53
119. Basil Lamb Shoulder with Pine Nuts 53
120. Lemon-Mint Grilled Lamb Chops................. 53
121. Beef and Onion Stuffed Zucchinis 54
122. Garlicky Lamb Chops in White Wine 54
123. Grilled Lamb Kebabs 54
124. Beef and Mushroom Cheeseburgers 54
125. Asian-Flavored Beef and Broccoli 55
126. Juicy Beef with Thyme and Rosemary 55
127. Traditional Italian Bolognese Sauce 55
128. Sirloin Steak Skewers with Ranch Dressing 55
129. Mascarpone Beef Balls with Cilantro 56
130. Veggie cauliflower rice with Beef Steak 56
131. Beef Ragout with Green Beans 56

132. Beef Sausage Casserole with Okra 57
133. Rack of Lamb with Pepper Butter Sauce ... 57
134. Beef Stew with Black Olives.......................... 57
135. Beef-Stuffed Zucchini Boats 58
136. Sirloin Steak with Sauce Diane 58
137. Beef Lasagna with Zucchinis 58
138. Beef Steaks with Mushrooms and Bacon .. 59
139. Balsamic Glazed Meatloaf 59
140. Buttery Habanero and Beef Balls................. 59
141. Beef Meatloaf with Balsamic Glaze............. 60
142. Smoked Paprika Beef Ragout 60
143. Rump Steak Salad 60
144. Grilled Beef Skewers with Fresh Salad 61
145. Balsamic Glazed Meatloaf 61
146. Beef Meatball Salad with Dilled Yogurt 61
147. Beef Chuck Roast with Veggies 62
148. Cheesy Beef Gratin 62
149. Flank Steak and Kale Roll.............................. 62
150. Beef Casserole with Cauliflower 62
151. Seared Ribeye Steak with Shitake
Mushrooms 63
152. Lemon-Mustard Beef Rump Steak.............. 63
153. Paprika Roast Beef Brisket............................ 63
154. Italian Beef Roast with Jalapeño 63
155. Beef and Cauliflower Curry with Cilantro .. 64
156. Garlicky Lamb Chops with Sage 64
157. Juicy Beef Meatballs with Parsley 64
158. Beef and Mushrooms in Red Wine 64
159. Beef-Cabbage Casserole 65
160. Three-Cheese Beef Sausage Casserole.... 65
161. Beef and Egg cauliflower rice Bowls.......... 65

Chapter 6 Fish and Seafood 67

162. Anchovies and Veggies Wraps 67
163. Haddock with Mediterranean Sauce........... 67
164. Tuna Fillet Salade Niçoise 67
165. Anchovies with Caesar Dressing................. 67
166. Seafood Chowder... 68
167. Gambas al Ajillo 68
168. Garlicky Mackerel Fillet................................... 68
169. Curry White Fish Fillet 68
170. Sardine Burgers... 69
171. Crispy Keto Creamy Fish Casserole............ 69
172. Asian Salmon and Veggies Salad 69
173. Cheesy Shrimp Stuffed Mushrooms........... 70
174. Tuna Niçoise Salad 70
175. White Chowder 70
176. Provençal Lemony Fish Stew....................... 71
177. Alaskan Cod Fillet 71
178. Sole Fish Jambalaya 71
179. Smoked Haddock Burgers............................. 72
180. Cajun Tilapia Fish Burgers 72
181. Shrimp Jambalaya 72
182. Tuna, Ham and Avocado Wraps 72
183. Grilled Salmon Steak 73

184. Old Bay Sea Bass Fillet 73
185. Swedish Herring and Spinach Salad 73
186. Spanish Cod à La Nage................................ 73
187. Thai Tuna Fillet 74
188. Italian Haddock Fillet.................................... 74
189. Mediterranean Halibut Fillet 74
190. Cod Patties with Creamed Horseradish 74
191. Red Snapper Fillet and Salad 75
192. Lemony Shrimp and Veggie Bowl............... 75
193. Goan Sole Fillet Stew................................... 75
194. Cod Fillet with Summer Salad 75
195. Cheesy Cod Fillet 76
196. Spicy Tiger Prawns 76
197. Baked Halibut Steaks................................... 76
198. Salmon Tacos with Guajillo Sauce 76
199. Dijon Sea Bass Fillet 77
200. Monkfish Mayonnaise Salad........................ 77
201. Cod Fillet and Mustard Greens 77
202. Mahi Mahi Ceviche 77
203. Salmon Fillet 78
204. Tilapia Fillet... 78
205. Cod Fillet with Lemony Sesame Sauce...... 78
206. Shrimp and Sea Scallop............................... 78
207. Herbed Monkfish Fillet................................. 79
208. Old Bay Prawns 79
209. New Orleans Halibut and Crabmeat............ 79
210. Catfish Flakes and Cauliflower Casserole . 80
211. Tilapia and Shrimp Soup 80
212. Curry Tilapia.. 80
213. Cod Fillet with Parsley Pistou 81
214. Scallops and Calamari 81
215. Cheesy Tilapia Omelet 81
216. Rosemary-Lemon Snapper Fillet 82
217. Asian Scallop and Vegetable 82
218. Haddock and Turkey Smoked Sausage...... 82
219. Chepala Vepudu 83
220. Goat Cheese Stuffed Squid 83
221. Halászlé with Paprikash 83
222. Mackerel Fillet and Clam.............................. 84
223. Stir-Fried Scallops with Cauliflower 84
224. Swordfish with Greek Yogurt Sauce 84

Chapter 7 Poultry 86

225. Tuscan Chicken Breast Sauté 86
226. Roasted Chicken Breasts with Capers....... 86
227. Herbed Turkey with Cucumber Salsa 87
228. Spiced Chicken Breast 87
229. Lemony Rosemary Chicken Thighs............ 87
230. Slow Cooked Chicken Cacciatore............... 87
231. Spiced Chicken Wings 88
232. Herbed Turkey Breast 88
233. Cheesy Chicken and Tomato Packets 88
234. Grilled Lemony Chicken Wings 89
235. Turkey and Pumpkin Ragout....................... 89
236. Classic Jerk Chicken.................................... 89

237. Spicy Chicken Skewers 89
238. Pesto Turkey with Zucchini Spaghetti........ 90
239. Roast Herbs Stuffed Chicken 90
240. Itanlian Chicken Cacciatore......................... 90
241. Basil Turkey Meatballs 90
242. Hungarian Chicken Thighs.......................... 91
243. Braised Chicken and Veggies 91
244. Cooked Chicken in Creamy Spinach Sauce 91
245. Lemony Chicken Wings................................ 91
246. Creamy-Lemony Chicken Thighs................ 92
247. Dijon Chicken Thighs 92
248. Browned Chicken and Mushrooms 92
249. Bacon-Wrapped Chicken with Asparagus 92
250. Baked Cheesy Chicken and Spinach........... 93
251. Ritzy Baked Chicken with Vegetable 93
252. Chicken Paella and Chorizo 93
253. Lemony Chicken Skewers 94
254. Hearty Stuffed Chicken................................ 94
255. Cheesy Spinach Stuffed Chicken 94
256. Chicken Fingers.. 95
257. Stir-Fried Chicken, Broccoli and Cashew . 95
258. Marinated Chicken with Peanut Sauce....... 95
259. Chicken with Mayo-Avocado Sauce 96
260. Baked Cheesy Chicken and Zucchini.......... 96
261. Baked Chicken and Chorizo Sausages 96
262. Baked Chicken Skewers and Celery Fries . 97
263. Chicken Garam Masala 97
264. Coconut-Chicken Breasts............................ 97
265. Chili Chicken Breast 98
266. Garlicky Sweet Chicken Skewers 98
267. Mexican Chicken Mole 98
268. Cheesy Spinach Stuffed Chicken 99
269. Paprika Chicken with Steamed Broccoli.... 99
270. Chicken Breast with Anchovy Tapenade.... 99
271. Bacon on Cheesy Chicken Breast 99
272. Baked Chicken in Tomato Purée................100
273. Bacon Fat Browned Chicken.......................100
274. Traditional Chicken Stroganoff 100
275. Garlicky Chicken Thighs.............................101
276. Homemade Poulet en Papillote...................101
277. Parma Ham-Wrapped Stuffed Chicken......101
278. oasted Chicken..102
279. Parmesan Chicken Wings with Yogurt Sauce 102
280. Chicken in Creamy Mushroom Sauce 102

Chapter 8 Vegan and Vegetarian 104

281. Cauliflower and Celery Soup......................104
282. Mushroom and Bell Pepper Omelet............104
283. Mushroom and Zucchini Stew.....................104
284. Double Cheese Kale Bake 104
285. Lemony Cucumber-Avocado Salad 105
286. Citrus Asparagus and Cherry Tomato Salad 105
287. Shirataki Mushroom Ramen 105
288. Peanut Butter Crêpes with Coconut...........105

289. Greek-Style Aubergine-Egg Casserole.......106
290. Cheesy Egg-Stuffed Avocados 106
291. Mexican-Flavored Stuffed Peppers............106
292. Halloumi Asparagus Frittata......................106
293. Cheesy Broccoli Bake 107
294. Swiss Zucchini Gratin................................107
295. Garlicky Creamed Swiss Chard 107
296. Broccoli-Cabbage Soup............................107
297. Cauliflower Chowder with Fresh Dill 108
298. Provolone Zucchini Lasagna.....................108
299. Creamy Broccoli and Zucchini Soup 108
300. Cheesy Veggie Fritters..............................109
301. Creamy Summer Stew with Chives............109
302. Vegetable Stir-Fry with Seeds 109
303. Spinach and Zucchini Chowder.................109
304. Easy Roasted Asparagus with Mayo Sauce 110
305. Spiced Mashed Cauliflower.......................110
306. Italian Broccoli and Spinach Soup 110
307. Braised Mushrooms with Parsley 110
308. Colby Broccoli Bake...................................111
309. Hearty Veggie Stir-Fry................................111
310. Braised Mushrooms and Cabbage 111
311. Balsamic Zucchini Salad............................112
312. Creamy Cabbage and Cauliflower 112
313. Peppery Omelet with Cheddar Cheese 112
314. Parmesan Zoodles with Avocado Sauce ...112
315. Chinese Cabbage Stir-Fry..........................113
316. Balsamic Broccoli Salad 113
317. Herbed Cheese Balls with Walnuts 113
318. Fried Veggies with Eggs 113
319. Creamy Broccoli-Spinach Soup 114
320. Mediterranean Cauliflower Quiche 114
321. Indian Tomato Soup with Raita 114
322. Traditional Thai Tom Kha Soup..................115
323. Italian Pepper and Mushrooms Stew 115
324. Homemade Coleslaw with Cauliflower.......115
325. Slow Cooked Spaghetti Squash..................115
326. Baked Stuffed Peppers with Olives 116
327. Greek Roasted Cauliflower with Feta Cheese116
328. Creamy Vegetable Chowder......................116
329. Double Cheese Braised Vegetables...........116
330. Broccoli Salad with Tahini Dressing 117
331. Spinach and Egg Salad..............................117
332. Garlicky Voodles with Avocado Sauce......117
333. Garlicky Cauliflower-Pecan Casserole 117
334. Spicy Roasted Eggplant with Avocado 118
335. Button Mushroom Stroganoff 118
336. Mozzarella Creamed Salad with Basil........118
337. Lebanese Tabbouleh Salad 119
338. Provençal Ratatouille Casserole................119
339. Gouda Cauli-Broccoli Casserole................119

Chapter 9 Soup 121

340. Rich Taco Soup..121
341. Creamy Turkey and Celery Soup 121
342. Rich Cheesy Bacon-Cauliflower Soup 121
343. Tangy Cucumber and Avocado Soup 121
344. Nacho Soup..122
345. Spiced-Pumpkin Soup 122
346. Saffron Coconut Shrimp Soup....................122
347. Creamy-Cheesy Cauliflower Soup.............123
348. Colden Gazpacho Soup.............................123
349. Cioppino...123
350. Creamy Tomato Soup.................................124
351. Cheesy Cauliflower Soup 124
352. Power Green Soup 124
353. Almond Soup with Sour Cream and Cilantro 124
354. Slow Cooked Faux Lasagna Soup..............125
355. Creamy-Lemony Chicken Soup 125
356. Coconut Cheesy Cauliflower Soup 125
357. Pork and Vegetable Soup 126
358. Green Minestrone Soup 126
359. Reuben Beef Soup.....................................126
360. Curry Green Beans and Shrimp Soup........126
361. Cheesy Broccoli Soup 127
362. Lush Vegetable Soup 127
363. Creamy Chicken Soup 127
364. Salsa Verde Chicken Soup 127
365. Creamy Cauliflower Soup with Sausage ...128
366. Spicy Chicken Soup 128
367. Red Curry Shrimp and Bean Soup 128
368. White Mushroom Cream Soup with Herbs 128
369. Turnip and Soup with Pork Sausage 129
370. Creamy Cauliflower and Leek Soup 129
371. Cheesy Broccoli and Spinach Soup...........129
372. Butternut Squash Soup 129
373. Heavy Cream-Cheese Broccoli Soup 130
374. Creamy Tomato Soup with Basil 130
375. Buffalo Cheese Chicken Soup 130
376. Cheesy Tomato and Onion Soup 130
377. Turkey and Veggies Soup 131
378. Asparagus Parmesan Soup 131
379. Cheesy Broccoli and Bacon Soup 131
380. Creamy Tomato Soup.................................131
381. Spiced Pumpkin Soup 132
382. Spinach Mozzarella Soup 132
383. Spiced Cucumber Soup 132

Chapter 10 Salad 134

384. Classic Greek Salad 134
385. Caesar Salad with Salmon and Egg 134
386. Tuna Salad with Olives and Lettuce 134
387. Lemony Prawn and Arugula Salad 134
388. Mediterranean Tomato and Avocado Salad 135
389. Salmon Fillet and Spinach Cobb Salad......135
390. Egg and Chicken Salad in Lettuce Cups ...135
391. Tuna Cheese Caprese Salad 136
392. Balsamic Brussels Sprouts Cheese Salad 136
393. Garlicky Chicken Salad 136
394. Shrimp Salad with Lemony Mayonnaise ...136

395. Mackerel and Green Bean Salad 137
396. Strawberry and Spinach Salad 137
397. Cheesy Pork Patties Salad 137
398. Bacon, Avocado, and Veggies Salad 137
399. Cheesy Green Salad with Bacon 138
400. Shrimp, Cauliflower and Avocado Salad ...138
401. Mozzarella Bacon and Tomato Salad 138
402. Skirt Steak, Veggies, and Pecan Salad.......138
403. Spring Vegetable Salad with Cheese Balls 139
404. Baby Arugula and Walnuts Salad 139
405. Ritzy Chicken Salad with Tzatziki Sauce....139
406. Tuscan Kale Salad with Lemony Anchovies 140
407. Caesar Salad with Chicken and Cheese 140
408. Tangy Squid and Veggies Salad 140
409. Mustard Eggs Salad 140
410. Skirt Steak and Pickled Peppers Salad 141
411. Lush Greek Salad 141
412. Dijon Broccoli Slaw Salad 141
413. Tangy Shrimp Ceviche Salad 141
414. Dijon Cauliflower Salad.................................142
415. Classic Caprese Salad 142
416. Cheesy Bacon Salad with Walnuts 142
417. Turkey and Walnuts Salad 143
418. Dijon Egg Salad 143
419. Vinegary Cucumber Salad 143
420. Homemade Albacore Tuna Salad................143

Chapter 11 Side Dishes 145

421. Roasted Cauliflower with Serrano Ham 145
422. Chicken-Stuffed Cucumber Bites 145
423. Roasted Brussels Sprouts with Balsamic Glaze...145
424. Cheddar Buffalo Chicken Bake 145
425. Chicken Breast Fritters with Dill Dip 146
426. Simple Buttery Broccoli.................................146
427. Classic Devilled Eggs with Sriracha Mayo 146
428. Cheesy Cauli Bake with Mayo 146
429. Mashed Cauliflower with Bacon and Chives 147
430. Baked Zucchini Sticks with Garlic Aioli 147
431. Crispy Chorizo with Parsley 147
432. Simple Boiled Stuffed Eggs 147
433. Garlicky Roasted Vegetable Mix 148
434. Avocado Crostini Nori with Walnuts...........148
435. Baked Spinach Cheese Balls 148
436. Pecorino Mushroom Burgers 148
437. Feta Zucchini and Pepper Gratin 149
438. Prosciutto-Wrapped Piquillo Peppers........149
439. Colby Bacon-Wrapped Jalapeño Peppers.149
440. Ricotta Spinach Gnocchi 149
441. Mascarpone Turkey Pastrami Pinwheels ...150
442. Scrambled Eggs with Swiss Chard Pesto .150
443. Parmesan Cauliflower Fritters.....................150
444. Garlicky Roasted Broccoli 150
445. Grilled Prosciutto-Chicken Wraps 151
446. Buttered Mushrooms with Sage 151
447. Tuna-Mayo Topped Dill Pickles 151
448. Parmesan Creamed Spinach.......................151
449. Mozzarella Prosciutto Wraps with Basil.....152
450. Fried Cauliflower Rice with Peppers 152
451. Zoodles with Almond-Basil Pesto 152
452. Smoked Mackerel and Turnip Patties 153
453. Spicy Onion Rings 153
454. Baked Broccoli Bites.....................................153
455. Herbed Roasted Radishes 153
456. Roasted Brussels Sprouts with Balsamic Glaze...154
457. Cheesy Ham Pizza Rolls 154
458. Duo-Cheese Lettuce Rolls 154
459. Liverwurst and Pistachio Balls 154
460. Spiced Baked Gruyere Crisps.....................155
461. Cauli Rice with Cheddar and Bacon 155
462. Oven Baked String Beans and Mushrooms 155
463. Avocado-Bacon Stuffed Eggs 155

Chapter 12 Appetizers and Snacks 157

464. Avocado and Ham Stuffed Eggs 157
465. Mini Bacon and Kale Muffins.......................157
466. Fajita Spareribs..157
467. Herbed Provolone Cheese Chips...............157
468. Crispy Five Seed Crackers 158
469. Traditional Walnut Fat Bombs.....................158
470. Avocado-Bacon Sushi..................................158
471. Bacon-Wrapped Enoki Mushrooms 158
472. Paprika Veggie Bites 159
473. Herbed Prawn and Veggie Skewers............159
474. Beef-Stuffed Peppers 159
475. Spicy Chicken Drumettes 159
476. Cheesy Ham-Egg Cups................................160
477. Chicken Wings with Ranch Dressing 160
478. Cheesy Ham and Chicken Bites.................160
479. Baked Romano Zucchini Rounds 160
480. Whiskey-Glazed Chicken Wings 161
481. Deviled Eggs with Roasted Peppers 161
482. Cheesy Prosciutto Balls 161
483. Crispy Fried Dill Pickles...............................161
484. Parmesan Crab Dip 162
485. Cheddar Anchovies Fat Bombs 162
486. Turkey and Avocado Roll-Ups.....................162
487. Deviled Eggs with Chives 162
488. Romano Cheese Meatballs 163
489. Chicken Wings in Spicy Tomato Sauce 163
490. Greek-Style Ricotta Olive Dip......................163
491. Classic Caprese Skewers 163
492. Baked Cocktail Franks 164
493. Bacon-Loaded Deviled Eggs 164
494. Lettuce Wraps with Ham and Tomato........164
495. Lime Brussels Sprout Chips 164
496. Mozzarella Meatballs....................................165
497. Hearty Burger Dip..165

498. Italian Cheddar Cheese Crisps 165
499. Ranch Chicken-Bacon Dip........................ 165
500. Cheesy Charcuterie Board 166
501. Cheese Crisps with Basil 166
502. Creamy Herb Dip 166
503. Fresh Homemade Guacamole 166
504. Lemony Bacon Chips 167
505. Mexican Shrimp-Stuffed Avocados 167
506. Blue Cheese and Ranch Dip 167
507. Italian Fried Mozzarella Sticks................... 167
508. Margherita Pizza with Mushrooms............. 168
509. Oven-Baked Prosciutto-Wrapped Asparagus... 168
510. Cheesy Bacon-Stuffed Jalapeño Poppers ..168

Chapter 13 Desserts 170

511. Coffee-Coconut Ice Pops......................... 170
512. Cheesy Lemonade Fat Bomb 170
513. Coconut-Fudge Ice Pops......................... 170
514. Chocolate-Coconut Shake....................... 170
515. Crispy Strawberry Chocolate Bark 171
516. Creamy Strawberry Shake....................... 171
517. Fresh Strawberry Cheesecake Mousse...... 171
518. Cheesecake Fat Bomb with Berries 171
519. Simple Peanut Butter Fat Bomb 172
520. Keto Peanut Butter Cookies 172
521. Baked Cheesecake Bites 172
522. Pumpkin Cheesecake Bites..................... 172
523. Chocolate Pecan-Berry Mascarpone Bowl 173
524. Chocolate Chip Ice Cream with Mint 173
525. Creamsicle Float.................................... 173
526. Creamy Chocolate Mousse...................... 173
527. Avocado-Chocolate Pudding 174
528. Slow Cooker Chocolate Pot De Crème 174
529. Lemon Custard 174
530. Ginger-Pumpkin Pudding 174
531. Pumpkin Compote with Mix Berries 175
532. Almond-Sour Cream Cheesecake............. 175
533. Almond-Peanut Butter Cheesecake........... 175
534. Blackberry Cobbler with Almonds 176
535. Almond Chocolate Cookies...................... 176
536. Citrus Raspberry Custard Cake 176
537. Peanut Butter Cupcake 177
538. Blueberry-Pecan Crisp............................ 177
539. Vanilla-Flavored Hazelnut Ice Cream 177
540. Tender Almond Pound Cake 178
541. Old-fashioned Gingerbread Cake 178
542. Pecan-Carrot Muffins 178
543. Chocolate Brownie Cake 179
544. Coconut Lemon Truffles with Pecans 179
545. Keto Almond Butter Fudge....................... 179
546. Super Easy Peanut Butter Mousse 179
547. Classic Almond Golden Cake................... 180
548. Almond Butter Fat Bombs........................ 180
549. Banana Fat Bombs................................. 180
550. Easy Dark Chocolate Fudge..................... 180
551. Simple Blueberry Fat Bombs 181
552. Almond Flour Crusted Cheesecake........... 181
553. Coconut-Vanilla Ice Pops......................... 181
554. Blueberry-Almond Muffins 182
555. Pumpkin-Almond Fat Bombs 182
556. Hazelnut Shortbread Cookies 182
557. Coconut-Chocolate Treats 182
558. Vanilla-Raspberry Cheesecake 183
559. Blueberry-Vanilla Pudding 183
560. Cream Cheese Chocolate Mousse............ 183
561. Keto Vanilla Ice Cream............................ 183
562. Spicy Almond Fat Bombs 184
563. Microwaved Rhubarb Cakes..................... 184
564. Chia Pudding with Blueberries 184
565. Almond and Cinnamon Truffles 184
566. Macadamia Nut and Chocolate Fat Bombs 185
567. Strawberry Popsicles 185
568. No-Bake Hemp Seeds and Chocolate Cookies.. 185
569. Cardamom Orange Bark 185
570. Gingersnap Nutmeg Cookies 186
571. Lemony Poppy Seed Cookies 186
572. Keto Matcha Brownies with Pistachios...... 186
573. Easy Peanut Butter Cookies.................... 187
574. Raspberry and Chocolate Fat Bombs 187
575. Strawberries in Chocolate 187
576. Healthy Blueberry Fat Bombs 187

Chapter 14 Smoothies 189

577. Avocado and Berry Smoothie 189
578. Blueberry-Almond Butter Smoothie 189
579. Morning Five Greens Smoothie 189
580. Spiced Pistachio-Lemon Smoothie 189
581. Easy Peanut Butter Smoothie 190
582. Classic PB and J Smoothie 190
583. Raspberry and Kale Smoothie.................. 190
584. Creamy Cashew Lemon Smoothie............ 190
585. Spinach and Cucumber Smoothie 190
586. Spinach-Cucumber Smoothie 191
587. Creamy Vanilla Smoothie 191
588. Vanilla Coconut Smoothie 191
589. Double-Berry Coconut Smoothie 191
590. Apple-Almond Butter Smoothie 191
591. Blueberry-Spinach Smoothie 191
592. Refreshing Green Smoothie 192
593. Avocado Smoothie with Mixed Berries 192
594. Lemony Berry Smoothie 192
595. Creamy Flaxseed-Ginger Smoothie 192
596. Coconut Strawberry Smoothie 193
597. Spinach and Hemp Heart Smoothie 193
598. Avocado and Almond Smoothie 193
599. Avocado and Seed Smoothie Bowl 193
600. Turmeric Avocado Smoothie 193

Appendix 1: Measurement Conversion Chart... 194
Appendix 2: Recipe Index..................... 195

Introduction

Are you struggling to find the best way to lose weight? Well, you can now sit and relax because that came to an end a few seconds ago. I am a living testimony that Keto diet is the ultimate problem solver and is 100% effective.

If you last saw me a year ago, and you see me right now, you would be surprised that I am a totally different person in terms of my size. In that time, I have shed off about half of my weight.

I must say that it's not easy to be overweight, or rather to weigh much more than the average person. To make you understand, let's do a flashback of me some years back.

"Janet, you are getting so fat". That was the statement from one of the girls in my class. Me? Fat? No way! "I am not fat", I tried to comfort myself. Honestly speaking, that statement struck me like a sword while deep down I knew it was true. Imagine a situation in school where the boys are trying to get girlfriend, you are told you are fat! Moreover, the words from a lady makes thing worse.

I just had to do something immediately that would make me cut my weight. I decided to cut the "fatty" foods that I thought greatly contributed to my weight. I was in college when I noticed that I was becoming "overweight".

Fast-forward three months later I was shocked when I realized

that instead of cutting my weight, I had gained two pounds. "How on earth did that happen?" I couldn't help but think that I had made such a joke of myself because the results were the opposite of what I expected. "There has to be a way out of this", I told myself.

In the process of finding a solution, my friend Anthony told me of keto diet. He told me that his mom used that diet and she lost her weight even without having to avoid "fatty" foods like me. That is the moment I made a decision that I will try this diet.

I must say that was the best decision I ever made in regard to my weight. I have managed to cut my weight while enjoying the delicious keto recipes. I wished I had earlier met someone to tell me about the amazing keto diet.

With keto diet, there is a wide variety of meals that you can eat. There are snacks, appetizers, poultry, meat and also drinks. You will enjoy the best recipes while you lose weight effortlessly. Who wouldn't want that? I know you want it too. This is the reason why you should go for keto diet and enjoy its full benefits.

This book is the ultimate guide to ketogenic diet. It has all the information that you need to know about keto. The recipes in this book are proven to work. I have cooked every one of them and they are the reason I have cut a lot of weight. Try them today and you will not regret.

Thanks for downloading my book! Enjoy reading!

Chapter 1 The Basics of the Keto Diet

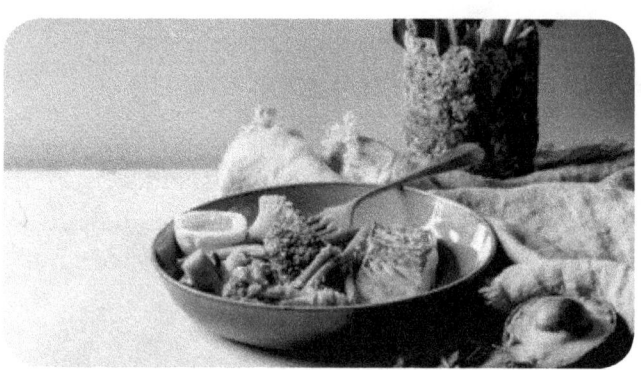

The name "ketogenic" diet comes from the word "ketone." Ketones are small molecules produced in the body and used for fuel when glucose is not available. They are produced in the liver from fat and can then be used throughout the body as a source of energy – they can even be used by the brain!

In order to switch your body from burning glucose for energy to producing ketones, you need to significantly reduce your carbohydrate intake and increase your fat intake, so you have energy stores to draw from.

This is the basis of the ketogenic diet – it is a low carb, high fat, moderate protein diet.

To help you understand how the ketogenic diet is different, you need to understand how your body is currently burning energy. If you follow the typical Western diet, you probably eat a lot of grain-based foods, processed carbohydrates, and added sugar. Each of these foods is broken down by the digestive system into their primary components which include glucose.

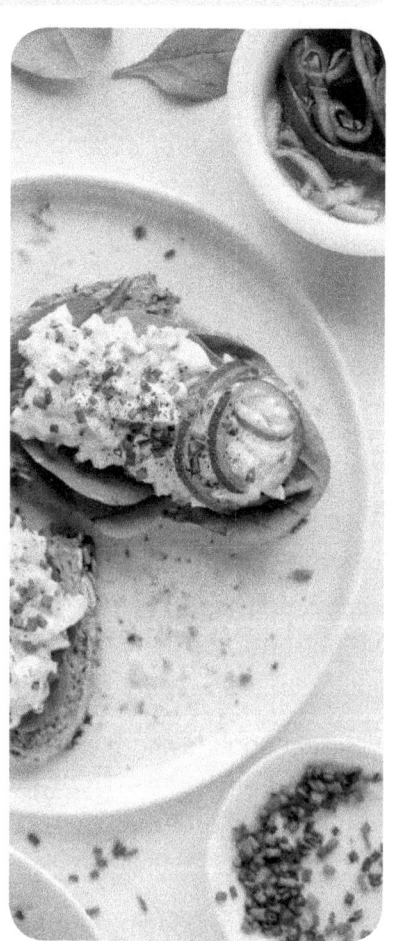

Glucose is a source of energy that is very easy for the body to burn. When you consume simple carbohydrates (things like processed carbs and sugar), your body breaks them down quickly and the glucose becomes available as a fast-burning source of energy.

When you have more glucose than your body can use in the moment, your body stores the excess in your cells in the form of glycogen. Later, when your body needs more energy, but you haven't eaten recently, it can tap into those glycogen stores to find the energy it needs. If you continue to restrict your carbohydrate intake, your body will burn through those glycogen stores at which point it will need to find another source of energy – that's when ketones come in.

In the absence of glucose, your body starts to burn through your fat stores in a process that produces ketones. Ketones are a highly efficient source of fuel that can be used by the whole body, including your brain.

When your body switches over from burning glucose as energy to burning fat instead, it enters a state of ketosis. The goal of the ketogenic diet is to enter and then maintain this metabolic state in which your body will burn your stored fat for fuel, helping you lose weight.

The longer you follow the ketogenic diet, the more your body adapts, and you will experience additional benefits. Keep reading to find out what they are.

The Benefits of the Ketogenic Diet

The primary benefit of the ketogenic diet is, of course, weight loss. If you stick to the diet for a while, however, you'll experience a wide range of other benefits. Here is a quick overview of some of the top health benefits associated with the keto diet:

- Fast weight loss without feeling hungry or deprived – fat keeps you feeling full longer than carbohydrates.

- Healthy fat consumption supports cardiovascular health and reduces risk factors such as high blood pressure and high cholesterol.

- The ketogenic diet offers neuroprotective benefits, helping slow down the progression of neurodegenerative disease and prevent conditions like Parkinson's and Alzheimer's.

- Could reduce the risk of cancer and may improve the efficacy of cancer treatments – may also reduce the severity of side effects from chemotherapy and radiation treatments.

- Improve microflora balance in the digestive tract for improved skin health – helps to fight chronic acne and other skin conditions.

- May reduce the frequency or severity of seizures in people with seizure disorders like epilepsy – particularly for children with epilepsy.

- Improve symptoms of polycystic ovary syndrome (PCOS) in women and may help treat the condition.

- Increase mental performance(e.g, improve concentration and focus)

- Regulate blood sugar levels to help improve or reverse type 2 diabetes by lowering blood sugar levels and regulating insulin.

- Improve health indicators to prevent chronic diseases.

- May help improve symptoms of mental health issues., For example, it may reduce anxiety and depression as well as mood swings.

The benefits you receive from the ketogenic diet depend on how well you stick to your macronutrient ratio and how long you follow the diet. There is nothing wrong with following the diet for a few months to meet your goals, but you should consider making the ketogenic diet your long-term eating plan because of all the wonderful health benefits listed above.

Though the ketogenic diet has the potential to provide a great many benefits, it is not the right choice for everyone. If you take medications for diabetes or hypertension, you may want to talk to your doctor before starting the diet.

How Keto Diet Works

For each activity that the body partakes in, there is a considerable amount of energy utilized. This energy comes from a wide range of sources in the body, high on the list being carbohydrates which are quickly converted into glucose –an ever-ready energy. Not only that, the body would also be fueled by fat and protein that is broken down into water soluble particles in the body. However, fat is not as easily digestible into the system as are carbohydrates. Excess fat ends up being stored within the body. For this reason, if you then want to reduce the amount of fat in your body, the idea is to systematically reduce the sugar and carbs in the diet. When the body runs out of ready-to make sugar, it seeks alternate sources of energy.

At this point, ketones come into play. Ketones are created from a combination of three main soluble compounds; acetoacetate, acetone and B-hydroxybutyrate, commonly known as BHB. These are produced by the liver in the absence of carbs for energy. All the stored fat and protein begin to be utilized, burnt and converted into ketones for the body to continue functioning well. Ketosis is the state you are in when this happens.

Ketosis can thus be deliberate or a result of starvation or continued fasting, this way ketosis can have both positive and negative effects on the body. The safest way to achieve a state of ketosis is the deliberate one, attained through a specially formulated diet which excludes starchy foods and increased protein. In medical scenarios, it has been known since the 1912s that a state where the body is fueled by energy proceeding from fat and protein and no carbs can be extremely beneficial for the body.

This was discovered after testing and observing patients to take a controlled ketogenic diet. After a couple of weeks, patients previously suffering from epileptic episodes showed signs of improvement, experiencing less seizures and better control of their mental faculties. Mayo Clinic's Dr. Russel Wilder then named the "ketogenic diet" and to date, it has been prescribed to some patients presenting epilepsy, autism, hypertension and many other ailments because the ketones that fuel the brain enhance brain functionality much better than the energy fueled by carbs.

8 Critical Tips for Entering Ketosis Quickly

Now that you know the benefits of the ketogenic diet and the secret to activate your body's fat-burning switch, all you have to do is take the necessary steps to enter ketosis. If you stick to your macros, you should be able to enter ketosis within 5 to 10 days. Here are some simple tips to expedite the process:

1. Minimize your carbohydrate intake – try to consume no more than 20 grams per day and focus on whole food sources like fresh veggies rather than processed carbohydrates.

2. Maximize your fat intake, focusing on healthy sources like coconut oil, avocado, and other sources of MCTs.

3. Start each day with a brisk 15 to 30 minute walk before breakfast to help burn through your glycogen stores.

4. Make fat the star of every meal and consume moderate amounts of protein with each meal – just try not to go overboard on protein.

5. Try intermittent fasting to encourage your body to enter a state of ketosis more quickly – one easy way is to stop eating at 8pm everyday then have your first meal at noon.

6. Start testing your ketones with a urine test after the first 3 days and make adjustments to your diet as needed.

7. Try taking exogenous ketone supplements to speed up the process of entering a state of ketosis.

8. Track your macros and try to stick within the recommended macronutrient range as much as possible.

* As you take the steps above to encourage your body to enter a state of ketosis, you may experience some negative side effects along the way. It takes time for your body to adjust to any major change you make to your diet or lifestyle, so be prepared.

Calculating and Tracking Your Macros

The beauty of the ketogenic diet is that it is not a typical crash diet – you don't have to severely restrict your calorie intake. In fact, you don't have to count calories at all!

The key to the ketogenic diet is maintaining the right macronutrient ratio. This simply means that you eat a specific amount of fat, protein, and carbs each day to maintain a specific ratio of macronutrients. As long as you stick to your macros, it doesn't matter all that much how many calories you consume.

But What is the Recommended Macronutrient Ratio For The Ketogenic Diet?

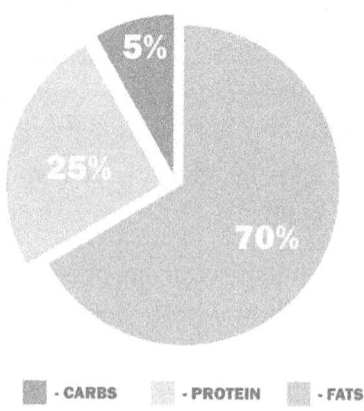

The idea is to consume most of your daily calories in the form of fat with moderate protein intake and low carb intake. Generally speaking, you aim for 70% to 75% of your daily calorie intake to come from fat, 20% to 25% from protein, and no more than 5% from carbohydrates. Some people like to limit their carb intake to 20g or 25g daily, but you have some wiggle room as long as you stick to the right ratio.

What if You Want To Stick To a Certain Calorie Range?

If your primary goal with the ketogenic diet is to lose weight, you may want to eat at a slight calorie deficit to help boost your results. You can find plenty of free calculators online to help you determine your ideal calorie range, and then you can use that information to determine how many grams of fat, protein, and carbs you can consume to stay within the right ratio.

Here's How to Calculate Your Macros:

1. Take your total daily calorie intake and multiply it by 70% (or 0.70) – this will tell you how many of your daily calories should come from fat.

2. Do the same with 75% to find the upper end of your fat intake range.

3. Take the total number of calories from fat (from Step 1) and divide it by 9 (each gram of fat contains 9 calories).

4. Repeat this with the value from Step 2 – now you know what range you want to stay within for your fat intake.

5. Repeat these four steps with your protein range – you'll need to divide your calories from protein by 4 instead of 9 (each gram of protein contains 4 calories).

6. Repeat with your 5% carbohydrate intake, dividing the total calories from carbs by 4 to determine your daily carb intake in grams.

To show you what this looks like, here is an example using a daily calorie intake of 1,600 calories:

- 1,600 x 70% (0.70) = 1,120 / 9 = 124 grams
- 1,600 x 75% (0.75) = 1,200 / 9 = 133 grams

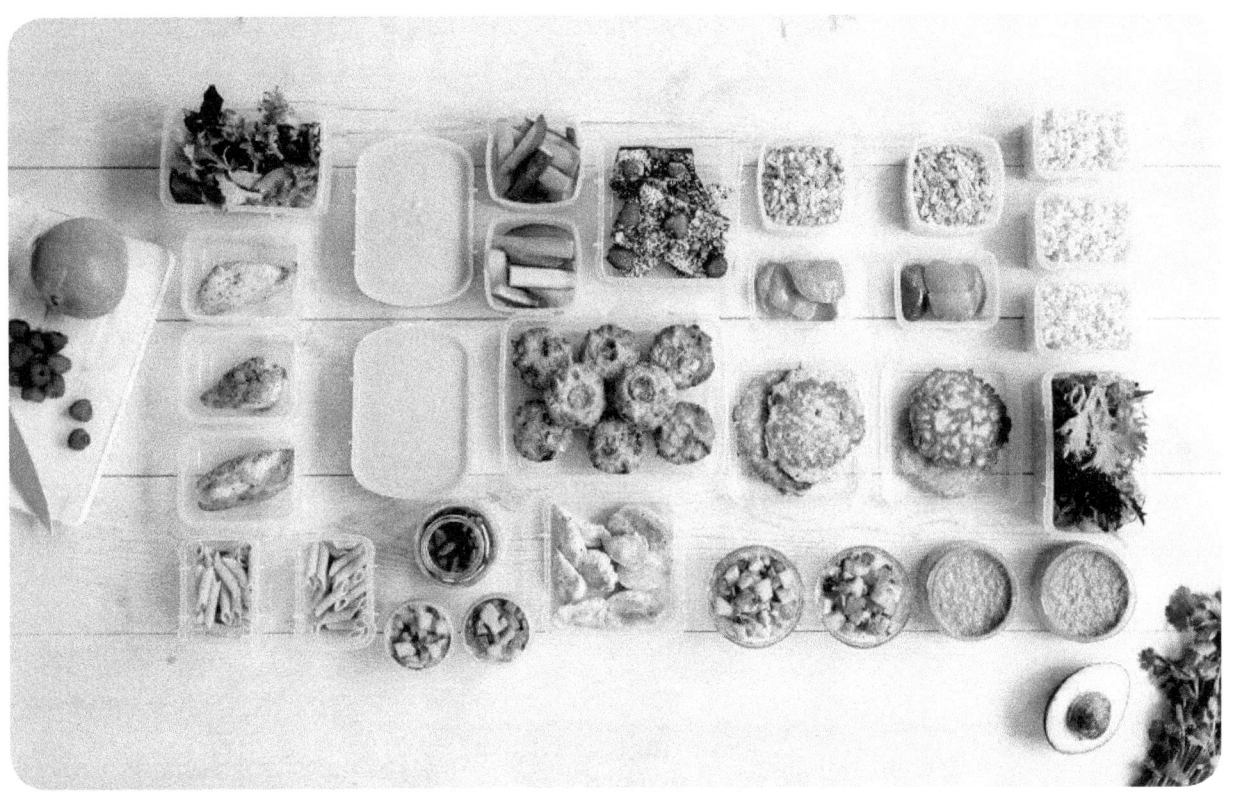

So, now you can see that your daily macro range for fat should be between 124 and 133 grams. You can do the same calculations for protein, dividing your total calories from protein by 4, and again for carbohydrates. Using these calculations, you can determine your individual macronutrient range based on your daily calorie goals.

By now you should have a thorough understanding of the ketogenic diet and how to make it work for you. All that is left now is to give it a try!

So, turn the page to check out the three weekly meal plans. Each week you'll be preparing easy ketogenic meals in a day-by-day plan designed to help you stick to your macros. Plus, each recipe features no more than 6 main ingredients which means that it is as simple as possible.

If you're ready to get started, just turn the page!

21-Day Meal Plan

	Breakfast	Lunch	Dinner	Snack/Dessert
1	Cheesy Omelet and Vegetables	Grilled Beef Skewers with Fresh Salad	Thai Tuna Fillet	Fresh Strawberry Cheesecake Mousse
2	Crustless Cheesy Quiche Lorraine	Italian Beef Roast with Jalapeño	Rosemary-Lemon Snapper Fillet	Chocolate-Peanut Butter Fudge
3	Yogurt and Swiss Cheese Soup	Balsamic Glazed Meatloaf	Grilled Salmon Steak	Chocolate-Coconut Shake
4	Mediterranean Shakshuka	Buttery Habanero and Beef Balls	Roast Herbs Stuffed Chicken	Pecan-Carrot Muffins
5	Prosciutto and Egg Muffins	Pork and Yellow Squash Traybake	Baked Halibut Steaks	Pumpkin Cheesecake Bites
6	Yogurt and Swiss Cheese Soup	Grilled Beef Skewers with Fresh Salad	Catfish Flakes and Cauliflower Casserole	Almond Flour Crusted Cheesecake
7	Cheesy Omelet and Vegetables	Pork and Yellow Squash Traybake	Braised Chicken and Veggies	Creamy Chocolate Mousse
8	Double-Berry Coconut Smoothie	Asian-Flavored Beef and Broccoli	Pork and Butternut Squash Stew	Creamy Chocolate Mousse
9	Egg and Bacon Muffins with Kale	Skirt Steak with Green Beans	Slow Cooked Chicken Cacciatore	Chocolate-Peanut Butter Fudge
10	Turmeric Avocado Smoothie	Veggie Cauliflower Rice with Beef Steak	Salmon Fillet	Old-fashioned Gingerbread Cake

11	Two-Cheese Sausage Balls	King Size Beef Burgers	Dijon Egg Salad	Vanilla-Flavored Hazelnut Ice Cream
12	Egg, Scallion, Jalapeño Pepper Salad	Pork Kofte with Cauliflower Mash	Roast Herbs Stuffed Chicken	Chocolate Pecan-Berry Mascarpone Bowl
13	Blueberry-Almond Butter Smoothie	Hearty Pork Stew Meat	New Orleans Halibut and Crabmeat	Cheesecake Fat Bomb with Berries
14	Yogurt and Swiss Cheese Soup	Mozzarella Beef Gratin	Baked Chicken in Tomato Purée	Blackberry Cobbler with Almonds
15	Apple-Almond Butter Smoothie	Italian Beef Roast with Jalapeño	Chepala Vepudu	Almond-Sour Cream Cheesecake
16	Mangalore-Style Egg Curry	Paprika Roast Beef Brisket	Roasted Chicken Breasts with Capers	Blackberry Cobbler with Almonds
17	Mediterranean Shakshuka	Lemon-Mustard Beef Rump Steak	Coconut-Chicken Breasts	Chocolate Pecan-Berry Mascarpone Bowl
18	Vanilla Coconut Smoothie	Juicy Beef Meatballs with Parsley	Traditional Chicken Stroganoff	Cheesecake Fat Bomb with Berries
19	Creamy Flaxseed-Ginger Smoothie	Creamy Reuben Soup with Sauerkraut	Red Snapper Fillet and Salad	Citrus Raspberry Custard Cake
20	Cheesy Tomato Frittata	Cheesy Pork Nachos	Three-Cheese Beef Sausage Casserole	Almond Flour Crusted Cheesecake
21	Easy Peanut Butter Smoothie	Beef and Mushrooms in Red Wine	Chicken Wings with Ranch Dressing	Blueberry-Vanilla Pudding

Foods to Eat

Healthy Fats

- Saturated fat (goose fat, tallow, clarified butter / ghee, coconut oil, duck fat, lard, butter, chicken fat)
- Monounsaturated (olive, macadamia and avocado oil)
- Polyunsaturated omega 3 (seafood and fatty fish)

Non-Starchy Vegetables

- Spinach
- Endive
- Bamboo Shoots
- Asparagus
- Lettuce
- Cucumber
- Kale
- Radishes
- Celery Stalk
- Chives
- Zucchini

Fruits

- avocado, berries

Nuts and Seeds

- Macadamia nuts, pine nuts, walnuts, sunflower seeds, sesame seeds, hemp seeds, pumpkin seeds, pecans, hazelnuts, almonds

Dairy Products

- Cream cheese
- Heavy whipping cream
- Whole milk yogurt (unsweetened)

Beverages

- Water
- Unsweetened herbal tea
- Unsweetened coconut milk
- Decaf coffee
- Unsweetened almond milk
- Unsweetened soy milk
- Unsweetened herbal tea

Protein

- **Fish:** cod, halibut, tuna, salmon, trout, flounder, mackerel, snapper, and catfish.
- **Meat:** Goat, Beef, Lamb, and other wild game
- **Poultry:** Chicken meat, duck meat, and quail meat
- **Shellfish:** Squid, Clams, scallops, lobster, mussels, crab, and oysters,
- Whole Eggs
- Pork products
- Sausage and bacon
- Peanut Butter

Dressings

- Balsamic Vinegar
- Ranch
- Blue Cheese
- Apple Cider Vinegar
- Creamy Caesar

Spices

- Oregano
- Black Pepper
- Rosemary
- Basil
- Thyme
- Sea salt
- Cumin
- Parsley
- Sage
- Cayenne Pepper

Foods to Avoid

Processed Foods

- **Artificial sweeteners:** sweeteners containing Aspartame, Equal, Sucralose, Acesulfame, Saccharin, Splenda
- **Refined fats / oils** e.g. grape seed, corn oil, sunflower
- **Alcoholic drinks:** beer, cocktails,
- **Tropical fruit:** papaya, banana, mango, pineapple

Tips for Successful and Happy Ketogenic Lifestyle

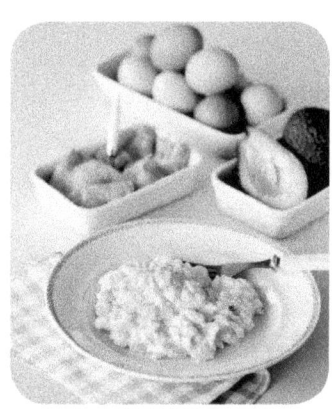

The ketogenic lifestyle is enjoyable. You get to enjoy amazingly delicious recipes as you cut your weight. You don't have to eat some nasty tasting foods to achieve your desired weight. Isn't that a win-win? Definitely yes! To make the keto journey happy and more enjoyable, there are some tips that you should follow. Below are the tips that will help you make the keto journey interesting.

Clear Carbohydrates From Your Kitchen

Most people will only stick to the ketogenic diet if they had access to healthy ketogenic foods. This will help you a lot in avoiding falling prey to the carbohydrate concentrated foods in your cabinet. Clean your kitchen from high-carbohydrate foods like pastry, bread, potatoes, soda, rice, and candy. This will help a long way in achieving the ketogenic diet. I must say this helped me a lot in achieving my weight goal.

Have Ketogenic Snacks At Hand

Cooking had been a hard thing for me. However, I had made the choice to lose weight and not even having to cook at home would stand on my way. Having to prepare a lot of homemade meals is a big challenge for people as regards the ketogenic diet. There is a solution for you: why not have ketogenic snacks instead whenever you are hungry and you are not at home?

You can buy ketogenic snacks like hard boiled eggs, beef jerky, pre-cooked bacon, pre-made guacamole and so on or you can have them on the go. You can prepare a lot of them and this will not allow you to buy carbohydrate-heavy snacks.

Buy a Food Scale

This might sound surprising but it is quite crucial. As it has been said, "Drops of water make an ocean." The amount of food you eat matters even to the tiniest form. Buy a food scale to measure your food and make sure you are eating the appropriate size because even the least can make a difference.

For example, 2 extra tablespoons of almond butter turn out to be an additional 200 calories and 6 grams of carbohydrates. It is not necessary for you to keep using the food scale till the end of your challenge. It is just for you to get the appropriate measurement then you can eyeball to measure it as you continue.

Exercise Frequently

I have mentioned a lot. Exercising allows your body to break down the glycogen it has in store. It also helps you to get fit and healthy. It also helps you in maintaining your muscle mass and strengthens you.

Try Intermittent Fasting

This is one of the most effective tips that can get you right on track to achieve your fitness goals. It helps you get into ketosis and lose weight. This means that you do not eat anything that contains calories for a given period of time. A study in Harvard has made it known that intermittent fasting manipulates your mitochondria in a way that the ketogenic diet also does and this elongates your lifespan. When you stop taking calories for some time, your body will start breaking down the excess glucose in your body obtained from consuming carbohydrates.

Include Coconut Oil Into Your Diet

Coconut oil contains fats called medium chain triglycerides which help you to quickly get into ketosis. Unlike other fats, the MCTs get quickly absorbed into the liver where they can be used for energy or they can be converted into ketones.

Some Effects You May Undergo During the Transition

- Headache
- Irritability
- Weakness
- Muscle cramps
- Dizziness
- Nausea
- Vomiting
- Diarrhea
- Poor concentration
- Stomach pain
- Muscle soreness
- Trouble sleeping
- Sugar cravings
- Dehydration

* To help reduce the severity of your keto flu symptoms, and to help you get through the transition phase as quickly as possible, make sure you stay hydrated and get plenty of rest. Avoid any strenuous exercise for now and eat some leafy greens and avocado to replace depleted electrolyte stores.

Ketogenic Diet and Weight-Loss

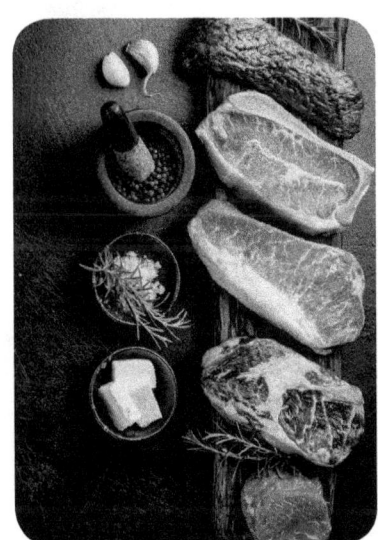

Ketogenic diet enables the breaking down of unwanted fats and stored substances by the body. It is one of the main bodybuilding solutions which helps in lowering fat content in the body while creating muscle. Many of the bodybuilders on keto diet regime set their everyday calorie intake to 20% more than their typical calorie level. The figure is not set but individuals can adjust it accordingly.

It is advised loading up on carbs for a three-day cycle while on keto plan. Eat about 1000 calories of carbs on the third day a couple of hours before exercising. For carb loading, there are two options:

i. eating what you like

ii. start with carbs with higher glycemic and then go to the lower ones.

Carb loading is good for intense workout because it enables endurance by enhancing glycogen in the muscles.

For instance, let us say you start off carb-loading on Friday. By Sunday, your muscle tissues will have a substantial amount of glycogen in them. This is the day you ought to exercise. It is optimal to only work out half of the body at this time with weights. Schedule your next exercise routine on Wednesday and be sure to consume 1000 calories worth of carbs prior to your routine. By Wednesday, your glycogen levels will likely be low, but the pre-workout carb load will allow you to work out intensely. This time you will perform exercises targeting the other half of your body.

The next exercise session should be scheduled on Friday at the beginning of the three-day cycle of loading up on carbohydrates. This training session has to be a complete overall body workout with 1-2 sets per workout completed until failure. Make barbell rows, bench presses, military presses, barbell/dumbbell curls, triceps pushups, squats, lunges, dead lifts, and reverse curls the focus of your training. The goal of this exercise session is to deplete your glycogen stores within the body completely. Nevertheless, keep cardio to a minimum. Ten-minute warm-ups in advance of each workout is fine, but do not go overload.

5 Weight Loss Tips During the Keto Journey

1. **Keep Your Carbs Very Low**

This is the most significant thing while on keto diet. Maintaining your carbs low helps to get the body into ketosis.

Do not cheat as that will hinder your success and slow the process of your body adapting to ketosis. I once tried cheating during the early stages of my keto journey but then swore never to do it again. "I had made the decision myself and therefore when I cheat, I am only doing to myself", I told myself. Therefore, I advise you to never cheat during your keto journey.

2. **Track Your Calories and Macros**

This is very important while on keto diet. Carbs are almost everywhere out there and you need to keep track of all that you eat.

3. **Watch Your Electrolytes**

Electrolytes are of great essence on keto diet as they are removed from the body system.

Ensure that you take enough potassium, magnesium and sodium to curb excessive hunger, cramps, water retention, headaches and cravings.

4. **Be Patient**

Losing weight does not come overnight. You must consistently work hard over a long period of time in order to achieve this goal. Keto diet is a great diet if you want to lose weight. However, you need to know that the weight cannot be lost in a fortnight. It took me more than a month to notice a change in my weight.

5. **Enough Sleep and Rest**

Stress levels in a person is also a factor in losing you weight. When you are more stressed, the level of cortisol increases, which in turn causes weight gain or retention.

Rest is also another factor that is very important. Most people require seven to nine hours of sleep for proper rest of the body each night.

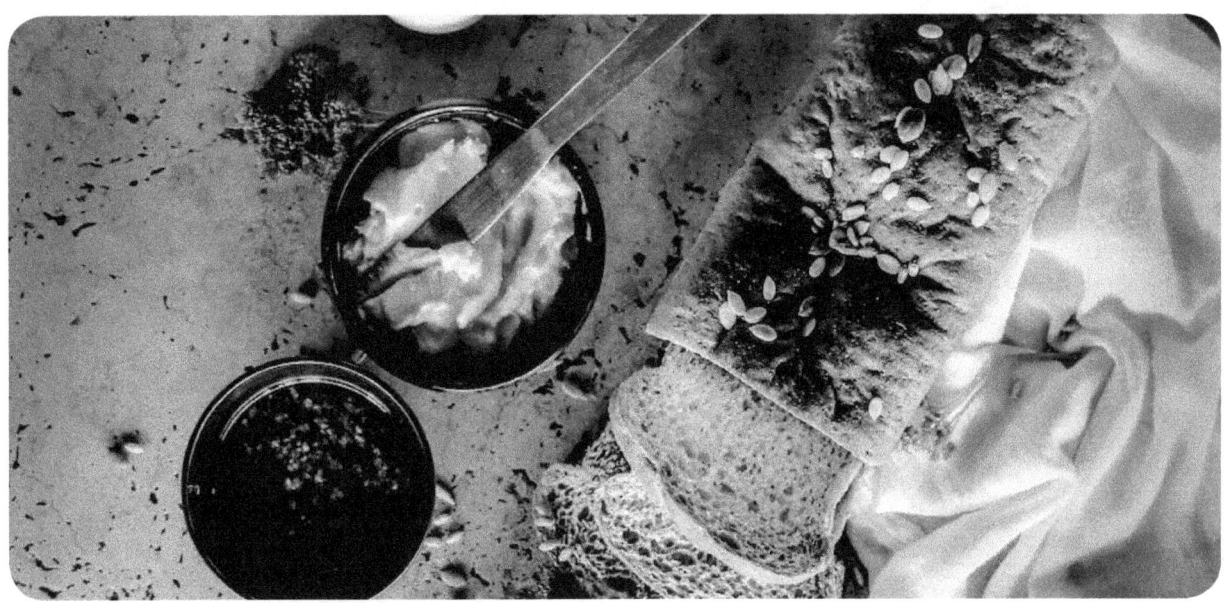

Frequently Asked Questions

Many people I meet ask me various questions about the ketogenic lifestyle. I have analyzed them and came up with the following most frequently asked questions. I answer every question according to my personal experience and interaction with people practicing the keto lifestyle. During my keto journey, I have met people who are practicing the lifestyle. My interaction with these different people has also added to my knowledge of this amazing diet and the many great things it can do.

1. Is Keto Same as Low-Carb?

Low-carb is any diet that has limited carbs. Keto is a type of low-carb meal. However, keto diet is a low-carb diet that is stricter.

2. Can I Drink Alcohol?

Yes, you can. I love drinking a glass or two of alcohol at least in every two days. Before I started the keto lifestyle, I was worried that alcohol may not be allowed. "Will I manage without even a glass?", I asked myself. However, when I came to learn that I can take a little, I was relieved.

Drinks that have high levels of carbs such as most beers, sweet wines and cocktails are a NO! You are only allowed to take pure liquor and only a maximum of three glasses.

3. Is Keto Good For Weight Loss?

Yes. I am a living testimony that keto diet is the best way to lose weight. You will lose your weight as you enjoy amazing recipes.

4. Can Pregnant Women Do The Ketogenic Diet?

The ketogenic has appeared safe due to the women that have done it and the doctors that have administered it to their patients during pregnancy. I cannot say I am right because there is no scientific research or study that has proved this. So, there is a lack of knowledge concerning this. The ketogenic diet may be very helpful in case of gestational diabetes. It is therefore advised that caution is to be exercised for a ketogenic diet during pregnancy unless there is a benefit you want to achieve while doing it in your own case.

5. Is Keto Diet Good For Kids?

It would be better to seek a doctor's advice before placing a child on any diet program that is strict. Keto diet has been found to take effect on cases of epilepsy and autism in children.

6. At What Level Should My Ketones Be During Ketosis?

Your ketones should be above 0.5mmol/l and this is general.

7. Is The Keto Diet For Vegan/Vegetarians?

Yes. Meat is among the staples of ketogenic diet. However, there are a lot of options for any person who is a vegetarian or vegan. I am a meat lover but I also enjoy other non-meat recipes.

8. Can I Develop Muscles While Doing My Ketogenic Diet?

Sure! It is even advised to do so but it is not compulsory. You can do this by going to the gym to work out; you can even buy the workout DVD if you do not have time to go to the gym. Like I said earlier, it is not compulsory.

9. While on Keto, Do I Have to Exercise?

It is not mandatory to exercise while under keto diet. However, if losing weight is your main objective, it's good for you to exercise.

10. How Long Can I Be On The Ketogenic Diet?

As long as you want! That is why the ketogenic diet is often referred to as a lifestyle. You can do it as long as you desire. It is now more than a year since I started the keto lifestyle and I can tell you that I do not intend to leave it. Not now, not ever! It has become my way of life.

11. How Long Does it Take To Be In Ketosis?

This is a popular question among those who are just starting the ketogenic diet. I have lost count for the times I have been asked this question. It actually varies from two weeks or more. People with more insulin resistance usually take a longer time before they get to ketosis. Lean and young people usually get to ketosis faster.

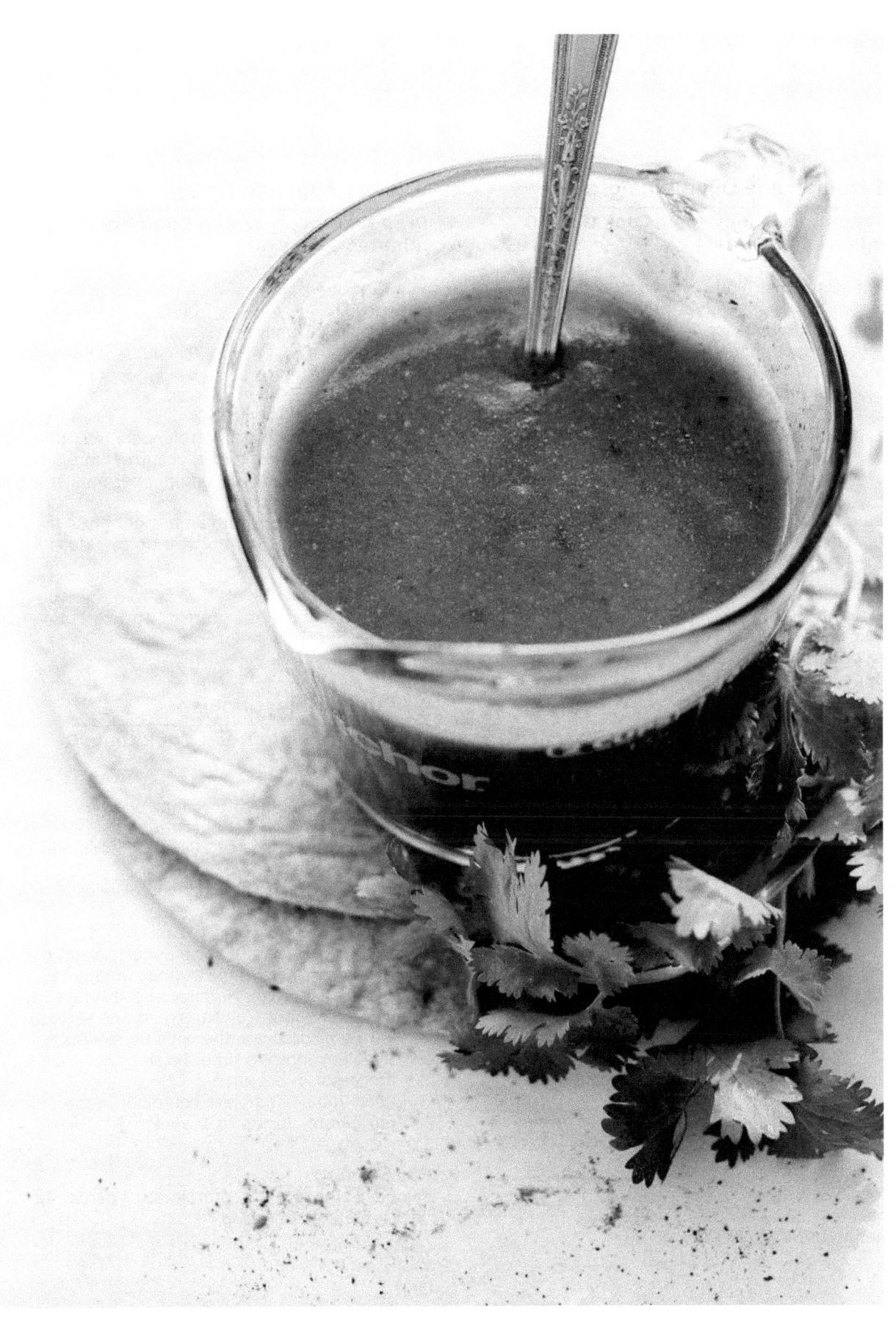

Chapter 2 Sauce and Dressing

1. Homemade Dijon Vinaigrette

Prep time: 5 minutes | Cook time: 0 minutes | Serves 4

2 tablespoons Dijon mustard
Juice of ½ lemon
1 garlic clove, finely minced
1½ tablespoons red wine vinegar
Pink Himalayan salt
Freshly ground black pepper, to taste
3 tablespoons olive oil

1. In a small bowl, whisk the mustard, lemon juice, garlic, and red wine vinegar until well combined. Season with pink Himalayan salt and pepper, and whisk again.
2. Slowly add the olive oil, a little bit at a time, whisking constantly.
3. Keep in a sealed glass container in the refrigerator for up to 1 week

Per Serving

calories: 99 | fat: 11g | protein: 1g | carbs: 1g net carbs: 1g | fiber: 0g

2. Creamy Caesar Dressing

Prep time: 5 minutes | Cook time: 0 minutes | Serves 4

½ cup mayonnaise
1 tablespoon Dijon mustard
Juice of ½ lemon
½ teaspoon Worcestershire sauce
Pinch pink Himalayan salt
Pinch freshly ground black pepper
¼ cup grated Parmesan cheese

1. In a medium bowl, whisk together the mayonnaise, mustard, lemon juice, Worcestershire sauce, pink Himalayan salt, and pepper until fully combined.
2. Add the Parmesan cheese, and whisk until creamy and well blended.
3. Keep in a sealed glass container in the refrigerator for up to 1 week.

Per Serving

calories: 222 | fat: 23g | protein: 2g | carbs: 2g net carbs: 2g | fiber: 0g

3. Tangy Avocado Crema

Prep time: 5 minutes | Cook time: 0 minutes | Serves 4

½ cup sour cream
½ avocado
1 garlic clove, finely minced
¼ cup fresh cilantro leaves
Juice of ½ lime
Pinch pink Himalayan salt
Pinch freshly ground black pepper

1. In a food processor (or blender), mix the sour cream, avocado, garlic, cilantro, lime juice, pink Himalayan salt, and pepper until smooth and fully combined.
2. Spoon the sauce into an airtight glass jar and keep in the refrigerator for up to 3 days.

Per Serving

calories: 87 | fat: 8g | protein: 1g | carbs: 4g net carbs: 2g | fiber: 2g

4. Avocado Mayonnaise

Prep time: 5 minutes | Cook time: 0 minutes | Serves 4

1 medium avocado, cut into chunks
½ teaspoon ground cayenne pepper
Juice of ½ lime
2 tablespoons fresh cilantro leaves (optional)
Pinch pink Himalayan salt
¼ cup olive oil

1. In a food processor (or blender), blend the avocado, cayenne pepper, lime juice, cilantro, and pink Himalayan salt until all the ingredients are well combined and smooth.
2. Slowly incorporate the olive oil, adding 1 tablespoon at a time, pulsing the food processor in between.
3. Keep in a sealed glass container in the refrigerator for up to 1 week.

Per Serving

calories: 58 | fat: 5g | protein: 1g | carbs: 4g net carbs: 1g | fiber: 3g

5. Chunky Lemony Blue Cheese

Prep time: 5 minutes | Cook time: 0 minutes | Serves 4

½ cup sour cream
½ cup mayonnaise
Juice of ½ lemon
½ teaspoon Worcestershire sauce
Pink Himalayan salt, to taste
Freshly ground black pepper, to taste
2 ounces (57 g) crumbled blue cheese

1. In a medium bowl, whisk the sour cream, mayonnaise, lemon juice, and Worcestershire sauce. Season with pink Himalayan salt and pepper, and whisk again until fully combined.
2. Fold in the crumbled blue cheese until well combined.
3. Keep in a sealed glass container in the refrigerator for up to 1 week.

Per Serving
calories: 306 | fat: 32g | protein: 7g | carbs: 3g net carbs: 3g | fiber: 0g

6. Bolognese Sauce

Prep time: 15 minutes | Cook time: 7 to 8 hours | Serves 10

3 tablespoons extra-virgin olive oil, divided
1 pound (454 g) ground pork
½ pound (227 g) ground beef
½ pound (227 g) bacon, chopped
1 sweet onion, chopped
1 tablespoon minced garlic
2 celery stalks, chopped
2 (28-ounce / 794-g) cans diced tomatoes
½ cup coconut milk
¼ cup apple cider vinegar

1. Lightly grease the insert of the slow cooker with 1 tablespoon of the olive oil.
2. In a large skillet over medium-high heat, heat the remaining 2 tablespoons of the olive oil. Add the pork, beef, and bacon, and sauté until cooked through, about 7 minutes.
3. Stir in the onion and garlic and sauté for an additional 2 minutes.
4. Transfer the meat mixture to the insert and add the celery, tomatoes, coconut milk, and apple cider vinegar.
5. Cover and cook on low for 7 to 8 hours.
6. Serve, or cool completely, and store in the refrigerator in a sealed container for up to 4 days or in the freezer for 1 month.

Per Serving (½ cup)
calories: 333 | fat: 23g | protein: 25g | carbs: 5g net carbs: 2g | fiber: 3g

7. Cheesy Hot Crab Sauce

Prep time: 10 minutes | Cook time: 5 to 6 hours | Makes 4 cups

8 ounces (227-g) cream cheese
8 ounces (227-g) goat cheese
1 cup sour cream
½ cup grated Asiago cheese
1 sweet onion, finely chopped
1 tablespoon granulated erythritol
2 teaspoons minced garlic
12 ounces (340-g) crabmeat, flaked
1 scallion, white and green parts, chopped

1. In a large bowl, stir together the cream cheese, goat cheese, sour cream, Asiago cheese, onion, erythritol, garlic, crabmeat, and scallion until well mixed.
2. Transfer the mixture to an 8-by-4-inch loaf pan and place the pan in the insert of the slow cooker.
3. Cover and cook on low for 5 to 6 hours.
4. Serve warm.

Per Serving (½ cup)
calories: 361 | fat: 28g | protein: 17g | carbs: 10g net carbs: 8g | fiber: 2g

8. Spicy Enchilada Sauce

Prep time: 10 minutes | Cook time: 7 to 8 hours | Makes 4 cups

¼ cup extra-virgin olive oil, divided
2 cups puréed tomatoes
1 cup water
1 sweet onion, chopped
2 jalapeño peppers, chopped
2 teaspoons minced garlic
2 tablespoons chili powder
1 teaspoon ground coriander

1. Lightly grease the insert of the slow cooker with 1 tablespoon of the olive oil.
2. Place the remaining 3 tablespoons of the olive oil, tomatoes, water, onion, jalapeño peppers, garlic, chili powder, and coriander in the insert.
3. Cover and cook on low 7 to 8 hours.
4. Serve over poultry or meat. After cooling, store the sauce in a sealed container in the refrigerator for up to 1 week.

Per Serving (½ cup)
calories: 92 | fat: 8g | protein: 2g | carbs: 4g net carbs: 2g | fiber: 2g

9. Basil Dressing

Prep time: 10 minutes | Cook time: 0 minutes | Makes 1 cup

1 avocado, peeled and pitted
¼ cup sour cream
¼ cup extra-virgin olive oil
¼ cup chopped fresh basil
1 tablespoon freshly squeezed lime juice
1 teaspoon minced garlic
Sea salt, to taste
Freshly ground black pepper, to taste

1. Place the avocado, sour cream, olive oil, basil, lime juice, and garlic in a food processor and pulse until smooth, scraping down the sides of the bowl once during processing.
2. Season the dressing with salt and pepper.
3. Keep the dressing in an airtight container in the refrigerator for 1 to 2 weeks.

Per Serving (1 tablespoon)

calories: 173 | fat: 17g | protein: 5g | carbs: 1g net carbs: 1g | fiber: 0g

10. Fettuccine Alfredo

Prep time: 5 minutes | Cook time: 10 minutes | Serves 2

4 tablespoons butter
2 ounces (57-g) cream cheese
1 cup heavy (whipping) cream
½ cup grated Parmesan cheese
1 garlic clove, finely minced
1 teaspoon dried Italian seasoning
Pink Himalayan salt, to taste
Freshly ground black pepper, to taste

1. In a heavy medium saucepan over medium heat, combine the butter, cream cheese, and heavy cream. Whisk slowly and constantly until the butter and cream cheese melt.
2. Add the Parmesan, garlic, and Italian seasoning. Continue to whisk until everything is well blended. Turn the heat to medium-low and simmer, stirring occasionally, for 5 to 8 minutes to allow the sauce to blend and thicken.
3. Season with pink Himalayan salt and pepper, and stir to combine.
4. Toss with your favorite hot, precooked, keto-friendly noodles and serve.
5. Keep this sauce in a sealed glass container in the refrigerator for up to 4 days.

Per Serving

calories: 294 | fat: 30g | protein: 5g | carbs: 2g net carbs: 2g | fiber: 0g

11. Bolognese Sauce

Prep time: 15 minutes | Cook time: 40 minutes | Serves 4

2 tablespoons good-quality olive oil
1 pound (454 g) grass-fed ground beef
1 onion, chopped
2 celery stalks, chopped
2 tablespoons minced garlic
1 (28-ounce / 794-g) can sodium-free diced tomatoes
¼ cup red wine
¼ cup tomato purée
2 teaspoons dried oregano
2 teaspoons dried basil
1 teaspoon dried parsley
½ teaspoon sea salt
¼ teaspoon red pepper flakes

1. Brown the beef. In a large pot over medium-high heat, warm the olive oil. Brown the ground beef, stirring it occasionally, until it's cooked through, about 6 minutes.
2. Sauté the vegetables. Stir in the onion, celery, and garlic and sauté them until they've softened, about 3 minutes.
3. Add the rest of the ingredients. Stir in the tomatoes, red wine, tomato purée, oregano, basil, parsley, salt, and red pepper flakes.
4. Cook the sauce. Bring the sauce to a boil, then reduce the heat to low and simmer it for 25 to 30 minutes, stirring occasionally.
5. Store. Cool the sauce completely and store in a sealed container in the refrigerator for up to four days or freeze for up to one month.

Per Serving

calories: 457 | fat: 35g | protein: 21g | carbs: 13g net carbs: 8g | fiber: 5g

12. Sriracha Mayonnaise

Prep time: 5 minutes | Cook time: 0 minutes | Serves 4

½ cup mayonnaise
2 tablespoons Sriracha sauce
½ teaspoon garlic powder
½ teaspoon onion powder
¼ teaspoon paprika

1. In a small bowl, whisk together the mayonnaise, Sriracha, garlic powder, onion powder, and paprika until well mixed.
2. Pour into an airtight glass container, and keep in the refrigerator for up to 1 week.

Per Serving

calories: 201 | fat: 22g | protein: 1g | carbs: 2g net carbs: 1g | fiber: 1g

13. Marinara Sauce

Prep time: 10 minutes | Cook time: 7 to 8 hours | Serves 12

3 tablespoons extra-virgin olive oil, divided
2 (28-ounce / 794-g) cans crushed tomatoes
½ sweet onion, finely chopped
2 teaspoons minced garlic
½ teaspoon salt
1 tablespoon chopped fresh basil
1 tablespoon chopped fresh oregano

1. Lightly grease the insert of the slow cooker with 1 tablespoon of the olive oil.
2. Add the remaining 2 tablespoons of the olive oil, tomatoes, onion, garlic, and salt to the insert, stirring to combine.
3. Cover and cook on low for 7 to 8 hours.
4. Remove the cover and stir in the basil and oregano.
5. Store the cooled sauce in a sealed container in the refrigerator for up to 1 week.

Per Serving (½ cup)
calories: 66 | fat: 5g | protein: 1g | carbs: 7g net carbs: 5g | fiber: 2g

14. Hollandaise Sauce

Prep time: 20 minutes | Cook time: 10 minutes | Makes 2 cups

1½ cups unsalted butter
4 large egg yolks
2 teaspoons cold water
Juice of 1 small lemon, about 4 teaspoons
Pinch sea salt

1. Place a medium heavy-bottomed saucepan over very low heat and melt the butter.
2. Remove the saucepan from the heat and let the melted butter stand for 5 minutes.
3. Carefully skim the foam from the top of the melted butter.
4. Very slowly pour the clarified part of the butter (it should be a clear yellow color) into a container, leaving the milky solids in the bottom of the saucepan.
5. Discard the milky solids and let the clarified butter cool in the container until it is just warm, about 15 minutes.
6. Put a medium saucepan with about 3 inches of water in it over medium heat until the water simmers gently.
7. In a large stainless steel bowl, add the egg yolks and 2 teaspoons of cold water and whisk them until they are foamy and light, about 3 minutes.
8. Add 3 or 4 drops of the lemon juice to the yolks and whisk for about 1 minute.
9. Place the bowl onto the mouth of the saucepan, making sure the bottom of the bowl does not touch the simmering water.
10. Whisk the yolks until they thicken a little, about 1 to 2 minutes, then remove the bowl from the simmering water.
11. In a very thin stream, add the clarified butter to the yolk mixture, whisking continuously, until you have used up all the butter and your sauce is thick and smooth. If you add the butter too quickly, the sauce will break.
12. Whisk in the remaining lemon juice and the salt.
13. This sauce should be used right away or held for only about 1 hour. Throw away any unused sauce.

Per Serving (1 tablespoon)
calories: 173 | fat: 17g | protein: 5g | carbs: 1g net carbs: 1g | fiber: 0g

15. Cheesy Spinach Basil Pesto

Prep time: 10 minutes | Cook time: 0 minutes | Serves 2 cups

2 cups fresh spinach
1 cup fresh basil leaves
3 garlic cloves, smashed
¼ cup pecans
¼ cup grated Parmesan cheese
½ cup good-quality olive oil
Sea salt, for seasoning
Freshly ground black pepper, for seasoning

1. Blend the base. Put the spinach, basil, garlic, pecans, and Parmesan in a blender and pulse until the mixture is finely chopped, scraping down the sides of the blender once.
2. Finish the pesto. While the blender is running, pour in the olive oil in a thin stream and blend until the pesto is smooth. Season it with salt and pepper.
3. Store. Store in a sealed container in the refrigerator for up to one week.
4. Swap: Pesto comes in many variations because this delectable creation is versatile. Try kale, basil, or cilantro in place of the spinach in the same amount.

Per Serving (2 tablespoons)
calories: 60 | fat: 6g | protein: 1g | carbs: 1g net carbs: 1g | fiber: 0g

16. Basil Kale Pesto

Prep time: 15 minutes | Cook time: 0 minutes | Makes 1½ cup

1 cup chopped kale
1 cup fresh basil leaves
3 garlic cloves
2 teaspoons nutritional yeast
¼ cup extra-virgin olive oil

1. Place the kale, basil, garlic, and yeast in a food processor and pulse until the mixture is finely chopped, about 3 minutes.
2. With the food processor running, drizzle the olive oil into the pesto until a thick paste forms, scraping down the sides of the bowl at least once.
3. Add a little water if the pesto is too thick.
4. Store the pesto in an airtight container in the refrigerator for up to 1 week

Per Serving (2 tablespoons)
calories: 44 | fat: 4g | protein: 1g | carbs: 1g net carbs: 1g | fiber: 0g

17. Spanish Queso Sauce

Prep time: 10 minutes | Cook time: 3 to 4 hours | Makes 4 cups

1 tablespoon extra-virgin olive oil
12 ounces (340-g) cream cheese
1 cup sour cream
2 cups salsa verde
1 cup monterey jack cheese, shredded

1. Lightly grease the insert of the slow cooker with the olive oil.
2. In a large bowl, stir together the cream cheese, sour cream, salsa verde, and Monterey Jack cheese, until blended.
3. Transfer the mixture to the insert.
4. Cover and cook on low for 3 to 4 hours.
5. Serve warm.

Per Serving (½ cup)
calories: 278 | fat: 25g | protein: 9g | carbs: 4g net carbs: 4g | fiber: 0g

18. Garlicky Mayonnaise

Prep time: 10 minutes | Cook time: 0 minutes | Serves 8

1 large egg
2 teaspoons Dijon mustard
1½ teaspoons minced garlic
1 cup olive oil
1 tablespoon freshly squeezed lemon juice
Sea salt, for seasoning

1. Combine the base. In a medium bowl, whisk together the egg, mustard, and garlic until they're well blended, about 2 minutes.
2. Add the oil. Slowly add the olive oil in a thin, continuous stream, whisking constantly until the aioli is thick. Whisk in the lemon juice and season the aioli with salt.
3. Store. Store the aioli in an airtight container in the refrigerator for up to four days.

Per Serving (1 tablespoon)
calories: 124 | fat: 14g | protein: 0g | carbs: 0g net carbs: 0g | fiber: 0g

19. Tzatziki Sauce

Prep time: 10 minutes | Cook time: 0 minutes | Serves 4

½ large English cucumber, unpeeled
1½ cups Greek yogurt (I use Fage)
2 tablespoons olive oil
Large pinch pink Himalayan salt
Large pinch freshly ground black pepper
Juice of ½ lemon
2 garlic cloves, finely minced
1 tablespoon fresh dill

1. Halve the cucumber lengthwise, and use a spoon to scoop out and discard the seeds.
2. Grate the cucumber with a zester or grater onto a large plate lined with a few layers of paper towels. Close the paper towels around the grated cucumber, and squeeze as much water out of it as you can. (This can take a while and can require multiple paper towels. You can also allow it to drain overnight in a strainer or wrapped in a few layers of cheesecloth in the fridge if you have the time.)
3. In a food processor (or blender), blend the yogurt, olive oil, pink Himalayan salt, pepper, lemon juice, and garlic until fully combined.
4. Transfer the mixture to a medium bowl, and mix in the fresh dill and grated cucumber.
5. I like to chill this sauce for at least 30 minutes before serving. Keep in a sealed glass container in the refrigerator for up to 1 week.

Per Serving
calories: 149 | fat: 11g | protein: 8g | carbs: 5g net carbs: 4g | fiber: 1g

20. Garlic Aioli Sauce

Prep time: 5 minutes | Cook time: 0 minutes | Serves 4

½ cup mayonnaise
2 garlic cloves, minced
Juice of 1 lemon
1 tablespoon chopped fresh flat-leaf Italian parsley
1 teaspoon chopped chives
Pink Himalayan salt, to taste
Freshly ground black pepper, to taste

1. In a food processor (or blender), combine the mayonnaise, garlic, lemon juice, parsley, and chives, and season with pink Himalayan salt and pepper. Blend until fully combined.
2. Pour into a sealed glass container and chill in the refrigerator for at least 30 minutes before serving. (This sauce will keep in the fridge for up to 1 week.)

Per Serving
calories: 204 | fat: 22g | protein: 1g | carbs: 3g | net carbs: 2g | fiber: 1g

21. Asian Peanut Sauce

Prep time: 5 minutes | Cook time: 0 minutes | Serves 4

½ cup creamy peanut butter (I use Justin's)
2 tablespoons coconut aminos
1 teaspoon Sriracha sauce
1 teaspoon toasted sesame oil
1 teaspoon garlic powder

1. In a food processor (or blender), blend the peanut butter, coconut aminos, Sriracha sauce, sesame oil, and garlic powder until thoroughly mixed.
2. Pour into an airtight glass container and keep in the refrigerator for up to 1 week.

Per Serving
calories: 185 | fat: 15g | protein: 7g | carbs: 8g | net carbs: 6g | fiber: 2g

22. Oregano Balsamic Vinegar

Prep time: 4 minutes | Cook time: 0 minutes | Makes 1 cup

1 cup extra-virgin olive oil
¼ cup balsamic vinegar
2 tablespoons chopped fresh oregano
1 teaspoon chopped fresh basil
1 teaspoon minced garlic
Sea salt, to taste
Freshly ground black pepper, to taste

1. Whisk the olive oil and vinegar in a small bowl until emulsified, about 3 minutes.
2. Whisk in the oregano, basil, and garlic until well combined, about 1 minute.
3. Season the dressing with salt and pepper.
4. Transfer the dressing to an airtight container, and store it in the refrigerator for up to 1 week. Give the dressing a vigorous shake before using it.

Per Serving (1 tablespoon)
calories: 83 | fat: 9g | protein: 0g | carbs: 0g | net carbs: 0g | fiber: 0g

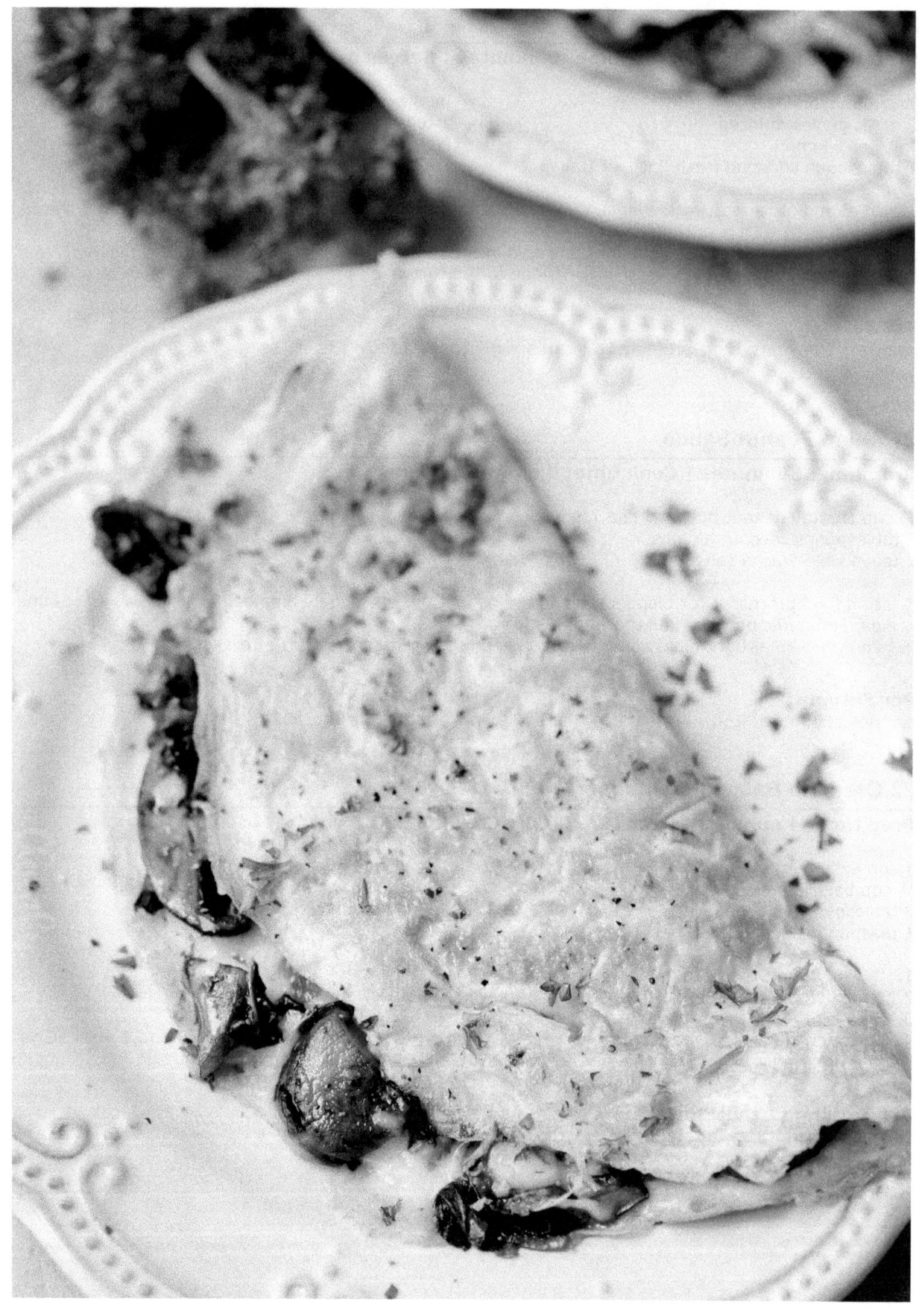

Chapter 3 Egg and Dairy

23. Double Cheese Stuffed Bell Peppers

Prep time: 10 minutes | Cook time: 17 minutes | Serves 4

4 summer bell peppers, divined and halved
1 clove garlic, minced
4 ounces (113 g) cream cheese
2 ounces (57 g) Mozzarella cheese, crumbled
2 tablespoons Greek-style yogurt

1. Cook the peppers in boiling water in a Dutch oven until just tender or approximately 7 minutes.
2. Mix the garlic, cream cheese, mozzarella, and yogurt until well combined. Then, stuff the peppers with the cheese mixture.
3. Arrange the stuffed peppers on a tinfoil-lined baking pan.
4. Bake in the preheated oven at 360ºF (182ºC) for 10 to 12 minutes. Serve at room temperature. Bon appétit!

Per Serving
calories: 140 | fat: 10g | protein: 8g | carbs: 6g
net carbs: 5g | fiber: 1g

24. Mediterranean Aïoli

Prep time: 10 minutes | Cook time: 0 minutes | Serves 6

2 egg yolks
1 teaspoon stone-ground mustard
½ teaspoon sea salt
A pinch of ground black pepper
1 teaspoon garlic, crushed
1 tablespoon lemon juice
½ cup extra-virgin olive oil
1 tablespoon fresh chives

1. Whisk the egg yolks and add them to your food processor.
2. Add in the mustard, salt, black pepper, garlic, and lemon juice; continue mixing until everything is well incorporated.
3. Now, with the machine running, add the oil to the egg yolk mixture in a steady stream. Mix until you reach your desired thickness.
4. Garnish with chives. Keep for about 1 week in the refrigerator. Bon appétit!

Per Serving
calories: 94 | fat: 9g | protein: 2g | carbs: 1g
net carbs: 1g | fiber: 0g

25. Egg Muffins

Prep time: 20 minutes | Cook time: 15 minutes | Serves 4

6 tablespoons almond flour
2 tablespoons flaxseed meal
¼ teaspoon baking soda
4 eggs
4 ounces (113 g) cheddar cheese, shredded

1. In a mixing bowl, thoroughly combine all of the above ingredients until well incorporated.
2. Line a muffin tin with non-stick baking cups. Scrape the batter into the prepared baking cups.
3. Bake in the preheated oven at 350ºF (180ºC) for 15 to 17 minutes.
4. Transfer to a wire rack to cool slightly before unmolding and serving. Bon appétit!

Per Serving
calories: 292 | fat: 23g | protein: 16g | carbs: 5g
net carbs: 2g | fiber: 3g

26. Herbed Cheese Balls

Prep time: 10 minutes | Cook time: 0 minutes | Serves 10

2 tablespoons mayonnaise
8 ounces (227 g) extra-sharp Cheddar cheese, shredded
6 ounces (170 g) cream cheese, softened
½ cup sour cream
½ teaspoon paprika
¼ teaspoon granulated garlic powder
1 teaspoon oregano
1 teaspoon basil
1 teaspoon rosemary
1 teaspoon mint
2 tablespoons chives, chopped

1. In a mixing bowl, thoroughly combine the mayonnaise, Cheddar cheese, cream cheese, and sour cream until smooth and uniform.
2. Wrap the cheese mixture in a plastic wrap and form into a ball. Refrigerate the cheese ball at least 2 hours.
3. Meanwhile, mix the remaining ingredients until well combined. Roll the cheese ball over the herb mixture. Serve well chilled with assorted keto veggies. Bon appétit!

Per Serving
calories: 176 | fat: 16g | protein: 7g | carbs: 2g
net carbs: 1g | fiber: 1g

27. Cheesy Omelet and Vegetables

Prep time: 15 minutes | Cook time: 5 minutes | Serves 2

2 teaspoons olive oil
2 scallion stalks, chopped
2 garlic cloves, minced
bell peppers, chopped
½ cup cauliflower florets
eggs
½ teaspoon cayenne pepper
Kosher salt and ground black pepper, to season
½ teaspoon dried Mexican oregano
½ teaspoon chili pepper flakes
½ teaspoon dried parsley flakes
2 ounces (57 g) Cotija cheese, crumbled

1. Heat the olive oil in a medium-sized pan over moderate heat. Sauté the scallions and garlic until just tender and fragrant.
2. Now, stir in the peppers and cauliflower and continue sautéing an additional 2 to 3 minutes.
3. Meanwhile, mix the eggs with the cayenne pepper, salt, black pepper, oregano, chili pepper flakes, and parsley.
4. Pour the egg mixture over the sautéed vegetables. Let it cook, tilting your pan so the raw parts can cook.
5. Add the Cotija cheese, fold over and leave for 1 minute before slicing and serving. Enjoy!

Per Serving
calories: 287 | fat: 20g | protein: 17g | carbs: 7g net carbs: 4g | fiber: 3g

28. French Scrambled Eggs

Prep time: 5 minutes | Cook time: 8 minutes | Serves 3

6 large eggs
1 tablespoon butter, at room temperature
¼ teaspoon ground black pepper
Sea salt, to taste
4 tablespoons crème fraîche

1. Crack the eggs into a bowl and beat them with a wire whisk until the yolks and whites are fully incorporated into each other.
2. Then, melt the butter in a nonstick skillet over a moderate flame. Once hot, add the egg mixture to the skillet.
3. The eggs will start to form curds. Stir until just set but still slightly wet or 8 to 10 minutes. Add in the black pepper, salt, and crème fraiche. Remove from the heat. Enjoy!

Per Serving
calories: 257 | fat: 21g | protein: 13g | carbs: 1g net carbs: 1g | fiber: 0g

29. Spicy Brown Mushroom Omelet

Prep time: 10 minutes | Cook time: 5 minutes | Serves 2

1 tablespoon olive oil
½ brown onion, thinly sliced
1 garlic clove, thinly sliced
1 green chili, minced
½ pound (227 g) brown mushrooms, sliced
4 eggs, whisked
1 tablespoon fresh coriander, chopped
Sea salt and ground black pepper, to taste
½ teaspoon Kashmiri chili powder
½ teaspoon garam masala

1. In a nonstick skillet, heat the olive oil until sizzling. Then, sauté the onion until translucent. Now, stir in the garlic, chili pepper, and mushrooms and continue sautéing until just tender and fragrant or about 2 minutes. Reserve.
2. Add in the whisked eggs, fresh coriander, salt, black pepper, Kashmiri chili powder, and garam masala. Give it a quick swirl to distribute the eggs evenly across the skillet. Cook for 2 to 3 minutes.
3. Flip your omelet over and cook an additional minute or so. Fill with the mushroom mixture, fold and serve immediately. Bon appétit!

Per Serving
calories: 217 | fat: 16g | protein: 14g | carbs: 5g net carbs: 4g | fiber: 1g

30. Scrambled Eggs and Baby Spinach

Prep time: 5 minutes | Cook time: 2 minutes | Serves 2

2 teaspoons olive oil
4 cups baby spinach
½ teaspoon garlic powder
4 eggs, well whisked
Sea salt cayenne pepper, to taste, to taste

1. Heat the olive oil in a frying pan over medium-high heat.
2. Add in the baby spinach and garlic powder; cook, until wilted, about 1 minute or so.
3. Now, add the whisked eggs to the pan and cook for 1 minute, stirring continuously to ensure even cooking.
4. Season with salt and cayenne pepper and serve immediately. Enjoy!

Per Serving
calories: 183 | fat: 13g | protein: 13g | carbs: 3g net carbs: 2g | fiber: 1g

31. Egg, Scallion, Jalapeño Pepper Salad

Prep time: 10 minutes | Cook time: 10 minutes | Serves 2

3 eggs
¼ cup scallions, chopped
1 jalapeño pepper, deseeded and minced
¼ cup mayonnaise
1 teaspoon Dijon mustard
Kosher salt and ground black pepper, to taste
1 tablespoon fresh parsley, roughly chopped
½ teaspoon sweet paprika

1. Arrange the eggs in a small saucepan. Pour in water (1-inch above the eggs) and bring to a boil.
2. Heat off and let it sit, covered, for 9 to 10 minutes.
3. When the eggs are cool enough to handle, peel away the shells, and rinse the eggs under running water. Chop the eggs and transfer them to a serving bowl.
4. Add in the scallions, jalapeno pepper, mayonnaise, mustard, salt, and black pepper.
5. Sprinkle fresh parsley and paprika over the salad and serve well chilled.

Per Serving
calories: 398 | fat: 35g | protein: 15g | carbs: 5g net carbs: 4g | fiber: 1g

32. Yogurt and Swiss Cheese Soup

Prep time: 10 minutes | Cook time: 13 minutes | Serves 2

2 tablespoons butter, at room temperature
½ cup shallots, chopped
½ cup cream of onion soup
½ cup water
1 cup yogurt
4 ounces (113 g) Swiss cheese, shredded

1. Melt the butter in a pot over a moderate flame; now, sauté the shallots until just tender and fragrant or about 3 minutes.
2. Stir in the cream of onion soup and water. Turn the heat to simmer and let it cook for 10 minutes more or until everything is heated through.
3. Heat off; fold in the yogurt and cheese. Whisk until everything is well incorporated and the cheese completely melts.
4. Ladle into individual bowls. Bon appétit!

Per Serving
calories: 365 | fat: 27g | protein: 21g | carbs: 7g net carbs: 6g | fiber: 1g

33. Italian Bacon Omelet

Prep time: 10 minutes | Cook time: 5 minutes | Serves 3

3 ounces (85 g) bacon, diced
2 garlic cloves, minced
1 Italian pepper, chopped
6 eggs, whisked
1 teaspoon Italian seasoning blend
Sea salt and ground black pepper, to season
½ cup goat cheese, shredded

1. Preheat a nonstick skillet over a medium-high flame. Now, cook the bacon until crisp or about 4 minutes; reserve.
2. Add in the garlic and Italian pepper; continue to sauté for a minute or so until aromatic. Pour the eggs into the skillet.
3. Sprinkle with the Italian seasoning blend, salt, and black pepper. Cook until the eggs are golden brown on top. Add the reserved bacon and goat cheese.
4. Fold your omelet in half and serve immediately. Bon appétit!

Per Serving
calories: 481 | fat: 43g | protein: 17g | carbs: 5g net carbs: 4g | fiber: 1g

34. Ham, Cheese and Egg Cups

Prep time: 10 minutes | Cook time: 5 minutes | Serves 6

6 thin slices ham
1 teaspoon mustard
6 eggs
4 ounces (113 g) cream cheese
½ teaspoon red pepper flakes, crushed
Garlic salt and ground black pepper, to taste
6 ounces (170 g) Colby cheese, shredded
2 tablespoons green onions, chopped

1. Spritz a muffin tin with nonstick cooking spray. Place the ham slices over each muffin cup and gently press down until a cup shape forms.
2. In a mixing dish, whisk the mustard, eggs, cream cheese, red pepper, garlic salt, and black pepper.
3. Divide the egg mixture between the cups. Top with the shredded Colby cheese. Bake in the preheated oven at 360ºF (182ºC) approximately 25 minutes.
4. Transfer the muffin tin to a wire rack before serving. Garnish with green onions and serve. Bon appétit!

Per Serving
calories: 258 | fat: 19g | protein: 18g | carbs: 3g net carbs: 3g | fiber: 0g

35. Jalapeño Pepper Cream Cheese Omelet

Prep time: 15 minutes | Cook time: 5 minutes | Serves 1

2 tablespoons cream cheese, softened at room temperature
4 tablespoons shredded cheddar cheese, divided into 2 tablespoons and 2 tablespoons
2 tablespoons cooked bacon bits
1½ teaspoons thinly sliced green onions
1½ teaspoons finely diced seeded jalapeño pepper (about ⅛ medium)
2 large eggs
2 tablespoons heavy cream
¼ teaspoon sea salt
⅛ teaspoon black pepper
1 tablespoon butter

1. In a medium bowl, mash together the cream cheese, 2 tablespoons of the cheddar, and the bacon bits. Stir in the green onions and jalapeño. Set the cream cheese mixture aside.
2. In another medium bowl, whisk together the eggs, heavy cream, sea salt, and black pepper.
3. In a medium skillet, melt the butter over medium heat. Pour in the egg mixture. Cover and cook for 1 to 2 minutes, until mostly cooked through. You can lift with a spatula to get more of the egg underneath if needed, but don't stir or scramble.
4. Drop dollops of the cream cheese mixture onto half of the omelet, distributing as evenly as possible. Use a spatula to fold the omelet over. Sprinkle the remaining 2 tablespoons cheddar cheese on top.
5. Reduce the heat to medium-low. Cover and cook for a couple of minutes, until the cheese melts on top and inside.

Per Serving
calories: 416 | fat: 35g | protein: 22g | carbs: 3g net carbs: 3g | fiber: 0g

36. Prosciutto and Egg Muffins

Prep time: 10 minutes | Cook time: 25 minutes | Serves 6

1 (12-ounce / 340-g) bag frozen spinach, thawed and drained
6 ounces (170 g) prosciutto, very thinly sliced (about 12 large, ultra-thin slices)
1 tablespoon avocado oil
6 cloves garlic, minced
¼ cup finely chopped sun-dried tomatoes
⅛ teaspoon sea salt
Pinch of black pepper, to taste
12 large eggs

1. Preheat the oven to 350ºF (180ºC).
2. Place the thawed spinach into a kitchen towel and squeeze well over the sink, getting rid of as much liquid as possible. Set aside.
3. Line 12 cups of a muffin tin with a thin layer of prosciutto, overlapping the prosciutto pieces slightly if necessary. Wrap around the sides first, then patch any holes and the bottom. Set aside.
4. In a large skillet, heat the oil over medium-high heat. Add the minced garlic and sauté for about 30 seconds, until fragrant. Add the spinach and sun-dried tomatoes. Season with the sea salt and black pepper. Sauté for 5 minutes.
5. Divide the spinach mixture evenly among the prosciutto-lined muffin cups. Crack an egg into each muffin cup.
6. Transfer the pan to the oven and bake until the eggs are done to your liking, approximately as follows:
7. a. Runny yolks: 13 to 15 minutes
8. b. Semi-firm yolks: 16 to 18 minutes
9. c. Firm yolks: 18 to 20 minutes
10. Allow the egg muffins to cool in the pan for a few minutes before removing.

Per Serving
calories: 314 | fat: 22g | protein: 20g | carbs: 7g net carbs: 5g | fiber: 2g

37. Greek Scrambled Eggs

Prep time: 6 minutes | Cook time: 6 minutes | Serves 3

2 tablespoons butter
4 tablespoons Greek yogurt
6 eggs
½ teaspoon cayenne pepper
½ teaspoon oregano
½ teaspoon basil
Sea salt and freshly ground black pepper, to taste
3 ounces (85 g) halloumi cheese, crumbled

1. Melt the butter in a frying pan over moderate heat.
2. Then, thoroughly combine the Greek yogurt, eggs, cayenne pepper, oregano, basil, salt, and black pepper.
3. Pour the yogurt/egg mixture into the frying pan. Continue to cook, stirring with a spatula, for about 6 minutes until thick and creamy curds form.
4. Top with halloumi cheese and serve warm. Enjoy!

Per Serving
calories: 313 | fat: 25g | protein: 19g | carbs: 2g net carbs: 2g | fiber: 0g

38. Boiled Eggs with Lemony Avocado

Prep time: 5 minutes | Cook time: 6 minutes | Serves 3

6 eggs
½ teaspoon kosher salt
½ teaspoon ground black pepper
½ teaspoon cayenne pepper
½ teaspoon dried dill weed
1 avocado, pitted and sliced
1 tablespoon lemon juice

1. Place the eggs in a pan of boiling water; then, cook over low heat for 6 minutes.
2. Peel and halve the eggs. Sprinkle the eggs with salt, black pepper, cayenne pepper, and dill.
3. Serve on individual plates; drizzle the avocado slices with fresh lemon juice and serve with eggs. Enjoy!

Per Serving

calories: 222 | fat: 17g | protein: 12g | carbs: 6g net carbs: 2g | fiber: 4g

39. Broccoli and Cauliflower Omelet

Prep time: 10 minutes | Cook time: 10 minutes | Serves 6

2 tablespoons butter
1 medium-sized leek, chopped
1 cup broccoli florets
1 cup cauliflower florets
8 eggs
4 tablespoons sour cream
¼ teaspoon garlic powder
½ teaspoon cayenne pepper
Sea salt and freshly ground black pepper, to taste
½ cup Greek feta cheese, crumbled

1. Melt the butter in a nonstick aluminum pan over a moderate flame. Now, sauté the leeks, broccoli and cauliflower for 5 minutes, until they've softened.
2. Thoroughly combine the eggs, sour cream, garlic powder, cayenne pepper, salt, and black pepper.
3. Pour the egg mixture over the vegetables in the pan. Move the pan around to spread it out evenly.
4. Continue to cook for about 5 minutes until the eggs are fully set and the surface is smooth. Top with feta cheese and serve immediately. Bon appétit!

Per Serving

calories: 266 | fat: 20g | protein: 15g | carbs: 6g net carbs: 5g | fiber: 1g

40. Paprika Egg Salad with Mayo

Prep time: 5 minutes | Cook time: 13 minutes | Serves 5

7 eggs
2 scallions, chopped
1 cup radishes, thinly sliced
1 bell pepper, chopped
⅓ cup mayonnaise
1 teaspoon stone-ground mustard
Kosher salt and ground black pepper, to taste
1 teaspoon paprika

1. Arrange the eggs in a saucepan. Pour in water (1-inch above the eggs) and bring to a boil. Heat off and let it sit, covered, for 13 minutes.
2. When the eggs are cool enough to handle, peel away the shells, and rinse the eggs under running water. Chop the eggs and transfer them to a salad bowl.
3. Add in the scallions, radishes, bell peppers, mayo, and mustard. Season with salt and black pepper to taste. Gently stir until everything is well incorporated.
4. Sprinkle paprika on top and serve well chilled. Bon appétit!

Per Serving

calories: 172 | fat: 14g | protein: 8g | carbs: 3g net carbs: 2g | fiber: 1g

41. Old-Fashioned Greek Tirokroketes

Prep time: 10 minutes | Cook time: 11 minutes | Serves 5

2 ounces (57 g) feta cheese, crumbled
3 ounces (85 g) smoked gouda cheese, grated
2 ounces (57 g) Cheddar cheese, grated
¼ teaspoon oregano
½ teaspoon basil
¼ teaspoon garlic powder
3 eggs, lightly beaten
¼ cup flaxseed meal
¼ cup almond flour
1 teaspoon baking powder

1. In a mixing bowl, combine all ingredients until everything is well incorporated.
2. Cover the bowl with a plastic wrap and place in your refrigerator at least 30 minutes.
3. Grab about a spoonful of the mixture and roll it into a ball using your hands.
4. Bake in the preheated oven at 390°F (199°C) for about 11 minutes. Serve immediately and enjoy!

Per Serving

calories: 247 | fat: 20g | protein: 14g | carbs: 5g net carbs: 2g | fiber: 3g

42. Mediterranean Shakshuka

Prep time: 10 minutes | Cook time: 0 minutes | Serves 3

1 tablespoon avocado oil
½ cup diced onion
2 cloves garlic, minced
1 (10-ounce / 283-g) can no-salt-added diced tomatoes with green chilies
½ cup tomato purée
1 teaspoon paprika
1 teaspoon ground cumin
½ teaspoon sea salt, plus more for taste
6 large eggs
2 tablespoons chopped fresh parsley

1. In a 12-inch sauté pan, heat the oil over medium-low heat. Add the diced onion and cook for about 10 minutes, until browned. Add the minced garlic and sauté for about 1 minute, until fragrant.
2. Add the diced tomatoes (with juices), tomato purée, paprika, and cumin and mix. Add the sea salt. Cover and simmer 12 to 15 minutes, until the tomato mixture has thickened and most of the liquid is gone. If needed, cook for a couple of minutes uncovered to reduce.
3. Crack the eggs into the pan so that each egg is surrounded by tomato mixture. If desired, you can create a little well for each egg first. Sprinkle the eggs lightly with more sea salt.
4. Cover and cook for 4 to 6 minutes, until the egg whites are opaque, but the yolks are still runny. If you prefer them more done, continue cooking the eggs to your liking.
5. Sprinkle with parsley to serve.

Per Serving

calories: 248 | fat: 15g | protein: 16g | carbs: 10g | net carbs: 8g | fiber: 2g

43. Crustless Cheesy Quiche Lorraine

Prep time: 10 minutes | Cook time: 0 minutes | Serves 6

6 slices bacon
½ cup half-moon sliced onion
6 large eggs
½ cup heavy cream
½ teaspoon sea salt
⅛ teaspoon cayenne pepper
2 tablespoons finely chopped fresh chives
1 cup shredded Swiss cheese, divided into ¾ cup and ¼ cup
1 cup shredded Gruyère cheese, divided into ¾ cup and ¼ cup

1. In a large sauté pan, fry the bacon over medium heat until crispy on both sides. Set aside to drain on paper towels, leaving the bacon grease in the pan.
2. Add the onion to the pan with the bacon grease and sauté over medium heat for about 10 minutes, until translucent and starting to brown. Set aside to cool slightly.
3. Preheat the oven to 350°F (180°C). Grease a 9-inch pie pan.
4. In a large bowl, whisk together the eggs, cream, sea salt, cayenne pepper, and chives. Stir in ¾ cup each of the Swiss and Gruyère cheeses.
5. Pour the egg mixture into the prepared pie pan. Sprinkle with the cooked onion. Cut the bacon into small pieces and sprinkle over the eggs. Push the onion and bacon into the eggs. Sprinkle with the remaining ¼ cup each of the Swiss and Gruyère cheeses.
6. Bake for 30 to 40 minutes, until a knife inserted in the center comes out clean.

Per Serving

calories: 405 | fat: 33g | protein: 22g | carbs: 3g | net carbs: 3g | fiber: 0g

44. Egg and Bacon Muffins with Kale

Prep time: 10 minutes | Cook time: 16 minutes | Serves 4

½ cup bacon
1 shallot, chopped
1 garlic clove, minced
1 cup kale
1 ripe tomato, chopped
6 eggs
1 cup Asiago cheese, shredded
Salt and black pepper, to taste
1 teaspoon dried rosemary
½ teaspoon dried basil
½ teaspoon dried marjoram

1. Start by preheating your oven to 390°F (199°C). Add muffin liners to a muffin tin.
2. Preheat your pan over medium heat. Cook the bacon for 3 to 4 minutes; now, chop the bacon and reserve.
3. Now, cook the shallots and garlic in the bacon fat until they are tender. Add the remaining ingredients and mix to combine well.
4. Pour the batter into muffin cups and bake for 13 minutes or until the edges are slightly browned.
5. Allow your muffins to stand for 5 minutes before removing from the tin. Bon appétit!

Per Serving

calories: 384 | fat: 30g | protein: 24g | carbs: 5g | net carbs: 4g | fiber: 1g

45. Goat Cheese Omelet

Prep time: 5 minutes | Cook time: 7 minutes | Serves 2

2 teaspoons butter, at room temperature
4 eggs, whisked
4 tablespoons goat cheese
1 teaspoon paprika
Sea salt and ground black pepper, to taste

1. Melt the butter in a pan over medium heat.
2. Add the whisked eggs to the pan and cover with the lid; reduce the heat to medium-low.
3. Cook for 4 minutes; now, stir in the cheese and paprika; continue to cook an additional 3 minutes or until cheese has melted.
4. Season with salt and pepper and serve immediately. Enjoy!

Per Serving
calories: 287 | fat: 23g | protein: 20g | carbs: 1g net carbs: 1g | fiber: 0g

46. Bacon Frittata with Olives and Herbs

Prep time: 10 minutes | Cook time: 19 minutes | Serves 4

6 eggs
½ cup heavy cream
2 tablespoons Greek-style yogurt
2 ounces (57 g) bacon, chopped
Sea salt and freshly ground black pepper, to taste
1 tablespoon olive oil
½ cup red onions, peeled and sliced
1 garlic clove, finely chopped
8 Kalamata olives, pitted and sliced
1 teaspoon dried oregano
½ teaspoon dried rosemary
½ teaspoon dried marjoram
4 ounces (113 g) feta cheese, crumbled

1. Preheat your oven to 360ºF (182ºC). Sprits a baking pan with a nonstick cooking spray.
2. Mix the eggs, cream, yogurt, bacon, salt, and black pepper.
3. Heat the oil in a skillet over medium-high heat. Now, cook the onion and garlic until tender and fragrant, about 3 minutes. Transfer the mixture to the prepared baking pan. Pour the egg mixture over the vegetables. Add olives, oregano, rosemary, and marjoram.
4. Bake approximately 13 minutes, until the eggs are set. Scatter feta cheese over the top and bake an additional 3 minutes. Let it sit for 5 minutes; slice into wedges and serve.

Per Serving
calories: 345 | fat: 29g | protein: 18g | carbs: 4g net carbs: 3g | fiber: 1g

47. Cheesy Tomato Frittata

Prep time: 5 minutes | Cook time: 25 to 33 minutes | Serves 4

⅓ cup Greek-style yogurt
6 eggs
⅔ cup Cheddar cheese, shredded
1 tomato, sliced
2 scallions, chopped

1. Start by preheating your oven to 355ºF (179ºC).
2. Then, mix the Greek-style yogurt and eggs until frothy. Add in ½ of cheese, tomato, and scallions. Spoon the mixture into a lightly oiled baking pan.
3. Scatter the remaining Cheddar cheese over the top.
4. Bake in the preheated oven for 25 to 33 minutes or until the edges appear cooked and the center jiggles just a bit. Remove your frittata to a cooling rack before slicing and serving.
5. Slice into four wedges and serve. Bon appétit!

Per Serving
calories: 299 | fat: 23g | protein: 20g | carbs: 3g net carbs: 3g | fiber: 0g

48. Fried Eggs with Canadian Bacon

Prep time: 5 minutes | Cook time: 5 minutes | Serves 2

2 slices Canadian bacon
4 eggs
¼ teaspoon ground black pepper
Salt, to season
8 cherry tomatoes, halves

1. Heat up a nonstick aluminum pan over a medium-high flame. Once hot, fry the bacon for 5 minutes until crispy; reserve, living the rendered fat in the pan.
2. Turn the heat to medium-low. Crack the eggs into the bacon grease. Cover the pan with a lid and fry the eggs until they are cooked through.
3. Salt and pepper to taste. Serve with the reserved bacon and cherry tomatoes on the side. Enjoy!

Per Serving
calories: 326 | fat: 13g | protein: 46g | carbs: 5g net carbs: 4g | fiber: 1g

49. Mangalore-Style Egg Curry

Prep time: 15 minutes | Cook time: 20 minutes | Serves 4

2 tablespoons olive oil
½ cup scallions, chopped
1 teaspoon Kashmiri chili powder
¼ teaspoon carom seeds
¼ teaspoon methi seeds
Kosher salt and ground black pepper, to taste
2 ripe tomatoes, puréed
2 teaspoons tamarind paste
½ cup chicken stock
4 boiled egg, peeled
1 teaspoon curry paste
2 tablespoons curry leaves
½ teaspoon cinnamon powder
½ cup coconut milk
1 tablespoon cilantro leaves

1. Heat the oil in a pan over medium heat. Now, cook the scallions and chili for 3 minutes, until tender and fragrant.
2. Add carom seeds, methi seeds, salt, pepper, and tomatoes; cook for a further 8 minutes.
3. Then, add the tamarind paste and chicken stock. Reduce the heat to medium-low and cook for 3 minutes more.
4. Add the eggs, curry paste, curry leaves, cinnamon powder, and coconut milk. Let it simmer for 6 minutes more. Garnish with cilantro leaves. Bon appétit!

Per Serving

calories: 305 | fat: 16g | protein: 32g | carbs: 6g net carbs: 5g | fiber: 1g

50. Two-Cheese Sausage Balls

Prep time: 5 minutes | Cook time: 18 minutes | Serves 3

½ pound (227 g) breakfast sausage
½ cup almond flour
½ cup Colby cheese, shredded
4 tablespoons Romano cheese, freshly grated
1 egg
1 garlic clove, pressed
2 tablespoons fresh chives, minced

1. Thoroughly combine all ingredients in a mixing bowl; mix until everything is well incorporated.
2. Shape the mixture into balls and arrange them on a parchment-lined cookie sheet. Bake in the preheated oven at 360ºF (182ºC) for about 18 minutes.
3. Serve warm or cold. Bon appétit!

Per Serving

calories: 412 | fat: 35g | protein: 20g | carbs: 5g net carbs: 5g | fiber: 0g

51. Sausage Frittatas with Goat Cheese

Prep time: 10 minutes | Cook time: 25 to 27 minutes | Serves 6

6 ounces (170 g) pork sausage, sliced
1 teaspoon fresh garlic
4 tablespoons green onions, chopped
1 bell pepper, chopped
⅓ cup heavy whipping cream
5 eggs
Flaky salt and ground black pepper, to season
½ teaspoon basil
½ teaspoon oregano
1⅓ cups goat cheese, crumbled

1. Heat up a lightly oiled nonstick skillet over a moderate flame. Then, sear the sausage, crumbling with a fork.
2. Then, cook the garlic, onions, and bell pepper in the pan drippings, stirring frequently to ensure even cooking. Add the sausage back to the skillet and stir to combine. Heat off.
3. Next, in a mixing dish, thoroughly combine the heavy whipping cream with the eggs; fold in the sausage/vegetable mixture. Season with salt, black pepper, basil, and oregano.
4. Divide the mixture between lightly greased muffin cups. Bake in the preheated oven at 360ºF (182ºC) approximately 20 minutes.
5. Top with the cheese and bake for 5 to 7 minutes longer or until they starting to get slightly browned on top.
6. You can store these mini frittatas in the refrigerator for up to 4 days and reheat when ready to eat. Bon appétit!

Per Serving

calories: 287 | fat: 24g | protein: 16g | carbs: 2g net carbs: 2g | fiber: 0g

52. Dilled Egg Salad with Dijon Mayo

Prep time: 5 minutes | Cook time: 12 minutes | Serves 3

4 eggs
1 teaspoon Dijon mustard
4 tablespoons mayonnaise
1 scallion, chopped
1 tablespoon fresh dill, minced

1. Place the eggs in a saucepan and fill with enough water. Bring the water to a rolling boil; heat off. Cover and allow the eggs to sit for about 12 minutes; let them cool.
2. Peel and chop the eggs; place them in a salad bowl; add in the mustard, mayonnaise, scallions, and dill. Salt and pepper to taste.
3. Serve well-chilled and enjoy!

Per Serving

calories: 212 | fat: 20g | protein: 8g | carbs: 1g net carbs: 1g | fiber: 0g

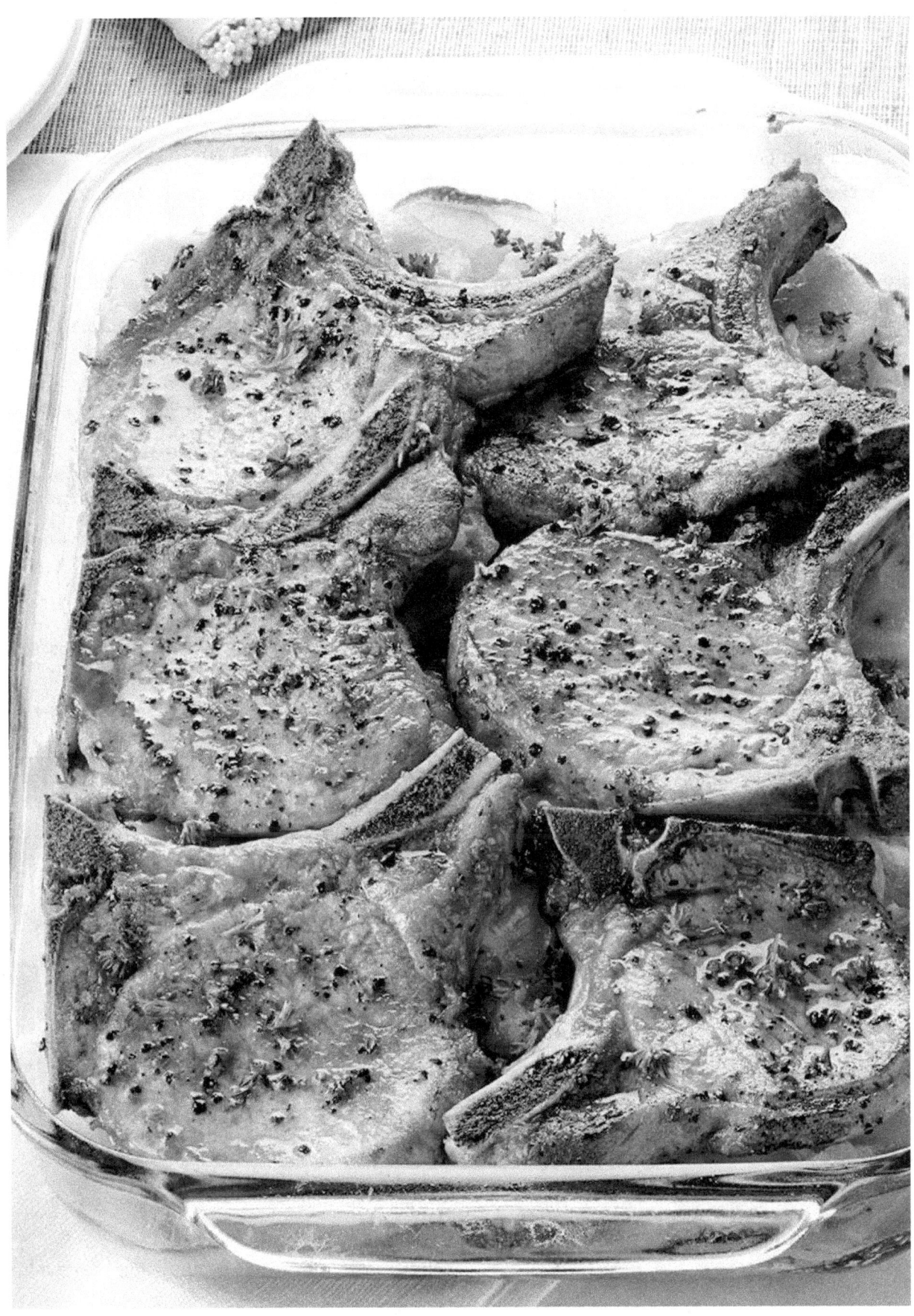

Chapter 4 Pork

53. Pork and Beef Meatballs

Prep time: 5 minutes | Cook time: 13 minutes | Serves 5

1 pound (454 g) ground pork	onion, chopped
½ pound (227 g) ground beef	garlic cloves, minced
	1 teaspoon Hungarian spice blend

1. In a mixing bowl, thoroughly combine all ingredients until they are well incorporated. Form the mixture into meatballs with oiled hands. Place your meatballs on a tinfoil-lined baking sheet.
2. Bake in the preheated oven at 395ºF (202ºC) for 12 to 14 minutes or until they are golden brown.
3. Arrange on a nice serving platter and serve. Bon appétit!

Per Serving
calories: 377 | fat: 24g | protein: 36g | carbs: 2g net carbs: 2g | fiber: 0g

54. Bacon and Pork Omelet

Prep time: 5 minutes | Cook time: 12 minutes | Serves 5

2 ounces (57 g) bacon, diced	1 shallot, chopped
1 pound (454 g) ground pork	1 teaspoon ginger-garlic paste
	6 eggs, whisked

1. Heat up a nonstick skillet over a moderate flame. Now, cook the bacon until it releases easily from the bottom of the skillet.
2. Then, add in the ground pork and shallot and cook for 4 to 5 minutes or until the pork is no longer pink; discard the excess fat.
3. Fold in the ginger-garlic paste and whisked eggs; partially cover and let it cook on mediumlow temperature for 4 minutes. Flip your omelet and cook on the other side for 3 minutes longer.
4. Slide your omelet onto a plate and serve right now. Bon appétit!

Per Serving
calories: 393 | fat: 28g | protein: 31g | carbs: 1g net carbs: 1g | fiber: 0g

55. Mustard Pork Meatballs

Prep time: 5 minutes | Cook time: 21 minutes | Serves 2

1 pound (454 g) ground pork	½ cup almond flour
Salt and black pepper, to taste	¼ cup mozzarella cheese, grated
1 tablespoon yellow mustard	¼ cup hot sauce
	1 egg

1. Preheat oven to 400ºF (205ºC) and line a baking tray with parchment paper.
2. In a bowl, combine the pork, pepper, mustard, flour, mozzarella cheese, salt, and egg. Form meatballs and arrange them on the baking tray.
3. Cook for 16 minutes, then pour over the hot sauce and bake for 5 more minutes.
4. Serve warm.

Per Serving
calories: 518 | fat: 22g | protein: 60g | carbs: 2g net carbs: 1g | fiber: 1g

56. Baked Cheesy Pork and Veggies

Prep time: 10 minutes | Cook time: 40 minutes | Serves 4

1 pound (454 g) ground pork	to taste
1 onion, chopped	1 zucchini, sliced
1 garlic clove, minced	¼ cup heavy cream
½ green beans, chopped	5 eggs
Salt and black pepper	½ cup Monterey Jack cheese, grated

1. In a bowl, mix onion, green beans, ground pork, garlic, black pepper and salt. Layer the meat mixture on the bottom of a small greased baking dish. Spread zucchini slices on top.
2. In a separate bowl, combine cheese, eggs and heavy cream. Top with this creamy mixture and bake for 40 minutes at 360ºF (182ºC), until the edges and top become brown.
3. Serve immediately.

Per Serving
calories: 335 | fat: 21g | protein: 28g | carbs: 4g net carbs: 4g | fiber: 0g

57. Cheesy Pork Nachos

Prep time: 5 minutes | Cook time: 10 minutes | Serves 4

1 bag low carb tortilla chips
2 cups leftover pulled pork
1 red bell pepper, seeded and chopped
1 red onion, diced
2 cups shredded Monterey Jack cheese

1. Preheat oven to 350ºF (180ºC).
2. Arrange the chips in a medium cast iron pan, scatter pork over, followed by red bell pepper, and onion, and sprinkle with cheese.
3. Place the pan in the oven and cook for 10 minutes until the cheese has melted. Allow cooling for 3 minutes and serve.

Per Serving
calories: 473 | fat: 25g | protein: 37g | carbs: 11g net carbs: 9g | fiber: 2g

58. Pork and Mashed Cauliflower Crust

Prep time: 15 minutes | Cook time: 1 hour | Serves 8

Crust:
1 egg
¼ cup butter
2 cups almond flour
¼ teaspoon xanthan gum
¼ cup mozzarella, shredded
A pinch of salt

Filling:
2 pounds (907 g) ground pork
⅓ cup onion, pureed
¾ teaspoon allspice
1 cup cauliflower, mashed
1 tablespoon ground sage
1 tablespoon butter

1. Preheat your oven to 350ºF (180ºC). Whisk together all of the crust ingredients in a bowl. Make two balls out of the mixture, and refrigerate for 10 minutes.
2. Melt the butter in a pan over medium heat and add the ground pork. Cook for about 10minutes, stirring occasionally. Remove to a bowl. Add in the other ingredients and mix to combine.
3. Roll out the tart crusts and place one at the bottom of a greased baking pan. Spread the filling over the crust. Top with the other coat. Bake for 50 minutes, then serve.

Per Serving
calories: 444 | fat: 19g | protein: 40g | carbs: 6g net carbs: 4g | fiber: 2g

59. Pork Chops and Bacon

Prep time: 5 minutes | Cook time: 11 minutes | Serves 6

7 strips bacon, chopped
6 pork chops
Pink salt and black pepper to taste
5 sprigs fresh thyme
¼ cup chicken broth
½ cup heavy cream

1. Cook bacon in a large skillet over medium heat for 5 minutes to crispy. Remove with a slotted spoon onto a paper towel-lined plate to soak up excess fat. Season pork chops with salt and black pepper, and brown in the bacon grease for 4 minutes on each side. Remove to the bacon plate.
2. Stir the thyme, chicken broth, and heavy cream in the same skillet, and simmer for 5 minutes. Season with salt and black pepper. Put the chops and bacon in the skillet, and cook further for another 2 minutes. Serve chops and a generous ladle of sauce with cauli mash.

Per Serving
calories: 435 | fat: 37g | protein: 22g | carbs: 4g net carbs: 3g | fiber: 1g

60. Pork Steaks with Chimichurri Sauce

Prep time: 10 minutes | Cook time: 5 minutes | Serves 4

1 garlic clove, minced
½ teaspoon white wine vinegar
1 tablespoon parsley leaves, chopped
1 tablespoon cilantro leaves, chopped
1 tablespoon extra-virgin olive oil
16 ounces (454 g) pork loin steaks
Salt and black pepper to season
1 tablespoon sesame oil

1. To make the sauce: in a bowl, mix the parsley, cilantro and garlic. Add the vinegar, extra-virgin olive oil, and salt, and combine well.
2. Preheat a grill pan over medium heat. Rub the pork with sesame oil, and season with salt and pepper. Grill the meat for 4 to 5 minutes on each side until no longer pink in the center. Put the pork on a serving plate and spoon chimichurri sauce over, to serve.

Per Serving
calories: 326 | fat: 21g | protein: 32g | carbs: 2g net carbs: 2g | fiber: 0g

61. Balsamic Pork Loin Chops

Prep time: 5 minutes | Cook time: 15 minutes | Serves 4

4 pork loin chops, boneless
1 tablespoon rosemary, chopped
1 tablespoon balsamic vinegar
1 garlic clove, minced
1 tablespoon olive oil
Salt and black pepper to taste

1. Put the pork in a deep dish. Add in the balsamic vinegar, rosemary, garlic, olive oil, salt, and black pepper, and toss to coat. Cover the dish with plastic wrap and marinate the pork for 1 to 2 hours.
2. Preheat grill to medium heat. Remove the pork when ready, reserve the marinade and grill covered for 10 minutes per side. Remove the pork chops and let them sit for 4 minutes on a serving plate.
3. In a saucepan over medium heat, pour in the reserved marinade, add in 1 tablespoon water and bring to a boil for 2-3 minutes until the liquid becomes thickened. Top the chops with the sauce and serve.

Per Serving

calories: 363 | fat: 21g | protein: 40g | carbs: 1g net carbs: 1g | fiber: 0g

62. Mediterranean Pork

Prep time: 10 minutes | Cook time: 35 minutes | Serves 4

1 garlic clove, minced
4 pork chops, bone-in
Salt and black pepper, to taste
1 teaspoon dried oregano
¼ cup kalamata olives, pitted and sliced
1 tablespoon olive oil
1 tablespoon vegetable broth
¼ cup feta cheese, crumbled

1. Preheat the oven to 425°F (220°C).
2. Rub pork chops with pepper and salt, and add in a roasting pan. Stir in the garlic, olives, olive oil, broth, and oregano, set in the oven and bake for 10 minutes. Reduce heat to 350°F (180°C) and roast for 25 minutes.
3. Slice the pork, divide among plates, and sprinkle with pan juices and feta cheese all over.
4. Serve immediately.

Per Serving

calories: 394 | fat: 24g | protein: 41g | carbs: 1g net carbs: 1g | fiber: 0g

63. Lemony Peanuts Pork Chops

Prep time: 10 minutes | Cook time: 30 minutes | Serves 4

⅓ cup cilantro
⅓ cup mint
1 onion, chopped
¼ cup peanuts
1 tablespoon olive oil
Salt, to taste
4 pork chops
2 garlic cloves, minced
Juice and zest from 1 lemon

1. Preheat oven to 250°F (121°C).
2. In a food processor, combine the cilantro with olive oil, mint, peanuts, salt, lemon zest, garlic, and onion. Rub the pork with this mixture, place in a bowl, and refrigerate for 1 hour while covered.
3. Remove to a greased baking dish, sprinkle with lemon juice, and bake for 30 minutes in the oven.
4. Serve immediately.

Per Serving

calories: 428 | fat: 26g | protein: 42g | carbs: 6g net carbs: 5g | fiber: 1g

64. Pork Shoulder and Sauerkraut Casserole

Prep time: 15 minutes | Cook time: 9 to 10 hours | Serves 6

3 tablespoons extra-virgin olive oil, divided
2 tablespoons butter
2 pounds (907 g) pork shoulder roast
1 (28-ounce / 794-g) jar sauerkraut, drained
1 cup chicken broth
½ sweet onion, thinly sliced
¼ cup granulated erythritol

1. Lightly grease the insert of the slow cooker with 1 tablespoon of the olive oil.
2. In a large skillet over medium-high heat, heat the remaining 2 tablespoons of the olive oil and the butter. Add the pork to the skillet and brown on all sides for about 10 minutes.
3. Transfer to the insert and add the sauerkraut, broth, onion, and erythritol.
4. Cover and cook on low for 9 to 10 hours.
5. Serve warm.

Per Serving

calories: 516 | fat: 42g | protein: 28g | carbs: 7g net carbs: 3g | fiber: 4g

65. Pork Chops with Broccoli

Prep time: 10 minutes | Cook time: 51 minutes | Serves 4

1 shallot, chopped
2 (10½-ounce / 298-g) cans mushroom soup
4 pork chops
½ cup sliced mushrooms
Salt and black pepper to taste
1 tablespoon parsley
½ head broccoli, cut into florets

1. Steam the broccoli in salted water over medium heat for 6-8 minutes until tender. Set aside.
2. Preheat the oven to 370ºF (188ºC). Season the pork chops with salt and pepper, and place in a greased baking dish. Combine the mushroom soup, mushrooms and onion, in a bowl. Pour this mixture over the pork chops. Bake for 45 minutes. Sprinkle with parsley and serve with broccoli.

Per Serving
calories: 434 | fat: 20g | protein: 40g | carbs: 7g net carbs: 5g | fiber: 2g

66. Pork and Veggies Burgers

Prep time: 10 minutes | Cook time: 5 minutes | Serves 6

2 pound (907 g) ground pork
Pink salt and chili pepper, to taste
1 tablespoon olive oil
1 tablespoon butter
1 white onion, sliced into rings
1 tablespoon balsamic vinegar
3 drops liquid stevia
6 low carb burger buns, halved
2 firm tomatoes, sliced into rings

1. Combine the pork, salt and chili pepper in a bowl, and mold out 6 patties.
2. Heat the olive oil in a skillet over medium heat, and fry the patties for 4 to 5 minutes on each side until golden brown on the outside. Remove onto a plate, and sit for 3 minutes.
3. Melt butter in a skillet over medium heat, sauté onions for 2 minutes, and stir in the balsamic vinegar and liquid stevia. Cook for 30 seconds stirring once, or twice until caramelized. In each bun, place a patty, top with some onion rings and 2 tomato rings.
4. Serve the burgers with cheddar cheese dip.

Per Serving
calories: 315 | fat: 23g | protein: 16g | carbs: 7g net carbs: 6g | fiber: 1g

67. Golden Pork Burgers

Prep time: 10 minutes | Cook time: 10 minutes | Serves 4

1 tablespoon olive oil
1 pound (454 g) ground pork
Salt and black pepper to taste
½ teaspoon chili pepper
1 tablespoon parsley
1 white onion, sliced into rings
½ tablespoon balsamic vinegar
1 drop liquid stevia
1 tomato, sliced into rings
1 tablespoon mayonnaise

1. Warm half of the oil in a skillet over medium heat, sauté onions for 2 minutes, and stir in the balsamic vinegar and liquid stevia. Cook for 30 seconds stirring once or twice until caramelized; remove to a plate. Combine the pork, salt, black pepper and chili pepper in a bowl, and mold out 2 patties.
2. Heat the remaining olive oil in a skillet over medium heat and fry the patties for 4 to 5 minutes on each side until golden brown on the outside. Remove to a plate and sit for 3 minutes.
3. In each tomato slice, place half of the mayonnaise and a patty, and top with some onion rings. Cover with another tomato slice and serve.

Per Serving
calories: 380 | fat: 27g | protein: 29g | carbs: 2g net carbs: 2g | fiber: 0g

68. Buttered Pork Chops

Prep time: 5 minutes | Cook time: 12 minutes | Serves 4

½ tablespoon olive oil
1 tablespoon butter
1 tablespoon rosemary
4 pork chops
Salt and black pepper, to taste
A pinch of paprika
½ teaspoon chili powder

1. Rub the pork chops with olive oil, salt, black pepper, paprika, and chili powder. Heat a grill over medium, add in the pork chops and cook for 10 minutes, flipping once halfway through.
2. Remove to a serving plate. In a pan over low heat, warm the butter until it turns nutty brown. Pour over the pork chops, sprinkle with rosemary and serve.
3. Serve immediately.

Per Serving
calories: 370 | fat: 22g | protein: 40g | carbs: 1g net carbs: 1g | fiber: 0g

69. Creamy Pork Chops and Canadian Ham

Prep time: 5 minutes | Cook time: 25 minutes | Serves 4

4 ounces (113 g) Canadian ham, chopped
4 pork chops
Salt and black pepper to taste
2 sprigs fresh thyme
1 tablespoon heavy cream
½ teaspoon Dijon mustard

1. Cook ham in a skillet over medium heat for 5 minutes. Remove to a plate. Season pork chops with salt and pepper, and brown in the bacon fat for 4 minutes on each side.
2. Remove to the bacon plate. Stir in thyme, 1 tablespoon of water, mustard, and heavy cream and simmer for 5 minutes. Return the chops and bacon, and cook for another 10 minutes. Garnish with thyme leaves.
3. Serve immediately.

Per Serving

calories: 373 | fat: 19g | protein: 40g | carbs: 1g net carbs: 1g | fiber: 0g

70. Pork Chops with Blackberry Gravy

Prep time: 10 minutes | Cook time: 10 minutes | Serves 4

1 tablespoon olive oil
1 pound (454 g) pork chops
Salt and black pepper to taste
1 cup blackberries
1 tablespoon chicken broth
½ tablespoon rosemary leaves, chopped
1 tablespoon balsamic vinegar
1 teaspoon Worcestershire sauce

1. Place the blackberries in a bowl and mash them with a fork until jam-like. Pour into a saucepan, add the chicken broth and rosemary. Bring to boil on low heat for 4 minutes. Stir in balsamic vinegar and Worcestershire sauce. Simmer for 1 minute.
2. Heat oil in a skillet over medium heat, season the pork with salt and black pepper, and cook for 5 minutes on each side. Put on serving plates and spoon sauce over the pork chops.

Per Serving

calories: 302 | fat: 18g | protein: 28g | carbs: 4g net carbs: 2g | fiber: 2g

71. Lemony Pork Loin and Brussels Sprouts

Prep time: 10 minutes | Cook time: 1¼ hours | Serves 4

½ pound (227 g) Brussels sprouts, chopped
1 tablespoon olive oil
Salt and black pepper, to taste
1½ pounds (680 g) pork loin
A pinch of dry mustard
1 teaspoon hot red pepper flakes
½ teaspoon ginger, minced
2 garlic cloves, minced
½ lemon sliced
¼ cup water

1. Preheat oven to 380ºF (193ºC). In a bowl, combine the ginger with salt, mustard, and black pepper.
2. Add in meat, toss to coat. Heat the oil in a saucepan over medium heat, brown the pork on all sides, for 8 minutes. Transfer to the oven and roast for 1 hour.
3. To the saucepan, add Brussels sprouts, lemon slices, garlic, and water; cook for 10 minutes. Serve on a platter, sprinkled with pan juices on top.

Per Serving

calories: 418 | fat: 22g | protein: 45g | carbs: 7g net carbs: 4g | fiber: 3g

72. Stewed Pork and Veggies

Prep time: 15 minutes | Cook time: 30 minutes | Serves 4

1 tablespoon olive oil
1 red bell pepper, chopped
1 pound (454 g) stewed pork, cubed
Salt and black pepper, to taste
2 cups cauliflower florets
2 cups broccoli florets
1 onion, chopped
14 ounces (397 g) canned diced tomatoes
¼ teaspoon garlic powder
1 tablespoon tomato puree
1½ cups water
1 tablespoon parsley, chopped

1. In a pan, heat olive oil and cook the pork over medium heat for 5 minutes, until browned.
2. Place in the bell pepper, and onion, and cook for 4 minutes. Stir in the water, tomatoes, broccoli, cauliflower, tomato purée, and garlic powder; bring to a simmer and cook for 20minutes while covered. Adjust the seasoning and serve sprinkled with parsley.

Per Serving

calories: 299 | fat: 13g | protein: 35g | carbs: 10g net carbs: 6g | fiber: 4g

73. Pork Medallions with Rosemary

Prep time: 10 minutes | Cook time: 20 minutes | Serves 4

2 onions, chopped
4 ounces (113 g) bacon, chopped
½ cup vegetable stock
Salt and black pepper, to taste
1 tablespoon fresh rosemary, chopped
1 pound (454 g) pork medallions

1. Fry the bacon in a pan over medium heat, until crispy, and remove to a plate. Add in onions, black pepper, and salt, and cook for 5 minutes; set to the same plate with bacon.
2. Add pork to the pan, brown for 3 minutes, turn, and cook for 7 minutes. Stir in stock and cook for 2 minutes. Return bacon and onions to the pan and cook for 1 minute. Garnish with rosemary.

Per Serving
calories: 258 | fat: 15g | protein: 23g | carbs: 8g net carbs: 6g | fiber: 2g

74. Lemony Pork Chops with Veggies

Prep time: 10 minutes | Cook time: 12 minutes | Serves 4

1 tablespoon olive oil
1 tablespoon lemon juice
1 garlic clove, pureed
4 pork loin chops
⅓ head cabbage, shredded
1 tomato, chopped
1 tablespoon white wine
Salt and black pepper to taste
¼ teaspoon cumin
¼ teaspoon ground nutmeg
1 tablespoon parsley

1. In a bowl, mix the lemon juice, garlic, salt, pepper and olive oil. Brush the pork with the mixture.
2. Preheat grill to high heat. Grill the pork for 2 to 3 minutes on each side until cooked through.
3. Remove to serving plates. Warm the remaining olive oil in a pan and cook in cabbage for 5 minutes.
4. Drizzle with white wine, sprinkle with cumin, nutmeg, salt and pepper. Add in the tomatoes, cook for another 5 minutes, stirring occasionally. Ladle the sautéed cabbage to the side of the chops and serve sprinkled with parsley.

Per Serving
calories: 382 | fat: 21g | protein: 41g | carbs: 6g net carbs: 4g | fiber: 2g

75. Pork with Raspberry Sauce

Prep time: 10 minutes | Cook time: 15 minutes | Serves 4

1 tablespoon olive oil
2 pound pork chops
Salt and black pepper to taste
2 cups raspberries
¼ cup water
1½ tablespoon Italian herb mix
1 tablespoon balsamic vinegar
1 teaspoon Worcestershire sauce

1. Heat oil in a skillet over medium heat, season the pork with salt and black pepper and cook for 5 minutes on each side. Put in serving plates, and reserve the pork drippings.
2. Mash raspberries with a fork in a bowl until jam-like. Pour into a saucepan, add water, and herb mix. Cook on low heat for 4 minutes. Stir in pork drippings, vinegar, and Worcestershire sauce. Simmer for 1 minute. Dish the pork chops, spoon sauce over, and serve with braised rapini.

Per Serving
calories: 413 | fat: 32g | protein: 26g | carbs: 5g net carbs: 1g | fiber: 4g

76. BBQ Grilled Pork Spare Ribs

Prep time: 10 minutes | Cook time: 50 minutes | Serves 4

1 tablespoon erythritol
Salt and black pepper, to taste
1 tablespoon olive oil
1 teaspoon chipotle powder
1 teaspoon garlic powder
1 pound (454 g) pork spare ribs
1 tablespoon sugar-free BBQ sauce + extra for serving

1. Mix the erythritol, salt, pepper, oil, chipotle, and garlic powder. Brush on the meaty sides of the ribs, and wrap in foil. Sit for 30 minutes to marinate.
2. Preheat oven to 400ºF (205ºC), place wrapped ribs on a baking sheet, and cook for 40 minutes to be cooked through. Remove ribs and aluminum foil, brush with BBQ sauce, and brown under the broiler for 10 minutes on both sides. Slice and serve with extra BBQ sauce and lettuce tomato salad.

Per Serving
calories: 294 | fat: 18g | protein: 28g | carbs: 3g net carbs: 3g | fiber: 0g

77. Pork Steaks with Broccoli

Prep time: 10 minutes | Cook time: 25 minutes | Serves 4

1 tablespoon olive oil
1 tablespoon butter
4 pork steaks, bone-in
½ cup water
Salt and black pepper, to taste
2 garlic cloves, minced
1 tablespoon fresh parsley, chopped
½ head broccoli, cut into florets
½ lemon, sliced

1. Heat oil and butter over high heat. Add in the pork steaks, season with pepper and salt, and cook until browned; set to a plate. In the same pan, add garlic and broccoli and cook for 4 minutes.
2. Pour the water, lemon slices, salt, and black pepper, and cook everything for 5 minutes.
3. Return the pork steaks to the pan and cook for 10 minutes. Serve the steaks sprinkled with sauce with parsley.

Per Serving

calories: 561 | fat: 39g | protein: 47g | carbs: 3g net carbs: 2g | fiber: 1g

78. Pork Lettuce Wraps

Prep time: 10 minutes | Cook time: 14 minutes | Serves 6

2 pound (907 g) ground pork
1 tablespoon ginger-garlic paste
Pink salt and chili pepper, to taste
1 teaspoon butter
1 fresh head iceberg lettuce
2 sprigs green onion, chopped
1 red bell pepper, chopped
½ cucumber, finely chopped

1. Put the pork with ginger-garlic, salt, and chili pepper seasoning in a saucepan. Cook for 10
2. minutes over medium heat while breaking any lumps until the beef is no longer pink.
3. Drain liquid and add the butter, melt, and brown the meat for 4 minutes with continuous stirring. Pat the lettuce dry with paper towel and in each leaf spoon two to three tablespoons of pork, top with green onions, bell pepper, and cucumber. Serve with soy drizzling sauce.

Per Serving

calories: 311 | fat: 24g | protein: 19g | carbs: 3g net carbs: 1g | fiber: 2g

79. Pork Loin Chops

Prep time: 10 minutes | Cook time: 13 minutes | Serves 2

½ tablespoon butter
½ tablespoon olive oil
4 pork loin chops
½ teaspoon Dijon mustard
½ tablespoon coconut aminos
½ teaspoon lemon juice
1 teaspoon cumin seeds
½ tablespoon water
Salt and black pepper, to taste
½ cup chives, chopped

1. Set a pan over medium heat and warm butter and olive oil, add in the pork chops, season with salt, and pepper, cook for 4 minutes, turn and cook for additional 4 minutes. Remove to a plate.
2. In a bowl, mix the water with lemon juice, cumin seeds, mustard and coconut aminos. Pour the mustard sauce in the same pan and simmer for 5 minutes. Spread over pork, top with chives and serve.

Per Serving

calories: 382 | fat: 21g | protein: 38g | carbs: 1g net carbs: 1g | fiber: 0g

80. Lemony Pork Chops and Brussel Sprouts

Prep time: 10 minutes | Cook time: 16 minutes | Serves 6

1 tablespoon lemon juice
3 cloves garlic, pureed
Salt and black pepper to taste
1 tablespoon olive oil
6 pork loin chops
1 tablespoon butter
1 pound (454 g) Brussel sprouts, halved
1 tablespoon white wine

1. Preheat grill to 400ºF (205ºC), and mix the lemon juice, garlic, salt, pepper, and oil in a bowl.
2. Brush the pork with mixture, place onto a baking sheet, and cook for 6 minutes on each side until browned. Share into 6 plates, and make the side dish.
3. Melt butter in a small wok, or pan and cook in Brussel sprouts for 5 minutes until tender.
4. Drizzle with white wine, sprinkle with salt and black pepper, and cook for another 5 minutes. Ladle Brussel sprouts to the side of the chops, and serve with a hot sauce.

Per Serving

calories: 400 | fat: 22g | protein: 36g | carbs: 7g net carbs: 4g | fiber: 3g

81. Tangy Pork Rib Roast

Prep time: 10 minutes | Cook time: 1 hour | Serves 6

¼ cup good-quality olive oil
Zest and juice of 1 lemon
Zest and juice of 1 lemon
4 rosemary sprigs, lightly crushed
4 thyme sprigs, lightly crushed
1 (4-bone) pork rib roast, about 2½ pounds
6 garlic cloves, peeled
Sea salt, for seasoning
Freshly ground black pepper, for seasoning

1. Make the marinade. In a large bowl, combine the olive oil, lemon zest, lemon juice, lemon zest, lemon juice, rosemary sprigs, and thyme sprigs.
2. Marinate the roast. Use a small knife to make six 1-inch-deep slits in the fatty side of the roast. Stuff the garlic cloves in the slits. Put the roast in the bowl with the marinade and turn it to coat it well with the marinade. Cover the bowl and refrigerate it overnight, turning the roast in the marinade several times.
3. Preheat the oven. Set the oven temperature to 350ºF (180ºC).
4. Roast the pork. Remove the pork from the marinade and season it with salt and pepper, then put it in a baking dish and let it come to room temperature. Roast the pork until it's cooked through (145- to 160-ºF / 63- to 71-ºC internal temperature), about 1 hour. Throw out any leftover marinade.
5. Serve. Let the pork rest for 10 minutes, then cut it into slices and arrange the slices on a platter. Serve it warm.

Per Serving
calories: 403 | fat: 30g | protein: 30g | carbs: 1g net carbs: 1g | fiber: 0g

82. Pork Chops with Greek Salsa

Prep time: 15 minutes | Cook time: 15 minutes | Serves 4

¼ cup good-quality olive oil, divided
1 tablespoon red wine vinegar
3 teaspoons chopped fresh oregano, divided
1 teaspoon minced garlic
4 (4-ounce / 113-g) boneless center-cut loin pork chops
½ cup halved cherry tomatoes
½ yellow bell pepper, diced
½ English cucumber, chopped
¼ red onion, chopped
1 tablespoon balsamic vinegar
Sea salt, for seasoning
Freshly ground black pepper, for seasoning

1. Marinate the pork. In a medium bowl, stir together 3 tablespoons of the olive oil, the vinegar, 2 teaspoons of the oregano, and the garlic. Add the pork chops to the bowl, turning them to get them coated with the marinade. Cover the bowl and place it in the refrigerator for 30 minutes.
2. Make the salsa. While the pork is marinating, in a medium bowl, stir together the remaining 1 tablespoon of olive oil, the tomatoes, yellow bell pepper, cucumber, red onion, vinegar, and the remaining 1 teaspoon of oregano. Season the salsa with salt and pepper. Set the bowl aside.
3. Grill the pork chops. Heat a grill to medium-high heat. Remove the pork chops from the marinade and grill them until just cooked through, 6 to 8 minutes per side.
4. Serve. Rest the pork for 5 minutes. Divide the pork between four plates and serve them with a generous scoop of the salsa.

Per Serving
calories: 277 | fat: 17g | protein: 25g | carbs: 4g net carbs: 3g | fiber: 1g

83. Tangy-Garlicky Pork Chops

Prep time: 10 minutes | Cook time: 15 minutes | Serves 4

1 pound (454 g) boneless center-cut pork chops, pounded to ¼ inch thick
Sea salt, for seasoning
Freshly ground black pepper, for seasoning
¼ cup good-quality olive oil, divided
¼ cup finely chopped fresh cilantro
1 tablespoon minced garlic
Juice of 1 lime

1. Marinate the pork. Pat the pork chops dry and season them lightly with salt and pepper. Place them in a large bowl, add 2 tablespoons of the olive oil, and the cilantro, garlic, and lime juice. Toss to coat the chops. Cover the bowl and marinate the chops at room temperature for 30 minutes.
2. Cook the pork. In a large skillet over medium-high heat, warm the remaining 2 tablespoons of olive oil. Add the pork chops in a single layer and fry them, turning them once, until they're just cooked through and still juicy, 6 to 7 minutes per side.
3. Serve. Divide the chops between four plates and serve them immediately.

Per Serving
calories: 249 | fat: 16g | protein: 25g | carbs: 2g net carbs: 2g | fiber: 0g

84. Pork and Butternut Squash Stew

Prep time: 15 minutes | Cook time: 45 minutes | Serves 6

1 cup butternut squash
2 pounds (907 g) pork, chopped
1 tablespoon peanut butter
1 tablespoon peanuts, chopped
1 garlic clove, minced
½ cup onion, chopped
½ cup white wine
1 tablespoon olive oil
1 teaspoon lemon juice
¼ cup sweetener, granulated
¼ teaspoon cardamom
¼ teaspoon all spice
2 cups chicken stock

1. Heat olive oil in a large pot. Add onions and sauté for 3 minutes until translucent. Add garlic, and cook for 30 more seconds. Add the pork, and cook until browned, about 5-6 minutes, stirring periodically. Pour in the wine, and cook for one minute. Throw in the remaining ingredients, except for the lemon juice and peanuts. Add two cups of water, bring the mixture to a boil, and cook for 5 minutes.
2. Reduce the heat to low, cover the pot, and let cook for about 30 minutes. Adjust seasoning.
3. Stir in the lemon juice before serving. Ladle into serving bowls, and serve topped with peanuts, and enjoy.

Per Serving
calories: 545 | fat: 33g | protein: 46g | carbs: 7g net carbs: 4g | fiber: 3g

85. Herbed Pork Chops with Cranberry Sauce

Prep time: 20 minutes | Cook time: 2⅔ hours | Serves 2

4 pork chops
½ teaspoon garlic powder
Salt and black pepper to taste
1 teaspoon fresh basil, chopped
A drizzle of olive oil
½ onion, chopped
½ cup white wine
Juice of ½ lemon
1 bay leaf
1 cup chicken stock
Fresh parsley, chopped, for serving
1 cup cranberries
½ teaspoon fresh rosemary, chopped
½ cup xylitol
½ cup water
½ teaspoon harissa paste sriracha sauce

1. Preheat oven to 360°F (182°C). In a bowl, combine the pork chops with basil, salt, garlic powder, and black pepper. Heat a pan with a drizzle of oil over medium heat, place in the pork, and cook until browned, about 4-5 minutes; set aside.
2. Stir in the onion and cook for 2 minutes. Place in the bay leaf and wine, and cook for 4 minutes. Pour in lemon juice, and chicken stock, and simmer for 5 minutes. Return the pork and cook for 10 minutes. Cover the pan and place it in the oven for 2 hours.
3. Set a pan over medium-high heat, add in the cranberries, rosemary, sriracha sauce, water and xylitol, and bring to a simmer for 15 minutes. Remove the pork chops from the oven and discard the bay leaf. Pour the sauce over the pork and serve sprinkled with parsley.

Per Serving
calories: 450 | fat: 24g | protein: 42g | carbs: 10g net carbs: 7g | fiber: 3g

86. Pork and Yellow Squash Traybake

Prep time: 15 minutes | Cook time: 31 minutes | Serves 4

1 pound (454 g) ground pork
1 large yellow squash, thinly sliced
Salt and black pepper to taste
1 garlic clove, minced
2 red onions, chopped
1 cup broccoli, chopped
1 (15 ounce / 425-g) can diced tomatoes
½ cup pork rinds, crushed
¼ cup parsley, chopped
2 cups cottage cheese
1 tablespoon olive oil
⅓ cup chicken broth

1. Heat the olive oil in a skillet over medium heat, add the pork, season it with salt and pepper, and cook for 3 minutes or until no longer pink. Stir occasionally while breaking any lumps apart.
2. Add the garlic, half of the red onions, broccoli, and 2 tablespoons of pork rinds. Continue cooking for 3 minutes. Stir in the tomatoes, half of the parsley, and chicken broth. Cook further for 3 minutes.
3. Mix the remaining parsley and cottage cheese and set aside. Sprinkle the bottom of a baking dish with 1 tablespoon of pork rinds; top with half of the squash and a season of salt, ⅔ of the pork mixture, and the cheese mixture. Repeat the layering process a second time to exhaust the ingredients.
4. Cover the baking dish with foil and put in the oven to bake for 20 minutes at 380°F (193°C). Remove the foil and brown the top of the casserole with the broiler side of the oven for 2 minutes.
5. Serve immediately.

Per Serving
calories: 531 | fat: 35g | protein: 49g | carbs: 10g net carbs: 3g | fiber: 7g

87. Hearty Pork Stew Meat

Prep time: 10 minutes | Cook time: 1 hour | Serves 5

2 tablespoons olive oil
2 pounds pork stew meat
1 yellow onion, chopped
1 garlic cloves, minced
¼ cup dry sherry wine
4 cups chicken bone broth
1 cup tomatoes, pureed
1 bay laurel
Sea salt and ground black pepper, to taste
1 tablespoon fresh cilantro, chopped

1. Heat the olive oil in a soup pot over a moderate flame. Sear the pork for about 5 minutes, stirring continuously to ensure even cooking; reserve.
2. Cook the yellow onion in the pan drippings until just tender and translucent. Stir in the garlic and continue to sauté for a further 30 seconds.
3. Pour in a splash of dry sherry to deglaze the pan.
4. Pour in the chicken bone broth and bring to a boil. Stir in the tomatoes and bay laurel. Season with salt and pepper to taste. Turn the heat to medium-low and continue to cook 10 minutes longer.
5. Add the reserved pork back to the pot, partially cover, and continue to simmer for 45 minutes longer. Garnish with cilantro and serve hot. Bon appétit!

Per Serving
calories: 332 | fat: 15g | protein: 41g | carbs: 4g net carbs: 3g | fiber: 1g

88. Pork Meatballs in Pasta Sauce

Prep time: 15 minutes | Cook time: 35 minutes | Serves 6

2 pound (907 g) ground pork
1 tablespoon olive oil
1 cup pork rinds, crushed
3 cloves garlic, minced
½ cup coconut milk
2 eggs, beaten
½ cup grated Parmesan cheese
½ cup grated asiago cheese
Salt and black pepper to taste
¼ cup chopped parsley
2 jars sugar-free marinara sauce
½ teaspoon Italian seasoning
1 cup Italian blend kinds of cheeses
Chopped basil to garnish

1. Preheat the oven to 400ºF (205ºC), line a cast iron pan with foil and oil it with cooking spray. Set aside.
2. Combine the coconut milk and pork rinds in a bowl. Mix in the ground pork, garlic, Asiago cheese, Parmesan cheese, eggs, salt, and pepper, just until combined. Form balls of the mixture and place them in the prepared pan. Bake in the oven for 20 minutes at a reduced temperature of 370ºF (188ºC).
3. Transfer the meatballs to a plate. Pour half of the marinara sauce in the baking pan. Place the meatballs back in the pan and pour the remaining marinara sauce all over them. Sprinkle with the Italian blend cheeses, drizzle with the olive oil, and then sprinkle with Italian seasoning.
4. Cover the pan with foil and put it back in the oven to bake for 10 minutes. After, remove the foil, and cook for 5 minutes. Once ready, take out the pan and garnish with basil. Serve on a bed of squash spaghetti.

Per Serving
calories: 716 | fat: 50g | protein: 50g | carbs: 5g net carbs: 4g | fiber: 1g

89. Baked Pork Sausage and Bell Pepper

Prep time: 10 minutes | Cook time: 45 minutes | Serves 4

12 pork sausages
5 large tomatoes, cut in rings
1 red bell pepper, seeded and sliced
1 yellow bell pepper, seeded and sliced
1 green bell pepper, seeded and sliced
1 sprig thyme, chopped
1 sprig rosemary, chopped
4 cloves garlic, minced
2 bay leaves
1 tablespoon olive oil
1 tablespoon balsamic vinegar

1. Preheat the oven to 350ºF (180ºC).
2. In the cast iron pan, add the tomatoes, bell peppers, thyme, rosemary, garlic, bay leaves, olive oil, and balsamic vinegar. Toss everything and arrange the sausages on top of the veggies.
3. Put the pan in the oven and bake for 20 minutes. After, remove the pan shake it a bit and turn the sausages over with a spoon. Continue cooking for 25 minutes or until the sausages have browned to your desired color. Serve with the veggie and cooking sauce with cauli rice.

Per Serving
calories: 465 | fat: 41g | protein: 15g | carbs: 8g net carbs: 4g | fiber: 4g

90. Pork Wraps with Veggies

Prep time: 10 minutes | Cook time: 10 minutes | Serves 4

1 tablespoon avocado oil	1 teaspoon butter
1 pound (454 g) ground pork	1 head Iceberg lettuce
1 tablespoon ginger paste	½ onion, sliced
Salt and black pepper to taste	1 red bell pepper, seeded and chopped
	2 dill pickles, finely chopped

1. Heat avocado oil in a pan over medium heat and put the in pork with ginger paste, salt, and pepper. Cook for 10 to 15 minutes over medium heat while breaking any lumps until the pork is no longer pink.
2. Pat the lettuce dry with a paper towel and in each leaf, spoon two to three tablespoons of the pork mixture, top with onion slices, bell pepper, and dill pickles.
3. Serve immediately.

Per Serving

calories: 424 | fat: 28g | protein: 31g | carbs: 4g net carbs: 1g | fiber: 3g

91. Spicy Pork and Capers with Olives

Prep time: 10 minutes | Cook time: 9 minutes | Serves 4

4 pork chops	Salt and black pepper, to taste
1 tablespoon olive oil	½ teaspoon hot pepper sauce
1 garlic clove, minced	¼ cup capers
¼ tablespoon chili powder	6 black olives, sliced
¼ teaspoon cumin	

1. Preheat grill over medium heat. In a mixing bowl, combine olive oil, cumin, salt, hot pepper sauce, pepper, garlic and chili powder. Place in the pork chops, toss to coat, and refrigerate for 4 hours.
2. Arrange the pork on a preheated grill, cook for 7 minutes, turn, add in the capers, and cook for another 2 minutes. Place onto serving plates and sprinkle with olives to serve.

Per Serving

calories: 300 | fat: 14g | protein: 40g | carbs: 2g net carbs: 1g | fiber: 1g

92. Roasted Stuffed Pork Loin Steak

Prep time: 15 minutes | Cook time: 30 minutes | Serves 4

1 tablespoon olive oil	to taste
Zest and juice from 1 lime	1 teaspoon cumin
1 garlic clove, minced	2 pork loin steaks
1 tablespoon fresh cilantro, chopped	1 pickle, chopped
1 tablespoon fresh mint, chopped	2 ounces (57 g) smoked ham, sliced
Salt and black pepper,	2 ounces (57 g) Gruyere cheese sliced
	1 tablespoon mustard

1. Start with making the marinade: combine the lime zest, oil, black pepper, cumin, cilantro, lime juice, garlic, mint and salt, in a food processor. Place the steaks in the marinade, and toss well to coat; set aside for some hours in the fridge.
2. Arrange the steaks on a working surface, split the pickles, mustard, cheese, and ham on them, roll, and secure with toothpicks. Heat a pan over medium heat, add in the pork rolls, cook each side for 2 minutes and remove to a baking sheet. Bake in the oven at 350ºF (180ºC) for 25 minutes.
3. Serve immediately.

Per Serving

calories: 433 | fat: 38g | protein: 30g | carbs: 5g net carbs: 4g | fiber: 1g

93. Parmesan Bacon-Stuffed Pork Roll

Prep time: 15 minutes | Cook time: 30 minutes | Serves 4

1 tablespoon olive oil	chopped
4 ounces (113 g) bacon, sliced	1 garlic clove, minced
1 tablespoon fresh parsley, chopped	1 tablespoon Parmesan cheese, grated
4 pork chops, boneless and flatten	5 ounces (142 g) canned diced tomatoes
1 cup ricotta cheese	Salt and black pepper to taste
1 tablespoon pine nuts	½ teaspoon herbes de Provence
1 spring onion,	

1. Put the pork chops on a flat surface. Set the bacon slices on top, then divide the ricotta cheese, pine nuts, and Parmesan cheese. Roll each pork piece and secure with a toothpick.
2. Set a pan over medium heat and warm oil. Cook the pork rolls until browned, and remove to a plate.
3. Add in the spring onion and garlic, and cook for 5 minutes. Place in the stock and cook for 3 minutes. Get rid of the toothpicks from the rolls and return them to the pan. Stir in the

black pepper, salt, tomatoes and herbes de Provence. Bring to a boil, set heat to medium-low, and cook for 20 minutes while covered. Sprinkle with parsley to serve.

Per Serving
calories: 568 | fat: 38g | protein: 51g | carbs: 6g net carbs: 3g | fiber: 2g

94. Tomato purée Pork Chops

Prep time: 10 minutes | Cook time: 37 minutes | Serves 4

4 pork chops
½ tablespoon fresh basil, chopped
1 garlic clove, minced
1 tablespoon olive oil
7 ounces (198 g) canned diced tomatoes
½ tablespoon tomato purée
Salt and black pepper, to taste
½ red chili, finely chopped

1. Season the pork with salt and black pepper. Set a pan over medium heat and warm oil, place in the pork chops, cook for 3 minutes, turn and cook for another 3 minutes; remove to a bowl. Add in the garlic and cook for 30 seconds.
2. Stir in the tomato purée, tomatoes, and chili; bring to a boil, and reduce heat to medium-low. Place in the pork chops, cover the pan and simmer everything for 30 minutes. Remove the pork chops to plates and sprinkle with fresh oregano to serve.

Per Serving
calories: 372 | fat: 21g | protein: 40g | carbs: 3g net carbs: 2g | fiber: 1g

95. Pork Kofte with Cauliflower Mash

Prep time: 15 minutes | Cook time: 30 minutes | Serves 4

1 pound (454 g) ground pork
1 tablespoon olive oil
1 tablespoon pork rinds, crushed
1 garlic clove, minced
1 shallot, chopped
1 small egg
⅓ teaspoon paprika
Salt and black pepper
to taste
1 tablespoon parsley, chopped
½ cup tomato purée, sugar-free
½ teaspoon oregano
⅓ cup Italian blend kinds of cheeses
1 tablespoon basil, chopped to garnish

1. In a bowl, mix the ground pork, shallot, pork rinds, garlic, egg, paprika, oregano, parsley, salt, and black pepper, just until combined. Form balls of the mixture and place them in an oiled baking pan; drizzle with olive oil. Bake in the oven for 18 minutes at 390ºF (199ºC).
2. Pour the tomato purée all over the meatballs. Sprinkle with the Italian blend cheeses, and put it back in the oven to bake for 10 to 15 minutes until the cheese melts. Once ready, take out the pan and garnish with basil. Delicious when served with cauliflower mash.

Per Serving
calories: 458 | fat: 30g | protein: 34g | carbs: 8g net carbs: 6g | fiber: 2g

96. Pork Pie

Prep time: 15 minutes | Cook time: 1 hour | Serves 8

Crust:
1 egg
¼ cup butter
2 cups almond flour
¼ teaspoon xanthan gum
¼ cup shredded mozzarella
A pinch of salt

Filling:
2 pounds ground pork
½ cup water
⅓ cup pureed onion
¾ teaspoon allspice
1 cup cooked and mashed cauliflower
1 tablespoon ground sage
1 tablespoon butter

1. Preheat your oven to 350ºF (180ºC).
2. Whisk together all crust ingredients in a bowl. Make two balls out of the mixture and refrigerate for 10 minutes. Combine the water, meat, and salt, in a pot over medium heat. Cook for about 15 minutes, place the meat along with the other ingredients in a bowl. Mix with your hands to combine.
3. Roll out the pie crusts and place one at the bottom of a greased pie pan. Spread the filling over the crust. Top with the other coat. Bake in the oven for 50 minutes then serve.

Per Serving
calories: 435 | fat: 31g | protein: 31g | carbs: 5g net carbs: 4g | fiber: 1g

97. Homemade Pork Osso Bucco

Prep time: 15 minutes | Cook time: 1¾ hours | Serves 6

1 tablespoon butter, softened
6 (16-ounce / 454-g) pork shanks
1 tablespoon olive oil
3 cloves garlic, minced

1 cup diced tomatoes
Salt and black pepper to taste
½ cup chopped onions
½ cup chopped celery
2 cups Cabernet Sauvignon
5 cups vegetable broth
½ cup chopped parsley, extra to garnish
1 teaspoon lemon zest

1. Melt the butter in a large saucepan over medium heat. Season the pork with salt and black pepper and brown it for 12 minutes; remove to a plate.
2. In the same pan, sauté 2 cloves of garlic and onions in the oil, for 3 minutes; return the pork shanks. Stir in the Cabernet, celery, tomatoes, and vegetable broth; season with salt and pepper. Cover the pan and let simmer on low heat for 1½ hours basting the pork every 15 minutes with the sauce.
3. In a bowl, mix the remaining garlic, parsley, and lemon zest to make a gremolata, and stir the mixture into the sauce when it is ready. Turn the heat off and dish the Osso Bucco.
4. Garnish with parsley and serve with creamy turnip mash.

Per Serving

calories: 533 | fat: 40g | protein: 34g | carbs: 4g | net carbs: 2g | fiber: 2g

98. Rosemary Lamb Chops

Prep time: 15 minutes | Cook time: 6 hours | Serves 4

3 tablespoons extra-virgin olive oil, divided
1½ pounds (1.1 kg) lamb shoulder chops
Salt, for seasoning
Freshly ground black pepper, for seasoning
½ cup chicken broth
1 sweet onion, sliced
2 teaspoons minced garlic
2 teaspoons dried rosemary
1 teaspoon dried thyme

1. Lightly grease the insert of the slow cooker with 1 tablespoon of the olive oil.
2. In a large skillet over medium-high heat, heat the remaining 2 tablespoons of the olive oil.
3. Season the lamb with salt and pepper. Add the lamb to the skillet and brown for 6 minutes, turning once.
4. Transfer the lamb to the insert, and add the broth, onion, garlic, rosemary, and thyme.
5. Cover and cook on low for 6 hours.
6. Serve warm.

Per Serving

calories: 380| fat: 27g | protein: 31g | carbs: 3g | net carbs: 2g | fiber: 1g

99. Lemony Pork Chops and Brussels Sprouts

Prep time: 10 minutes | Cook time: 15 minutes | Serves 6

1 tablespoon lemon juice
3 cloves garlic, pureed
1 tablespoon olive oil
6 pork loin chops
1 tablespoon butter
1 pound (454 g) brussels sprouts, trimmed and halved
1 tablespoon white wine
Salt and black pepper, to taste

1. Preheat broiler to 400ºF (205ºC) and mix the lemon juice, garlic, salt, black pepper, and oil in a bowl.
2. Brush the pork with the mixture, place in a baking sheet, and cook for 6 minutes on each side until browned. Share into 6 plates and make the side dish.
3. Melt butter in a small wok or pan and cook in brussels sprouts for 5 minutes until tender. Drizzle with white wine, sprinkle with salt and black pepper and cook for another 5 minutes. Ladle brussels sprouts to the side of the chops and serve with a hot sauce.

Per Serving

calories: 400 | fat: 25g | protein: 40g | carbs: 6g | net carbs: 3g | fiber: 3g

100. Balsamic Pork Loin Chops

Prep time: 5 minutes | Cook time: 10 minutes | Serves 6

6 pork loin chops, boneless
1 tablespoon erythritol
¼ cup balsamic vinegar
3 cloves garlic, minced
¼ cup olive oil
⅓ teaspoon salt
Black pepper, to taste

1. Put the pork in a plastic bag. In a bowl, mix the erythritol, balsamic vinegar, garlic, olive oil, salt, pepper, and pour the sauce over the pork. Seal the bag, shake it, and place in the refrigerator.
2. Marinate the pork for 2 hours. Preheat the grill to medium heat, remove the pork when ready, and grill covered for 10 minutes on each side. Remove and let sit for 4 minutes, and serve immediately.

Per Serving

calories: 419 | fat: 26g | protein: 40g | carbs: 2g | net carbs: 2g | fiber: 0g

101. Pork Tenderloin with Lemon Chimichurri

Prep time: 10 minutes | Cook time: 50 minutes | Serves 6

Lemon Chimichurri:
1 lemon, juiced
¼ cup chopped mint leaves
¼ cup chopped oregano leaves
2 cloves garlic, minced
¼ cup olive oil
Salt to taste

Pork:
1 (4-pound / 1.8-kg) pork tenderloin
Salt and black pepper to season
Olive oil for rubbing

1. Make the lemon chimichurri to have the flavors incorporate while the pork cooks.
2. In a bowl, mix the mint, oregano, and garlic. Then, add the lemon juice, olive oil, and salt, and combine well. Set the sauce aside at room temperature.
3. Preheat the charcoal grill to 450ºF (235ºC) in medium heat creating a direct heat area and indirect heat area. Rub the pork with olive oil, season with salt and pepper. Place the meat over direct heat and sear for 3 minutes on each side, after which, move to the indirect heat area. Close the lid and cook for 25 minutes on one side, then open, turn the meat, and grill for 20 minutes on the other side. Remove the pork from the grill and let it sit for 5 minutes before slicing. Spoon lemon chimichurri over the pork and serve with fresh salad.

Per Serving
calories: 400 | fat: 17g | protein: 28g | carbs: 2g net carbs: 2g | fiber: 0g

102. Herbed Pork Chops with Raspberry Sauce

Prep time: 10 minutes | Cook time: 10 minutes | Serves 4

1 tablespoon olive oil, extra for brushing
2 pound (907 g) pork chops
Pink salt and black pepper to taste
2 cups raspberries
¼ cup water
1½ tablespoon Italian Herb mix
1 tablespoon balsamic vinegar
1 teaspoon sugar-free Worcestershire sauce

1. Heat oil in a skillet over medium heat, season the pork with salt and black pepper and cook for 5 minutes on each side. Put on serving plates and reserve the pork drippings.
2. Mash the raspberries with a fork in a bowl until jam-like. Pour into a saucepan, add the water, and herb mix. Bring to boil on low heat for 4 minutes. Stir in pork drippings, vinegar, and Worcestershire sauce. Simmer for 1 minute. Spoon sauce over the pork chops and serve with braised rapini.

Per Serving
calories: 413 | fat: 32g | protein: 26g | carbs: 5g net carbs: 1g | fiber: 4g

103. Pork with Cranberry Sauce

Prep time: 20 minutes | Cook time: 2⅔ hours | Serves 4

4 pork chops
1 teaspoon garlic powder
Salt and black pepper, to taste
1 teaspoon fresh basil, chopped
A drizzle of olive oil
1 shallot, chopped
1 cup white wine
1 bay leaf
2 cups vegetable stock
Fresh parsley, chopped, for serving
2 cups cranberries
½ teaspoon fresh rosemary, chopped
½ cup Swerve
Juice of 1 lemon
1 cup water
1 teaspoon harissa paste

1. In a bowl, combine the pork chops with 1 teaspoon of basil, salt, garlic powder and black pepper. Heat a pan with a drizzle of oil over medium heat, place in the pork and cook until browned; set aside.
2. Stir in the shallot, and cook for 2 minutes. Place in the bay leaf and wine, and cook for 4 minutes. Pour in juice from ½ lemon, and vegetable stock, and simmer for 5 minutes. Return the pork, and cook for 10 minutes. Cover the pan, and place in the oven to bake at 350ºF (180ºC) for 2 hours.
3. Set a pan over medium heat, add cranberries, rosemary, harissa paste, water, 1 teaspoon basil, Swerve, and juice from ½ lemon, simmer for 15 minutes. Remove the pork chops from the oven, remove and discard the bay leaf. Split among plates, spread over with the cranberry sauce, sprinkle with parsley to serve.

Per Serving
calories: 450 | fat: 34g | protein: 26g | carbs: 12g net carbs: 6g | fiber: 6g

104. Garlicky Pork and Bell Peppers

Prep time: 10 minutes | Cook time: 25 minutes | Serves 4

1 tablespoon butter
4 pork steaks, bone-in
1 cup chicken stock
Salt and black pepper, to taste
A pinch of lemon pepper
1 tablespoon olive oil
6 garlic cloves, minced
1 tablespoon fresh parsley, chopped
4 bell peppers, sliced
1 lemon, sliced

1. Heat a pan with 2 tablespoons oil and 2 tablespoons butter over medium heat. Add in the pork steaks, season with black pepper and salt, and cook until browned; remove to a plate. In the same pan, warm the rest of the oil and butter, add garlic and bell peppers and cook for 4 minutes.
2. Pour the chicken stock, lemon slices, salt, lemon pepper, and black pepper, and cook everything for 5 minutes. Return the pork steaks to the pan and cook for 10 minutes. Split the sauce and steaks among plates and sprinkle with parsley to serve.

Per Serving

calories: 580 | fat: 39g | protein: 48g | carbs: 7g net carbs: 6g | fiber: 1g

105. Classic Carnitas

Prep time: 15 minutes | Cook time: 9 to 10 hours | Serves 8

3 tablespoons extra-virgin olive oil, divided
2 pounds pork shoulder, cut into 2-inch cubes
2 cups diced tomatoes
2 cups chicken broth
½ sweet onion, chopped
2 fresh chipotle peppers, chopped
Juice of 1 lime
1 teaspoon ground coriander
1 teaspoon ground cumin
½ teaspoon salt
1 avocado, peeled, pitted, and diced, for garnish
1 cup sour cream, for garnish
2 tablespoons chopped cilantro, for garnish

1. Lightly grease the insert of the slow cooker with 1 tablespoon of the olive oil.
2. In a large skillet over medium-high heat, heat the remaining 2 tablespoons of the olive oil.
3. Add the pork and brown on all sides for about 10 minutes.
4. Transfer to the insert and add the tomatoes, broth, onion, peppers, lime juice, coriander, cumin, and salt.
5. Cover and cook on low for 9 to 10 hours.
6. Shred the cooked pork with a fork and stir the meat into the sauce.
7. Serve topped with the avocado, sour cream, and cilantro.

Per Serving

calories: 508 | fat: 41g | protein: 29g | carbs: 7g net carbs: 4g | fiber: 3g

106. Cranberry Pork Roast

Prep time: 15 minutes | Cook time: 7 to 8 hours | Serves 6

3 tablespoons extra-virgin olive oil, divided
2 tablespoons butter
2 pounds (907 g) pork shoulder roast
1 teaspoon ground cinnamon
¼ teaspoon allspice
¼ teaspoon salt
⅛ teaspoon freshly ground black pepper
½ cup cranberries
½ cup chicken broth
½ cup granulated erythritol
2 tablespoons dijon mustard
Juice and zest of ½ lemon
1 scallion, white and green parts, chopped, for garnish

1. Lightly grease the insert of the slow cooker with 1 tablespoon of the olive oil.
2. In a large skillet over medium-high heat, heat the remaining 2 tablespoons of the olive oil and the butter.
3. Lightly season the pork with cinnamon, allspice, salt, and pepper. Add the pork to the skillet and brown on all sides for about 10 minutes. Transfer to the insert.
4. In a small bowl, stir together the cranberries, broth, erythritol, mustard, and lemon juice and zest, and add the mixture to the pork.
5. Cover and cook on low for 7 to 8 hours.
6. Serve topped with the scallion.

Per Serving

calories: 492 | fat: 40g | protein: 26g | carbs: 4g net carbs: 3g | fiber: 1g

107. Pork Patties with Caramelized Onion Rings

Prep time: 10 minutes | Cook time: 10 minutes | Serves 6

2 pound (907 g) ground pork
Pink salt and chili pepper to taste
1 tablespoon olive oil
1 tablespoon butter
1 white onion, sliced into rings
1 tablespoon balsamic vinegar
3 drops liquid stevia
6 low carb burger buns, halved
2 firm tomatoes, sliced into rings

1. Combine the pork, salt and chili pepper in a bowl and mold out 6 patties.
2. Heat the olive oil in a skillet over medium heat and fry the patties for 4 to 5 minutes on each side until golden brown on the outside. Remove onto a plate and sit for 3 minutes.
3. Melt butter in a skillet over medium heat, sauté onions for 2 minutes, and stir in the balsamic vinegar and liquid stevia. Cook for 30 seconds stirring once or twice until caramelized. In each bun, place a patty, top with some onion rings and 2 tomato rings.
4. Serve the burgers with cheddar cheese dip.

Per Serving
calories: 490 | fat: 35g | protein: 35g | carbs: 7g | net carbs: 7g | fiber: 0g

108. Lemony Pork Loin Roast

Prep time: 15 minutes | Cook time: 7 to 8 hours | Serves 6

3 tablespoons extra-virgin olive oil, divided
1 tablespoon butter
2 pounds pork loin roast
½ teaspoon salt
¼ teaspoon freshly ground black pepper
¼ cup chicken broth
Juice and zest of 1 lemon
1 tablespoon minced garlic
½ cup heavy (whipping) cream

1. Lightly grease the insert of the slow cooker with 1 tablespoon of the olive oil.
2. In a large skillet over medium-high heat, heat the remaining 2 tablespoons of the olive oil and the butter.
3. Lightly season the pork with salt and pepper. Add the pork to the skillet and brown the roast on all sides for about 10 minutes. Transfer it to the insert.
4. In a small bowl, stir together the broth, lemon juice and zest, and garlic.
5. Add the broth mixture to the roast.
6. Cover, and cook on low for 7 to 8 hours.
7. Stir in the heavy cream and serve.

Per Serving
calories: 448 | fat: 31g | protein: 39g | carbs: 1g | net carbs: 1g | fiber: 0g

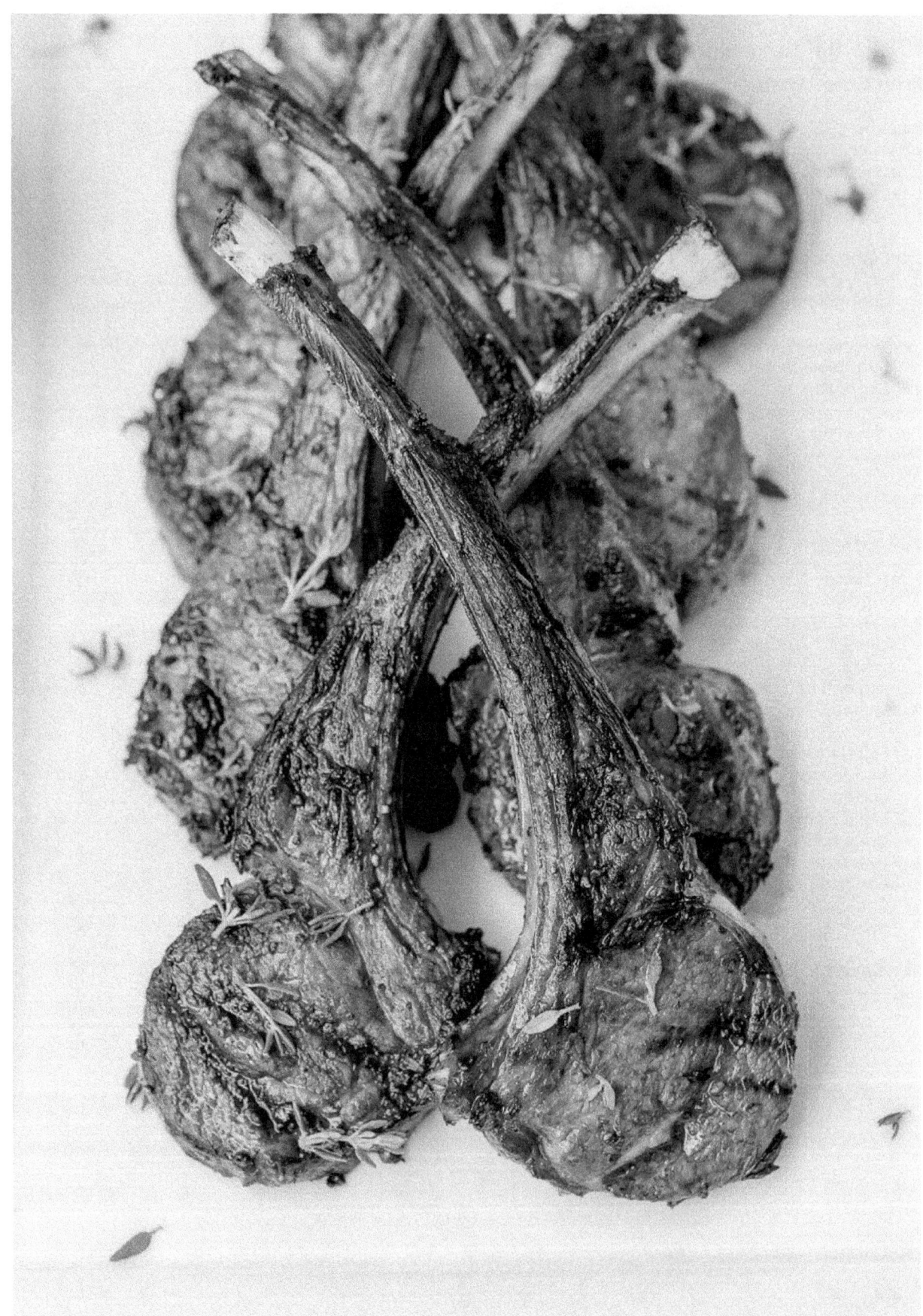

Chapter 5 Beef and Lamb

109. Skirt Steak with Green Beans

Prep time: 5 minutes | Cook time: 13 minutes | Serves 4

3 cups green beans, chopped
2 cups cauliflower rice
2 tablespoons butter
1 tablespoon olive oil
1 pound (454 g) skirt steak
Salt and black pepper, to taste
4 fresh eggs
Hot sauce (sugar-free) for topping (optional)

1. Put cauliflower rice and green beans in a bowl, sprinkle with a little water, and steam in the microwave for 90 seconds. Share into bowls. Warm butter and olive oil in a skillet, season the beef with salt and pepper, and brown for 5 minutes on each side. Ladle the meat onto the vegetables.
2. Wipe out the skillet and return to medium heat, crack in an egg, season with salt and pepper and cook until the egg white has set, but the yolk is still runny, for 3 minutes. Remove egg onto the vegetable bowl and fry the remaining 3 eggs. Add to the other bowls. Drizzle with hot sauce (if desired) and serve.

Per Serving
calories: 409 | fat: 25g | protein: 40g | carbs: 8g net carbs: 5g | fiber: 3g

110. Zoodles with Beef Bolognese Sauce

Prep time: 10 minutes | Cook time: 25 to 27 minutes | Serves 4

2 cups zoodles
1 pound (454 g) ground beef
2 garlic cloves
1 onion, chopped
1 teaspoon oregano
1 teaspoon sage
1 teaspoon rosemary
7 ounces (198 g) canned chopped tomatoes
2 tablespoons olive oil

1. Cook the zoodles in warm olive oil over medium heat for 3-4 minutes and remove to a serving plate. To the same pan, add onion and garlic and cook for 3 minutes. Add beef and cook until browned, about 4-5 minutes. Stir in the herbs and tomatoes. Cook for 15 minutes and serve over the zoodles.

Per Serving
calories: 371 | fat: 30g | protein: 20g | carbs: 5g net carbs: 3g | fiber: 2g

111. Creole Beef Tripe Stew with Onions

Prep time: 5 minutes | Cook time: 22 minutes | Serves 6

1½ pounds (680 g) beef tripe
4 cups coconut milk
Pink salt
2 teaspoons Creole seasoning
3 tablespoons olive oil
2 onions, sliced
3 tomatoes, diced

1. Put tripe in a bowl, and cover with coconut milk. Refrigerate for 3 hours to extract bitterness and gamey taste. Remove from coconut milk, pat dry with paper towels, and season with salt and creole seasoning.
2. Heat 2 tablespoons of oil in a skillet over medium heat and brown the tripe on both sides for 6 minutes in total. Remove, and set aside. Add the remaining oil, and sauté onions for 3 minutes. Include the tomatoes and cook for 10 minutes. Put the tripe in the sauce, and cook for 3 minutes.

Per Serving
calories: 284 | fat: 16g | protein: 20g | carbs: 14g net carbs: 12g | fiber: 2g

112. King Size Beef Burgers

Prep time: 5 minutes | Cook time: 18 minutes | Serves 4

2 tablespoons olive oil
1 pound (454 g) ground beef
2 green onions, chopped
1 garlic clove, minced
1 tablespoon thyme
2 tablespoons almond flour
2 tablespoons beef broth
½ tablespoon chopped parsley
½ tablespoon Worcestershire sauce

1. Grease a baking dish with the olive oil. Combine all ingredients except for the parsley in a bowl. Mix well with your hands and make 2 patties out of the mixture. Arrange on a lined baking sheet. Bake at 370ºF (188ºC), for about 18 minutes, until nice and crispy. Serve sprinkled with parsley.

Per Serving
calories: 371 | fat: 30g | protein: 20g | carbs: 5g net carbs: 4g | fiber: 1g

113. Ground Beef and Cauliflower Curry

Prep time: 5 minutes | Cook time: 21 minutes | Serves 6

1 tablespoon olive oil
1½ pounds (680 g) ground beef
1 tablespoon ginger-garlic paste
1 teaspoon garam masala
1 (7-ounce / 198-g) can whole tomatoes
1 small head cauliflower, cut into florets
Pink salt and chili pepper, to taste
¼ cup water

1. Heat oil in a saucepan over medium heat, add in beef, ginger-garlic paste and season with garam masala. Cook for 5 minutes while breaking any lumps. Stir in tomatoes and cauliflower, season with salt and chili pepper, and cook for 6 minutes. Add the water and bring to a boil over medium heat for 10 minutes, or until the liquid has reduced by half.
2. Adjust taste with salt. Serve with shirataki rice.

Per Serving
calories: 255 | fat: 17g | protein: 23g | carbs: 4g net carbs: 2g | fiber: 2g

114. Basil Feta Flank Steak Pinwheels

Prep time: 5 minutes | Cook time: 15 minutes | Serves 6

1½ pounds (680 g) beef flank steak
Salt and black pepper, to season
⅔ cup feta cheese, crumbled
½ loose cup baby spinach
1 jalapeño pepper, chopped
¼ cup basil leaves, chopped

1. Preheat oven to 400°F (205°C). Grease a baking sheet with cooking spray.
2. Wrap the steak in plastic wrap, place on a flat surface, and gently run a rolling pin over to flatten. Take off the wraps. Sprinkle with half of the feta cheese, top with spinach, jalapeño, basil leaves, and the remaining cheese. Carefully roll the steak over on the stuffing and secure with toothpicks.
3. Place in the greased baking sheet, and cook for 15 minutes, flipping once until nicely browned on the outside and the cheese melted within. Cool for 3 minutes, slice into pinwheels, and serve.

Per Serving
calories: 199 | fat: 9g | protein: 27g | carbs: 1g net carbs: 1g | fiber: 0g

115. Creamy Reuben Soup with Sauerkraut

Prep time: 10 minutes | Cook time: 20 minutes | Serves 6

1 onion, diced
7 cups beef stock
1 teaspoon caraway seeds
2 celery stalks, diced
2 garlic cloves, minced
¾ teaspoon black pepper
2 cups heavy cream
1 cup sauerkraut
1 pound (454 g) corned beef, chopped
3 tablespoons butter
1½ cups Swiss cheese
Salt and black pepper, to taste

1. Melt the butter in a large pot. Add onions and celery, and fry for 3 minutes until tender. Add garlic, and cook for another minute.
2. Pour the broth over and stir in sauerkraut, salt, caraway seeds, and add a pinch of pepper. Bring to a boil. Reduce the heat to low, and add the corned beef. Cook for about 15 minutes.
3. Adjust the seasoning. Stir in heavy cream and cheese, and cook for 1 minute.

Per Serving
calories: 567 | fat: 46g | protein: 29g | carbs: 12g net carbs: 9g | fiber: 3g

116. Beef and cauliflower rice Casserole

Prep time: 5 minutes | Cook time: 26 minutes | Serves 6

2 pounds (907 g) ground beef
Pink salt and black pepper, to taste
1 cup cauliflower rice
2 cups cabbage, chopped
1 (14-ounce / 397-g) can diced tomatoes
¼ cup water
1 cup Colby Jack cheese, shredded

1. Preheat oven to 375°F (190°C) and grease a baking dish with cooking spray.
2. Put beef in a pot and season with salt and pepper and cook over medium heat for 6 minutes until no longer pink. Drain grease. Add cauliflower rice, cabbage, tomatoes, and water. Stir and bring to boil covered for 5 minutes to thicken the sauce. Adjust taste with salt and black pepper.
3. Spoon the beef mixture into the baking dish. Sprinkle with cheese, and bake in the oven for 15 minutes until cheese has melted and golden brown. Remove, cool for 4 minutes, and serve.

Per Serving
calories: 501 | fat: 38g | protein: 33g | carbs: 6g net carbs: 3g | fiber: 3g

117. Beef Brisket with Red Wine

Prep time: 10 minutes | Cook time: 2 hours | Serves 4

1 tablespoon olive oil
1 pound (454 g) brisket
1 red onion, quartered
2 stalks celery, cut into chunks
1 garlic clove, minced
Salt and black pepper, to taste
1 bay leaf
1 tablespoon fresh thyme, chopped
1 cup red wine

1. Season the brisket with salt and pepper. Brown the meat on both sides in warm olive oil over medium heat for 6-8 minutes. Transfer to a deep casserole dish.
2. In the dish, arrange the onion, garlic, celery, and bay leaf around the brisket and pour the wine all over it. Cover the pot and cook the ingredients in the oven for 2 hours at 370ºF (188ºC). When ready, remove the casserole. Transfer the beef to a chopping board and cut it into thick slices. Serve the beef and vegetables with a drizzle of the sauce.

Per Serving
calories: 203 | fat: 9g | protein: 25g | carbs: 3g net carbs: 2g | fiber: 1g

118. Grilled Ribeye Steaks with Green Beans

Prep time: 5 minutes | Cook time: 12 to 13 minutes | Serves 4

4 ribeye steaks
2 tablespoons unsalted butter
1 teaspoon olive oil
½ cup green beans, sliced
Salt and ground pepper, to taste
1 tablespoon fresh thyme, chopped
1 tablespoon fresh rosemary, chopped
1 tablespoon fresh parsley, chopped

1. Brush the steaks with olive oil and season with salt and pepper. Preheat a grill pan over high heat and cook the steaks for about 4 minutes per side; set aside. Steam the green beans for 3-4 minutes until tender. Season with salt. Melt the butter in the pan and stir-fry the herbs for 1 minute; then mix in the green beans. Transfer over the steaks and serve.

Per Serving
calories: 516 | fat: 33g | protein: 49g | carbs: 6g net carbs: 5g | fiber: 1g

119. Basil Lamb Shoulder with Pine Nuts

Prep time: 10 minutes | Cook time: 50 minutes | Serves 4

1 pound (454 g) rolled lamb shoulder, boneless
1½ cups basil leaves, chopped
5 tablespoons pine nuts, chopped
½ cup green olives, pitted and chopped
3 cloves garlic, minced
Salt and black pepper, to taste

1. Preheat the oven to 450ºF.
2. In a bowl, combine the basil, pine nuts, olives, and garlic. Season with salt and pepper. Untie the lamb flat onto a chopping board, spread the basil mixture all over, and rub the spices onto the meat.
3. Roll the lamb over the spice mixture and tie it together using 3 to 4 strings of butcher's twine. Place the lamb onto a baking dish and cook in the oven for 10 minutes. Reduce the heat to 350ºF and continue cooking for 40 minutes. When ready, transfer the meat to a cleaned chopping board; let it rest for 10 minutes before slicing. Serve with roasted root vegetables.

Per Serving
calories: 391 | fat: 33g | protein: 21g | carbs: 3g net carbs: 2g | fiber: 1g

120. Lemon-Mint Grilled Lamb Chops

Prep time: 10 minutes | Cook time: 6 minutes | Serves 4

8 lamb chops
2 tablespoons favorite spice mix
2 tablespoons olive oil
Sauce:
¼ cup olive oil
1 teaspoon red pepper flakes
2 tablespoons lemon juice
2 tablespoons fresh mint
3 garlic cloves, pressed
2 tablespoons lemon zest
¼ cup parsley
½ teaspoon smoked paprika

1. Rub lamb with olive oil and sprinkle with the seasoning. Preheat the grill to medium. Grill the lamb chops for about 3 minutes per side. Whisk together the sauce ingredients. Serve the lamb with sauce.

Per Serving
calories: 488 | fat: 31g | protein: 49g | carbs: 5g net carbs: 3g | fiber: 2g

121. Beef and Onion Stuffed Zucchinis

Prep time: 5 minutes | Cook time: 21 minutes | Serves 4

4 zucchinis
2 tablespoons olive oil
1½ pounds (680 g) ground beef
1 medium red onion, chopped
2 tablespoons pimiento rojo, chopped
Pink salt and black pepper, to taste
1 cup yellow Cheddar cheese, grated

1. Preheat oven to 350°F (180°C).
2. Lay the zucchinis on a flat surface, trim off the ends, and cut in half lengthwise. Scoop out pulp from each half with a spoon to make shells. Chop the flesh.
3. Heat oil in a skillet; add the ground beef, red onion, pimiento, and zucchini pulp, and season with salt and black pepper. Cook for 6 minutes while stirring to break up lumps until beef is no longer pink. Spoon the beef into the boats, and sprinkle with Cheddar cheese.
4. Place on a greased baking sheet, and cook to melt the cheese for 15 minutes until zucchini boats are tender. Take out, cool for 2 minutes, and serve warm with a mixed green salad.

Per Serving

calories: 535 | fat: 40g | protein: 42g | carbs: 4g net carbs: 3g | fiber: 1g

122. Garlicky Lamb Chops in White Wine

Prep time: 5 minutes | Cook time: 1 hour 9 minutes | Serves 6

6 lamb chops
1 tablespoon sage
1 teaspoon thyme
1 onion, sliced
3 garlic cloves, minced
2 tablespoons olive oil
½ cup white wine
Salt and black pepper, to taste

1. Heat the olive oil in a pan. Add onion and garlic and cook for 3 minutes, until soft. Rub the sage and thyme over the lamb chops. Cook the lamb for about 3 minutes per side. Set aside.
2. Pour the white wine and 1 cup of water into the pan, bring the mixture to a boil. Cook until the liquid is reduced by half. Add the chops in the pan, reduce the heat, and let simmer for 1 hour.

Per Serving

calories: 392 | fat: 35g | protein: 18g | carbs: 2g net carbs: 1g | fiber: 1g

123. Grilled Lamb Kebabs

Prep time: 5 minutes | Cook time: 10 minutes | Serves 4

1 pound (454 g) ground lamb
¼ teaspoon cinnamon
1 egg
1 onion, grated
Salt and ground black pepper, to taste

1. Place all ingredients in a bowl. Mix with your hands to combine well. Divide the meat into 4 pieces. Shape all meat portions around previously-soaked skewers.
2. Preheat grill to medium and grill the kebabs for about 5 minutes per side.

Per Serving

calories: 246 | fat: 15g | protein: 25g | carbs: 3g net carbs: 2g | fiber: 1g

124. Beef and Mushroom Cheeseburgers

Prep time: 5 minutes | Cook time: 11 to 13 minutes | Serves 4

2 tablespoons olive oil
1 pound (454 g) ground beef
½ teaspoon fresh parsley, chopped
½ teaspoon Worcestershire sauce
Salt and black pepper, to taste
2 slices Mozzarella cheese
2 portobello mushroom caps

1. In a bowl, mix the beef, parsley, Worcestershire sauce, salt and black pepper with your hands until evenly combined. Make medium-sized patties out of the mixture.
2. Preheat a grill to 400°F (205°C) and coat the mushroom caps with olive oil, salt and black pepper.
3. Lay portobello caps, rounded side up and burger patties onto the hot grill pan and cook for 5 minutes. Turn the mushroom caps and continue cooking for 1 minute.
4. Lay a Mozzarella slice on top of each patty. Continue cooking until the mushroom caps are softened, 4-5 minutes. Flip the patties and top with cheese. Cook for another 2-3 minutes until the cheese melts onto the meat. Remove the patties and sandwich into two mushroom caps each.

Per Serving

calories: 397 | fat: 32g | protein: 24g | carbs: 2g net carbs: 1g | fiber: 1g

125. Asian-Flavored Beef and Broccoli

Prep time: 10 minutes | Cook time: 24 minutes | Serves 4

- ½ cup coconut milk
- 2 tablespoons coconut oil
- ¼ teaspoon garlic powder
- ¼ teaspoon onion powder
- ½ tablespoon coconut aminos
- 1 pound (454 g) beef steak, cut into strips
- Salt and black pepper, to taste
- 1 head broccoli, cut into florets
- ½ tablespoon Thai green curry paste
- 1 teaspoon ginger paste
- 1 tablespoon cilantro, chopped
- ½ tablespoon sesame seeds

1. Warm coconut oil in a pan over medium heat, add in beef, season with garlic powder, pepper, salt, ginger paste, and onion powder and cook for 4 minutes. Mix in the broccoli and stir-fry for 5 minutes.
2. Pour in the coconut milk, coconut aminos, and Thai curry paste and cook for 15 minutes.
3. Serve sprinkled with cilantro and sesame seeds.

Per Serving

calories: 350 | fat: 22g | protein: 30g | carbs: 13g net carbs: 8g | fiber: 5g

126. Juicy Beef with Thyme and Rosemary

Prep time: 15 minutes | Cook time: 17 minutes | Serves 4

- 2 garlic cloves, minced
- 2 tablespoons butter
- 2 tablespoons olive oil
- 1 tablespoon fresh rosemary, chopped
- 1 pound (454 g) beef rump steak, sliced
- Salt and black pepper, to taste
- 1 shallot, chopped
- ½ cup heavy cream
- ½ cup beef stock
- 1 tablespoon mustard
- 2 teaspoons coconut aminos
- 2 teaspoons lemon juice
- 1 teaspoon xylitol
- A sprig of rosemary
- A sprig of thyme

1. Set a pan to medium heat, warm in a tablespoon of olive oil and stir in the shallot; cook for 3 minutes. Stir in the stock, coconut aminos, xylitol, thyme sprig, cream, mustard and rosemary sprig, and cook for 8 minutes. Stir in butter, lemon juice, pepper and salt. Get rid of the rosemary and thyme. Set aside.
2. In a bowl, combine the remaining oil with black pepper, garlic, rosemary, and salt. Toss in the beef to coat, and set aside for some minutes.
3. Heat a pan over medium-high heat, place in the beef steak, cook for 6 minutes, flipping halfway through; set aside and keep warm. Plate the beef slices, sprinkle over the sauce, and enjoy.

Per Serving

calories: 339 | fat: 25g | protein: 26g | carbs: 3g net carbs: 2g | fiber: 1g

127. Traditional Italian Bolognese Sauce

Prep time: 5 minutes | Cook time: 22 minutes | Serves 5

- 1 pound (454 g) ground beef
- 2 garlic cloves
- 1 onion, chopped
- 1 teaspoon oregano
- 1 teaspoon sage
- 1 teaspoon rosemary
- 7 ounces (198 g) canned chopped tomatoes
- 1 tablespoon olive oil

1. Heat olive oil in a saucepan. Add onion and garlic and cook for 3 minutes. Add beef and cook until browned, about 4-5 minutes. Stir in the herbs and tomatoes. Cook for 15 minutes. Serve with zoodles.

Per Serving

calories: 216 | fat: 14g | protein: 18g | carbs: 4g net carbs: 3g | fiber: 1g

128. Sirloin Steak Skewers with Ranch Dressing

Prep time: 5 minutes | Cook time: 13 minutes | Serves 4

- 1 pound (454 g) sirloin steak, boneless, cubed
- ¼ cup ranch dressing, divided
- Chopped scallions, for garnish

1. Preheat the grill on medium heat to 400°F and thread the beef cubes on the skewers, about 4 to 5 cubes per skewer. Brush half of the ranch dressing on the skewers (all around) and place them on the grill grate to cook for 6 minutes. Turn the skewers once and cook further for 6 minutes.
2. Brush the remaining ranch dressing on the meat and cook them for 1 more minute on each side. Plate, garnish with the scallions, and serve with a mixed veggie salad, and extra ranch dressing.

Per Serving

calories: 278 | fat: 19g | protein: 24g | carbs: 1g net carbs: 1g | fiber: 0g

129. Mascarpone Beef Balls with Cilantro

Prep time: 15 minutes | Cook time: 33 minutes | Serves 4

1 garlic clove, minced
1 pound (454 g) ground beef
1 small onion, chopped
1 jalapeño pepper, chopped
2 teaspoons cilantro
½ teaspoon allspice
1 teaspoon cumin
Salt and black pepper, to taste
1 tablespoon butter plus 1½ tablespoon, melted
½ cup mascarpone cheese, at room temperature
¼ teaspoon turmeric
¼ teaspoon baking powder
1 cup flax meal
¼ cup coconut flour

1. Purée onion with garlic, jalapeño pepper, and ¼ cup water in a blender. Set a pan over medium heat, add in 1 tablespoon butter and cook the beef for 3 minutes. Stir in the onion mixture, and cook for 2 minutes. Stir in cilantro, salt, cumin, turmeric, allspice, and black pepper, and cook for 3 minutes.
2. In a bowl, combine coconut flour, flax meal, and baking powder. In a separate bowl, combine the melted butter with the mascarpone cheese. Combine the 2 mixtures to obtain a dough. Form balls from this mixture, set them on a parchment paper, and roll each into a circle.
3. Split the beef mix on one-half of the dough circles, cover with the other half, seal edges, and lay on a lined sheet. Bake for 25 minutes in the oven at 350ºF (180ºC).

Per Serving
calories: 668 | fat: 44g | protein: 32g | carbs: 17g net carbs: 13g | fiber: 4g

130. Veggie cauliflower rice with Beef Steak

Prep time: 5 minutes | Cook time: 9 minutes | Serves 4

2 cups cauliflower rice
3 cups mixed vegetables
3 tablespoons butter
1 pound (454 g) beef skirt steak
Salt and black pepper, to taste
4 fresh eggs
Hot sauce (sugar-free) for topping (optional)

1. Mix the cauliflower rice with mixed vegetables in a bowl, sprinkle with a little water, and steam in the microwave for 1 minute to tender. Share into 4 serving bowls.
2. Melt the butter in a skillet, season the beef with salt and pepper, and brown in the butter for 5 minutes on each side. Use a perforated spoon to ladle the meat onto the vegetables.
3. Wipe out the skillet and return to medium heat, crack in an egg, season with salt and pepper, and cook until the egg white has set, but the yolk is still runny, for 3 minutes. Remove egg onto the vegetable bowl, and fry the remaining 3 eggs. Add to the other bowls. Drizzle the beef bowl with hot sauce (if desired) and serve.

Per Serving
calories: 791 | fat: 47g | protein: 65g | carbs: 22g net carbs: 14g | fiber: 8g

131. Beef Ragout with Green Beans

Prep time: 15 minutes | Cook time: 1 hour 48 minutes | Serves 4

2 tablespoons olive oil
1 pound (454 g) chuck steak, cubed
Salt and black pepper, to taste
2 tablespoons almond flour
4 green onions, diced
½ cup dry white wine
1 yellow bell pepper, diced
1 cup green beans, chopped
2 teaspoons Worcestershire sauce
4 ounces (113 g) tomato purée
3 teaspoons smoked paprika
1 cup beef broth
Parsley leaves, for garnish

1. Dredge the meat in the almond flour and set aside.
2. Place a large skillet over medium heat, add 1 tablespoon of oil to heat and then sauté the green onion, green beans, and bell pepper for 3 minutes. Stir in the paprika and the remaining olive oil.
3. Add the beef and cook for 10 minutes while turning them halfway. Stir in white wine, let it reduce by half, about 3 minutes, and add Worcestershire sauce, tomato purée, and beef broth.
4. Let the mixture boil for 2 minutes, then reduce the heat to lowest and let simmer for 1½ hours; stirring now and then. Adjust the taste and dish the ragout. Serve garnished with parsley leaves.

Per Serving
calories: 302 | fat: 17g | protein: 27g | carbs: 12g net carbs: 9g | fiber: 3g

132. Beef Sausage Casserole with Okra

Prep time: 15 minutes | Cook time: 25 minutes | Serves 4

1 cup okra, trimmed
1 tablespoon olive oil
1 celery stalk, chopped
¼ cup almond flour
1 egg
1 pound (454 g) beef sausage, chopped
Salt and black pepper, to taste
½ tablespoon dried parsley
¼ teaspoon red pepper flakes
¼ cup Parmesan cheese, grated
2 green onions, chopped
½ teaspoon garlic powder
¼ teaspoon dried oregano
½ cup ricotta cheese
½ cup marinara sauce, sugar-free
1 cup Cheddar cheese, shredded

1. In a bowl, combine the sausage, pepper, pepper flakes, oregano, egg, Parmesan cheese, green onions, almond flour, salt, parsley, celery, and garlic powder. Form balls, lay them on a lined baking sheet, place in the oven at 390°F (199°C), and bake for 15 minutes.
2. Remove the balls from the oven and cover with half of the marinara sauce and okra. Pour ricotta cheese all over followed by the rest of the marinara sauce. Scatter the Cheddar cheese and bake in the oven for 10 minutes. Allow the meatballs casserole to cool before serving.

Per Serving
calories: 611 | fat: 44g | protein: 36g | carbs: 14g net carbs: 12g | fiber: 2g

133. Rack of Lamb with Pepper Butter Sauce

Prep time: 15 minutes | Cook time: 21 minutes | Serves 4

1 pound (454 g) rack of lamb
Salt, to taste
3 cloves garlic, minced
Sauce:
2 tablespoons olive oil
1 large red bell pepper, seeded and diced
2 cloves garlic, minced
⅓ cup olive oil
⅓ cup white wine
6 sprigs fresh rosemary

1 cup chicken broth
2 ounces (57 g) butter
Salt and white pepper, to taste

1. Fill a large bowl with water and soak in the lamb for 30 minutes. Drain the meat after and season with salt. Let the lamb sit on a rack to drain completely and then rinse it afterward. Put in a bowl.
2. Mix the olive oil with wine and garlic, and brush the mixture all over the lamb. Drop the rosemary sprigs on it, cover the bowl with plastic wrap, and place in the refrigerator to marinate the meat.
3. The next day, preheat the grill to 450°F and cook the lamb for 6 minutes on both sides. Remove after and let rest for 4 minutes.
4. Heat the olive oil in a frying pan and sauté the garlic and bell pepper for 5 minutes. Pour in the chicken broth and continue cooking the ingredients until the liquid reduces by half, about 10 minutes. Add the butter, salt, and white pepper. Stir to melt the butter and turn the heat off.
5. Use the stick blender to purée the ingredients until very smooth and strain the sauce through a fine mesh into a bowl. Slice the lamb, serve with the sauce, and your favorite red wine.

Per Serving
calories: 601 | fat: 56g | protein: 22g | carbs: 5g net carbs: 4g | fiber: 1g

134. Beef Stew with Black Olives

Prep time: 15 minutes | Cook time: 1 hour 5 minutes | Serves 4

1 onion, chopped
2 tablespoons olive oil
1 teaspoon ginger paste
1 teaspoon coconut aminos
1 pound (454 g) beef stew meat, cubed
1 red bell pepper, seeded and chopped
½ scotch bonnet pepper, chopped
2 green chilies, chopped
1 cup tomatoes, chopped
1 tablespoon fresh cilantro, chopped
1 garlic clove, minced
¼ cup vegetable broth
Salt and black pepper, to taste
¼ cup black olives, chopped
1 teaspoon jerk seasoning

1. Brown the beef on all sides in warm olive oil over medium heat; remove and set aside. Stir-fry in the red bell peppers, green chilies, jerk seasoning, garlic, scotch bonnet pepper, onion, ginger paste, and coconut aminos, for about 5-6 minutes. Pour in the tomatoes and broth, and cook for 1 hour.
2. Stir in the olives, adjust the seasonings and serve sprinkled with fresh cilantro.

Per Serving
calories: 254 | fat: 12g | protein: 27g | carbs: 11g net carbs: 9g | fiber: 2g

135. Beef-Stuffed Zucchini Boats

Prep time: 20 minutes | Cook time: 33 minutes | Serves 4

2 garlic cloves, minced
1 teaspoon cumin
1 tablespoon olive oil
1 pound (454 g) ground beef
½ cup onions, chopped
1 teaspoon smoked paprika
Salt and black pepper, to taste
4 zucchinis
¼ cup fresh cilantro, chopped
½ cup Monterey Jack cheese, shredded
1½ cups enchilada sauce
1 avocado, chopped, for serving
Green onions, chopped, for serving
Tomatoes, chopped, for serving

1. Set a pan over high heat and warm the oil. Add the onions, and cook for 2 minutes. Stir in the beef, and brown for 4-5 minutes. Stir in the paprika, pepper, garlic, cumin, and salt; cook for 2 minutes.
2. Slice the zucchini in half lengthwise and scoop out the seeds. Set the zucchini in a greased baking pan, stuff each with the beef, scatter enchilada sauce on top, and spread with the Monterey cheese.
3. Bake in the oven at 350ºF for 20 minutes while covered. Uncover, spread with cilantro, and bake for 5 minutes. Top with tomatoes, green onions and avocado, place on serving plates and enjoy.

Per Serving

calories: 520 | fat: 36g | protein: 34g | carbs: 20g net carbs: 13g | fiber: 7g

136. Sirloin Steak with Sauce Diane

Prep time: 15 minutes | Cook time: 18 minutes | Serves 6

Sirloin Steak:
1½ pounds (680 g) sirloin steak
Salt and black pepper, to taste
1 teaspoon olive oil

Sauce Diane:
1 tablespoon olive oil
1 clove garlic, minced
1 cup sliced porcini mushrooms
1 small onion, finely diced
2 tablespoons butter
1 tablespoon Dijon mustard
2 tablespoons Worcestershire sauce
¼ cup whiskey
2 cups heavy whipping cream
Salt and black pepper, to taste

1. Put a grill pan over high heat and as it heats, brush the steak with oil, sprinkle with salt and pepper, and rub the seasoning into the meat with your hands. Cook the steak in the pan for 4 minutes on each side for medium rare and transfer to a chopping board to rest for 4 minutes before slicing. Reserve the juice.
2. Heat the oil in a frying pan over medium heat and sauté the onion for 3 minutes. Add the butter, garlic, and mushrooms, and cook for 2 minutes.
3. Add the Worcestershire sauce, the reserved juice, and mustard. Stir and cook for 1 minute. Pour in the whiskey and cook further 1 minute until the sauce reduces by half. Swirl the pan and add the cream. Let it simmer to thicken for about 3 minutes. Adjust the taste with salt and pepper. Spoon the sauce over the steaks slices and serve with celeriac mash.

Per Serving

calories: 436 | fat: 34g | protein: 25g | carbs: 6g net carbs: 5g | fiber: 1g

137. Beef Lasagna with Zucchinis

Prep time: 15 minutes | Cook time: 44 minutes | Serves 4

2 tablespoons olive oil
½ red chili, chopped
1 pound (454 g) ground beef
3 large zucchinis, sliced lengthwise
2 garlic cloves, minced
1 shallot, chopped
1 cup tomato purée
Salt and black pepper, to taste
2 teaspoons sweet paprika
1 teaspoon dried thyme
1 teaspoon dried basil
1 cup Mozzarella cheese, shredded
1 cup chicken broth

1. Heat the oil in a skillet and cook the beef for 4 minutes while breaking any lumps as you stir. Top with shallot, garlic, chili, tomatoes, salt, paprika and black pepper. Stir and cook for 5 more minutes.
2. Lay ⅓ of the zucchinis slices in a greased baking dish. Top with ⅓ of the beef mixture and repeat the layering process two more times with the same quantities. Season with basil and thyme. Pour in the chicken broth. Sprinkle the Mozzarella cheese on top and tuck the baking dish in the oven. Bake for 35 minutes at 380ºF (193ºC). Remove the lasagna and let it rest for 10 minutes before serving.

Per Serving

calories: 412 | fat: 30g | protein: 30g | carbs: 6g net carbs: 4g | fiber: 2g

138. Beef Steaks with Mushrooms and Bacon

Prep time: 10 minutes | Cook time: 40 minutes | Serves 4

2 ounces (57 g) bacon, chopped
1 cup mushrooms, sliced
1 garlic clove, chopped
1 shallot, chopped
1 cup heavy cream
1 pound (454 g) beef steaks
1 teaspoon ground nutmeg
¼ cup coconut oil
Salt and black pepper, to taste
1 tablespoon parsley, chopped

1. In a frying pan over medium heat, cook the bacon for 2-3 minutes and set aside. In the same pan, warm the oil, add in the onions, garlic and mushrooms, and cook for 4 minutes.
2. Stir in the beef, season with salt, black pepper and nutmeg, and sear until browned, about 2 minutes per side.
3. Preheat oven to 360°F (182°C) and insert the pan in the oven to bake for 25 minutes. Remove the beef steaks to a bowl and cover with foil.
4. Place the pan over medium heat, pour in the heavy cream over the mushroom mixture, add in the reserved bacon and cook for 5 minutes; remove from heat. Spread the bacon/mushroom sauce over beef steaks, sprinkle with parsley and serve.

Per Serving
calories: 447 | fat: 37g | protein: 27g | carbs: 3g net carbs: 2g | fiber: 1g

139. Balsamic Glazed Meatloaf

Prep time: 15 minutes | Cook time: 1 hour 10 minutes | Serves 12

3 pounds (1.4 kg) ground beef
½ cup onion, chopped
½ cup almond flour
2 garlic cloves, minced
1 cup mushrooms, sliced
3 eggs
Salt and black pepper, to taste
2 tablespoons parsley, chopped
¼ cup bell peppers, chopped
⅓ cup Parmesan cheese, grated
1 teaspoon balsamic vinegar
Glaze:
2 cups balsamic vinegar
1 tablespoon sweetener
2 tablespoons tomato purée

1. Combine all of the meatloaf ingredients in a large bowl. Press the mixture into greased loaf pan. Bake at 375°F (190°C) for about 30 minutes.
2. Make the glaze by combining all of the ingredients in a saucepan over medium heat.
3. Simmer for 20 minutes, until the glaze is thickened. Pour ¼ cup of the glaze over the meatloaf. Save the extra for future use. Put the meatloaf back in the oven, and cook for 20 more minutes.

Per Serving
calories: 375 | fat: 25g | protein: 23g | carbs: 13g net carbs: 12g | fiber: 1g

140. Buttery Habanero and Beef Balls

Prep time: 20 minutes | Cook time: 34 minutes | Serves 6

3 garlic cloves, minced
1 pound (454 g) ground beef
1 small onion, chopped
2 habanero peppers, chopped
1 teaspoon dried thyme
2 teaspoons cilantro
½ teaspoon allspice
2 teaspoons cumin
Pinch of ground cloves
Salt and black pepper, to taste
2 tablespoons butter
3 tablespoons butter, melted
6 ounces (170 g) cream cheese
1 teaspoon turmeric
¼ teaspoon stevia
½ teaspoon baking powder
1½ cups flax meal
½ cup coconut flour

1. In a blender, mix onion with garlic, habaneros, and ½ cup water. Set a pan over medium heat, add in 2 tablespoons butter and cook the beef for 3 minutes. Stir in the onion mixture, and cook for 2 minutes.
2. Stir in cilantro, cloves, salt, cumin, ½ teaspoon turmeric, thyme, allspice, and black pepper, and cook for 3 minutes. In a bowl, combine the remaining turmeric, with coconut flour, stevia, flax meal, and baking powder. In a separate bowl, combine the melted butter with the cream cheese.
3. Combine the 2 mixtures to obtain a dough. Form 12 balls from this mixture, set them on a parchment paper, and roll each into a circle. Split the beef mix on one-half of the dough circles, cover with the other half, seal edges, and lay on a lined sheet. Bake for 25 minutes in the oven at 350°F.

Per Serving
calories: 570 | fat: 41g | protein: 25g | carbs: 18g net carbs: 13g | fiber: 5g

141. Beef Meatloaf with Balsamic Glaze

Prep time: 15 minutes | Cook time: 50 minutes | Serves 4

Meatloaf:
1 pound (454 g) ground beef
½ onion, chopped
1 tablespoon almond milk
1 tablespoon almond flour
1 garlic clove, minced
1 cup sliced mushrooms
1 small egg
Salt and black pepper, to taste
1 tablespoon parsley, chopped
⅓ cup Parmesan cheese, grated

Glaze:
⅓ cup balsamic vinegar
¼ tablespoon xylitol
¼ teaspoon garlic powder
¼ teaspoon onion powder
1 tablespoon plus ¼ teaspoon tomato purée

1. Grease a loaf pan with cooking spray and set aside. Preheat oven to 390°F (199°C). Combine all meatloaf ingredients in a large bowl. Press this mixture into the prepared loaf pan. Bake for about 30 minutes.
2. To make the glaze, whisk all ingredients in a bowl. Pour the glaze over the meatloaf. Put the meatloaf back in the oven and cook for 20 more minutes. Let meatloaf sit for 10 minutes before slicing.

Per Serving
calories: 377 | fat: 26g | protein: 24g | carbs: 10g net carbs: 9g | fiber: 1g

142. Smoked Paprika Beef Ragout

Prep time: 15 minutes | Cook time: 1 hour 48 minutes | Serves 4

1 pound (454 g) chuck steak, trimmed and cubed
2 tablespoons olive oil
Salt and black pepper, to taste
2 tablespoons almond flour
1 medium onion, diced
½ cup dry white wine
1 red bell pepper, seeded and diced
2 teaspoons Worcestershire sauce
4 ounces (113 g) tomato purée
3 teaspoons smoked paprika
1 cup beef broth
Thyme leaves, for garnish

1. First, lightly dredge the meat in the almond flour and set aside. Place a large skillet over medium heat, add 1 tablespoon of oil to heat and then sauté the onion, and bell pepper for 3 minutes. Stir in the paprika, and add the remaining olive oil.
2. Add the beef and cook for 10 minutes in total while turning them halfway. Stir in white wine, let it reduce by half, about 3 minutes, and add Worcestershire sauce, tomato purée, and beef broth.
3. Let the mixture boil for 2 minutes, then reduce the heat to lowest and let simmer for 1½ hours; stirring now and then. Adjust the taste and dish the ragout. Serve garnished with thyme leaves.

Per Serving
calories: 299 | fat: 17g | protein: 27g | carbs: 11g net carbs: 9g | fiber: 2g

143. Rump Steak Salad

Prep time: 15 minutes | Cook time: 29 minutes | Serves 4

½ pound (227 g) rump steak, excess fat trimmed
3 green onions, sliced
3 tomatoes, sliced
1 cup green beans, steamed and sliced
2 kohlrabi, peeled and chopped
½ cup water
2 cups mixed salad greens
Salt and black pepper, to season

Salad Dressing:
2 teaspoons Dijon mustard
1 teaspoon erythritol
Salt and black pepper, to taste
3 tablespoons olive oil, plus more for drizzling
1 tablespoon red wine vinegar

1. Preheat the oven to 400°F. Place the kohlrabi on a baking sheet, drizzle with olive oil and bake in the oven for 25 minutes. After cooking, remove, and set aside to cool.
2. In a bowl, mix the Dijon mustard, erythritol, salt, black pepper, vinegar, and olive oil. Set aside.
3. Then, preheat a grill pan over high heat while you season the meat with salt and black pepper. Place the steak in the pan and brown on both sides for 4 minutes each. Remove to rest on a chopping board for 4 more minutes before slicing thinly.
4. In a salad bowl, add green onions, tomatoes, green beans, kohlrabi, salad greens, and steak slices. Drizzle the dressing over and toss with two spoons. Serve the steak salad warm with chunks of low carb bread.

Per Serving
calories: 232 | fat: 14g | protein: 15g | carbs: 13g net carbs: 7g | fiber: 6g

144. Grilled Beef Skewers with Fresh Salad

Prep time: 10 minutes | Cook time: 13 minutes | Serves 4

1 pound (454 g) sirloin steak, boneless, cubed
¼ cup ranch dressing
1 red onion, sliced
½ tablespoon white wine vinegar
1 tablespoon extra-virgin olive oil
2 ripe tomatoes, sliced
2 tablespoons fresh parsley, chopped
1 cucumber, sliced
Salt, to taste

1. Thread the beef cubes on the skewers, about 4-5 cubes per skewer. Brush half of the ranch dressing on the skewers (all around). Preheat grill to 400°F (205°C) and place the skewers on the grill grate to cook for 6 minutes. Turn the skewers once and cook further for 6 minutes.
2. Brush the remaining ranch dressing on the meat and cook them for 1 more minute on each side.
3. In a salad bowl mix together red onion, tomatoes, and cucumber, sprinkle with salt, vinegar, and extra-virgin olive oil; toss to combine. Top the salad with skewers and scatter the parsley all over.

Per Serving
calories: 357 | fat: 23g | protein: 25g | carbs: 12g net carbs: 10g | fiber: 2g

145. Balsamic Glazed Meatloaf

Prep time: 20 minutes | Cook time: 1 hour 10 minutes | Serves 6

1 cup white mushrooms, chopped
2 pounds (907 g) ground beef
2 tablespoons fresh parsley, chopped
2 garlic cloves, minced
1 onion, chopped
1 red bell pepper, seeded and chopped
½ cup almond flour
⅓ cup Parmesan cheese, grated
2 eggs
Salt and black pepper, to taste
1 teaspoon plus 2 cups balsamic vinegar, divided
1 tablespoon Swerve natural sweetener
1 tablespoon coconut aminos
2 tablespoons tomato purée

1. In a bowl, combine the beef with salt, mushrooms, bell pepper, Parmesan cheese, 1 teaspoon vinegar, parsley, garlic, black pepper, onion, almond flour, salt, and eggs. Set this into a loaf pan, and bake for 30 minutes in the oven at 370°F.
2. Meanwhile, heat a small pan over medium heat, add in the 2 cups vinegar, Swerve, coconut aminos, and tomato purée, and cook for 20 minutes. Remove the meatloaf from the oven, spread the glaze over the meatloaf, and bake in the oven for 20 more minutes. Allow the meatloaf to cool, slice, and enjoy.

Per Serving
calories: 469 | fat: 22g | protein: 35g | carbs: 14g net carbs: 12g | fiber: 2g

146. Beef Meatball Salad with Dilled Yogurt

Prep time: 15 minutes | Cook time: 8 minutes | Serves 6

¼ cup almond milk
2 pounds (907 g) ground beef
1 onion, grated
5 zero carb bread slices, torn
1 egg, whisked
¼ cup fresh parsley, chopped
Salt and black pepper, to taste
2 garlic cloves, minced
¼ cup fresh mint, chopped
2½ teaspoons dried oregano
¼ cup olive oil
1 cup cherry tomatoes, halved
1 cucumber, sliced
1 cup baby spinach
1½ tablespoons lemon juice
1 cup dilled Greek yogurt

1. Place the torn bread in a bowl, add in the milk, and set aside for 3 minutes. Squeeze the bread, chop, and place into a bowl. Stir in the beef, salt, mint, onion, parsley, pepper, egg, oregano, and garlic.
2. Form balls out of this mixture and place on a working surface. Set a pan over medium heat and warm half of the oil; fry the meatballs for 8 minutes. Flip occasionally, and set aside in a tray.
3. In a salad plate, combine the spinach with the cherry tomatoes and cucumber. Mix in the remaining oil, lemon juice, black pepper, and salt. Spread dilled yogurt over, and top with meatballs to serve.

Per Serving
calories: 568 | fat: 41g | protein: 32g | carbs: 17g net carbs: 12g | fiber: 5g

147. Beef Chuck Roast with Veggies

Prep time: 15 minutes | Cook time: 1 hour 35 minutes | Serves 4

2 tablespoons olive oil
1 pound (454 g) beef chuck roast, cubed
1 cup canned diced tomatoes
Salt and black pepper, to taste
½ pound (227 g) mushrooms, sliced
1 celery stalk, chopped
1 bell pepper, sliced
1 onion, chopped
1 bay leaf
½ cup beef stock
1 tablespoon fresh rosemary, chopped
½ teaspoon dry mustard
1 tablespoon almond flour

1. Preheat oven to 350ºF (180ºC). Set a pot over medium heat, warm olive oil and brown the beef on each side for 4-5 minutes. Stir in tomatoes, onion, mustard, mushrooms, bell pepper, celery, and stock. Season with salt and pepper.
2. In a bowl, combine ½ cup of water with flour and stir in the pot. Transfer to a baking dish and bake for 90 minutes, stirring at intervals of 30 minutes. Scatter the rosemary over and serve warm.

Per Serving

calories: 329 | fat: 17g | protein: 34g | carbs: 8g net carbs: 4g | fiber: 4g

148. Cheesy Beef Gratin

Prep time: 15 minutes | Cook time: 25 minutes | Serves 4

2 tablespoons olive oil
1 onion, chopped
1 pound (454 g) ground beef
2 garlic cloves, minced
Salt and black pepper, to taste
1 cup Mozzarella cheese, shredded
1 cup fontina cheese, shredded
1 (14-ounce / 397-g) canned tomatoes, chopped
2 tablespoons sesame seeds, toasted
20 dill pickle slices

1. Preheat the oven to 390ºF (199ºC). Heat olive oil in a pan over medium heat, place in the beef, garlic, salt, onion, and black pepper, and cook for 5 minutes. Remove and set to a baking dish, stir in half of the tomatoes and Mozzarella cheese. Lay the pickle slices on top, spread over the fontina cheese and sesame seeds, and place in the oven to bake for 20 minutes.

Per Serving

calories: 620 | fat: 49g | protein: 36g | carbs: 9g net carbs: 6g | fiber: 3g

149. Flank Steak and Kale Roll

Prep time: 10 minutes | Cook time: 30 minutes | Serves 4

1 pound (454 g) flank steak
Salt and black pepper, to taste
½ cup ricotta cheese, crumbled
½ cup baby kale, chopped
1 serrano pepper, chopped
1 tablespoon basil leaves, chopped

1. Wrap the steak in plastic wraps, place on a flat surface, and gently run a rolling pin over to flatten. Take off the wraps. Sprinkle with half of the ricotta cheese, top with kale, serrano pepper, and the remaining cheese. Roll the steak over on the stuffing and secure with toothpicks.
2. Place in the greased baking sheet and cook for 30 minutes at 390ºF (199ºC), flipping once until nicely browned on the outside and the cheese melted within. Cool for 3 minutes, slice and serve with basil.

Per Serving

calories: 211 | fat: 10g | protein: 28g | carbs: 1g net carbs: 1g | fiber: 0g

150. Beef Casserole with Cauliflower

Prep time: 10 minutes | Cook time: 24 minutes | Serves 4

2 tablespoons olive oil
1 pound (454 g) ground beef
Salt and black pepper, to taste
½ cup cauliflower rice
1 tablespoon parsley, chopped
½ teaspoon dried oregano
1 cup kohlrabi, chopped
1 (5-ounce / 142-g) can diced tomatoes
¼ cup water
½ cup Mozzarella cheese, shredded

1. Put beef in a pot and season with salt and pepper; cook over medium heat for 6 minutes until no longer pink. Add cauliflower rice, kohlrabi, tomatoes, and water. Stir and bring to boil for 5 minutes to thicken the sauce. Spoon the beef mixture into the baking dish and spread evenly. Sprinkle with cheese and bake in the oven for 15 minutes at 380ºF (193ºC) until cheese has melted and it's golden brown. Remove and cool for 4 minutes, and serve sprinkled with parsley.

Per Serving

calories: 409 | fat: 33g | protein: 24g | carbs: 5g net carbs: 3g | fiber: 2g

151. Seared Ribeye Steak with Shitake Mushrooms

Prep time: 5 minutes | Cook time: 12 minutes | Serves 1

6 ounces (170 g) ribeye steak
2 tablespoons butter
1 teaspoon olive oil
½ cup shitake mushrooms, sliced
Salt and black pepper, to taste

1. Heat the olive oil in a pan over medium heat. Rub the steak with salt and black pepper and cook about 4 minutes per side; set aside. Melt the butter in the pan and cook the shitakes for 4 minutes. Pour the butter and mushrooms over the steak to serve.

Per Serving
calories: 569 | fat: 47g | protein: 34g | carbs: 4g net carbs: 3g | fiber: 1g

152. Lemon-Mustard Beef Rump Steak

Prep time: 20 minutes | Cook time: 17 minutes | Serves 4

2 tablespoons olive oil
1 tablespoon fresh rosemary, chopped
2 garlic cloves, minced
1½ pounds (680 g) beef rump steak, thinly sliced
Salt and black pepper, to taste
1 shallot, chopped
½ cup heavy cream
½ cup beef stock
1 tablespoon mustard
2 teaspoons Worcestershire sauce
2 teaspoons lemon juice
1 teaspoon erythritol
2 tablespoons butter
A sprig of rosemary
A sprig of thyme

1. In a bowl, combine 1 tablespoon of oil with black pepper, garlic, rosemary, and salt. Toss in the beef to coat, and set aside for some minutes. Heat a pan with the rest of the oil over medium heat, place in the beef steak, cook for 6 minutes, flipping halfway through; set aside and keep warm.
2. Set the pan to medium heat, stir in the shallot, and cook for 3 minutes; stir in the stock, Worcestershire sauce, erythritol, thyme, cream, mustard, and rosemary, and cook for 8 minutes.
3. Stir in the butter, lemon juice, black pepper, and salt. Get rid of the rosemary and thyme, and remove from heat. Arrange the beef slices on serving plates, sprinkle over the sauce, and enjoy.

Per Serving
calories: 600 | fat: 49g | protein: 35g | carbs: 4g net carbs: 3g | fiber: 1g

153. Paprika Roast Beef Brisket

Prep time: 10 minutes | Cook time: 1 hour | Serves 4

2 pounds (907 g) beef brisket
½ teaspoon celery salt
1 teaspoon chili powder
2 tablespoons olive oil
1 tablespoon sweet paprika
Pinch of cayenne pepper
½ teaspoon garlic powder
½ cup beef stock
3 onions, cut into quarters
¼ teaspoon dry mustard

1. Grease a baking dish with cooking spray and preheat oven to 360ºF (182ºC). In a bowl, combine the paprika with dry mustard, chili powder, salt, garlic powder, cayenne pepper, and celery salt. Rub the meat with this mixture.
2. Set a pan over medium heat and warm olive oil, place in the beef, and sear until brown.
3. Remove to the baking dish. Pour in the stock, add onions and bake for 60 minutes.
4. Set the beef to a cutting board, and leave to cool before slicing. Take the juices from the baking dish and strain, sprinkle over the meat to serve.

Per Serving
calories: 601 | fat: 41g | protein: 36g | carbs: 19g net carbs: 16g | fiber: 3g

154. Italian Beef Roast with Jalapeño

Prep time: 5 minutes | Cook time: 1 hour 15 minutes | Serves 4

3½ pounds (1.5 kg) beef roast
4 ounces (113 g) mushrooms, sliced
12 ounces (340 g) beef stock
1 ounce (28 g) onion soup mix
½ cup Italian dressing
2 jalapeño peppers, shredded

1. In a bowl, combine the stock with the Italian dressing and onion soup mixture. Place the beef roast in a pan, stir in the stock mixture, mushrooms, and jalapeños; cover with aluminum foil.
2. Set in the oven at 300ºF, and bake for 1 hour. Take out the foil and continue baking for 15 minutes. Allow the roast to cool, slice, and serve alongside a topping of the gravy.

Per Serving
calories: 616 | fat: 26g | protein: 88g | carbs: 9g net carbs: 8g | fiber: 1g

155. Beef and Cauliflower Curry with Cilantro

Prep time: 10 minutes | Cook time: 21 minutes | Serves 4

1 tablespoon olive oil
½ pound (227 g) ground beef
1 garlic clove, minced
1 teaspoon turmeric
1 tablespoon cilantro, chopped
1 tablespoon ginger paste
½ teaspoon garam masala
5 ounces (142 g) canned whole tomatoes
1 head cauliflower, cut into florets
Salt and chili pepper, to taste
¼ cup water

1. Heat oil in a saucepan over medium heat, add the beef, garlic, ginger paste, and garam masala. Cook for 5 minutes while breaking any lumps.
2. Stir in the tomatoes and cauliflower, season with salt, turmeric, and chili pepper, and cook covered for 6 minutes. Add the water and bring to a boil over medium heat for 10 minutes or until the water has reduced by half. Spoon the curry into serving bowls and serve sprinkled with cilantro.

Per Serving

calories: 201 | fat: 15g | protein: 11g | carbs: 6g net carbs: 4g | fiber: 2g

156. Garlicky Lamb Chops with Sage

Prep time: 10 minutes | Cook time: 1 hour 10 minutes | Serves 6

6 lamb chops
1 tablespoon sage
1 teaspoon thyme
1 onion, sliced
1 cup water
3 garlic cloves, minced
2 tablespoons olive oil
½ cup white wine
Salt and black pepper, to taste

1. Heat the olive oil in a pan. Add onions and garlic, and cook for 4 minutes, until soft. Rub the sage and thyme over the lamb chops. Cook the lamb for about 3 minutes per side. Set aside. Pour the white wine and water into the pan, bring the mixture to a boil. Cook until the liquid is reduced by half. Add the chops in the pan, reduce the heat, and let simmer for 1 hour.

Per Serving

calories: 215 | fat: 13g | protein: 23g | carbs: 3g net carbs: 2g | fiber: 1g

157. Juicy Beef Meatballs with Parsley

Prep time: 10 minutes | Cook time: 21 minutes | Serves 4

1 pound (454 g) ground beef
Salt and black pepper, to taste
½ teaspoon garlic powder
1¼ tablespoons coconut aminos
1 cup beef stock
¾ cup almond flour
1 tablespoon fresh parsley, chopped
1 onion, sliced
2 tablespoons butter
1 tablespoon olive oil
¼ cup sour cream

1. Preheat the oven to 390°F (199°C) and grease a baking dish. In a bowl, combine beef with salt, garlic powder, almond flour, parsley, 1 tablespoon of coconut aminos, black pepper, ¼ cup of beef stock. Form patties and place on the baking sheet. Bake for 18 minutes.
2. Set a pan with the butter and olive oil over medium heat, stir in the onion, and cook for 3 minutes. Stir in the remaining beef stock, sour cream, and remaining coconut aminos, and bring to a simmer. Adjust the seasoning with black pepper and salt. Serve the meatballs topped with onion sauce.

Per Serving

calories: 519 | fat: 36g | protein: 24g | carbs: 18g net carbs: 16g | fiber: 2g

158. Beef and Mushrooms in Red Wine

Prep time: 15 minutes | Cook time: 10 minutes | Serves 4

3 tablespoons olive oil
1 tablespoon parsley, chopped
1 cup red wine
1 teaspoon dried thyme
Salt and black pepper, to taste
1 bay leaf
1 cup beef stock
1 pound (454 g) stewed beef, cubed
12 pearl onions, halved
1 tomato, chopped
2 ounces (57 g) pancetta, chopped
2 garlic cloves, minced
½ pound (227 g) mushrooms, chopped

1. Heat a pan over high heat, stir in the pancetta and beef and cook until lightly browned; set aside.
2. Place in the onions, mushrooms, and garlic, and cook for 5 minutes. Pour in the wine to deglaze the bottom of the pan and add beef stock, bay leaf, and tomato. Season with salt, black pepper and thyme. Return the meat and pancetta, cover and cook for 50 minutes.
3. Serve sprinkled with parsley.

Per Serving

calories: 468 | fat: 22g | protein: 46g | carbs: 23g net carbs: 18g | fiber: 5g

159. Beef-Cabbage Casserole

Prep time: 5 minutes | Cook time: 26 minutes | Serves 6

2 pounds (907 g) ground beef
Salt and black pepper, to taste
1 cup cauliflower rice
2 cups chopped cabbage
1 (14-ounce / 397-g) can diced tomatoes
1 cup shredded Colby jack cheese

1. Preheat oven to 370°F and grease a baking dish with cooking spray. Put beef in a pot and season with salt and black pepper and cook over medium heat for 6 minutes until no longer pink. Drain the grease. Add cauliflower rice, cabbage, tomatoes, and ¼ cup water. Stir and bring to boil covered for 5 minutes to thicken the sauce. Adjust taste with salt and black pepper.
2. Spoon the beef mixture into the baking dish and spread evenly. Sprinkle with cheese and bake in the oven for 15 minutes until cheese has melted and it's golden brown. Remove and cool for 4 minutes and serve with low carb crusted bread.

Per Serving
calories: 402 | fat: 27g | protein: 36g | carbs: 6g net carbs: 4g | fiber: 2g

160. Three-Cheese Beef Sausage Casserole

Prep time: 20 minutes | Cook time: 25 minutes | Serves 8

⅓ cup almond flour
2 eggs
2 pounds (907 g) beef sausage, chopped
Salt and black pepper, to taste
1 tablespoon dried parsley
¼ teaspoon red pepper flakes
¼ cup Parmesan cheese, grated
¼ teaspoon onion powder
½ teaspoon garlic powder
¼ teaspoon dried oregano
1 cup ricotta cheese
1 cup sugar-free marinara sauce
1½ cups Cheddar cheese, shredded

1. In a bowl, combine the sausage, black pepper, pepper flakes, oregano, eggs, Parmesan cheese, onion powder, almond flour, salt, parsley, and garlic powder. Form balls, lay them on a greased baking sheet, place in the oven at 370°F, and bake for 15 minutes.
2. Remove the balls from the oven and cover with half of the marinara sauce. Pour ricotta cheese all over followed by the rest of the marinara sauce. Scatter the Cheddar cheese and bake in the oven for 10 minutes. Allow the meatballs casserole to cool before serving.

Per Serving
calories: 505 | fat: 36g | protein: 33g | carbs: 12g net carbs: 11g | fiber: 1g

161. Beef and Egg cauliflower rice Bowls

Prep time: 5 minutes | Cook time: 14 minutes | Serves 4

2 cups cauliflower rice
3 cups frozen mixed vegetables
3 tablespoons butter
1 pound (454 g) skirt steak
Salt and black pepper, to taste
4 eggs
Hot sauce, for topping (optional)

1. Mix the cauliflower rice and mixed vegetables in a bowl, sprinkle with a little water, and steam in the microwave for 1 minute until tender. Share into 4 serving bowls.
2. Melt the butter in a skillet, season the beef with salt and black pepper, and brown for 5 minutes on each side. Use a perforated spoon to ladle the meat onto the vegetables.
3. Wipe out the skillet and return to medium heat, crack in an egg, season with salt and pepper and cook until the egg white has set, but the yolk is still runny 3 minutes. Remove egg onto the vegetable bowl and fry the remaining 3 eggs. Add to the other bowls. Drizzle the beef bowls with hot sauce (if desired) and serve.

Per Serving
calories: 470 | fat: 25g | protein: 42g | carbs: 21g net carbs: 14g | fiber: 7g

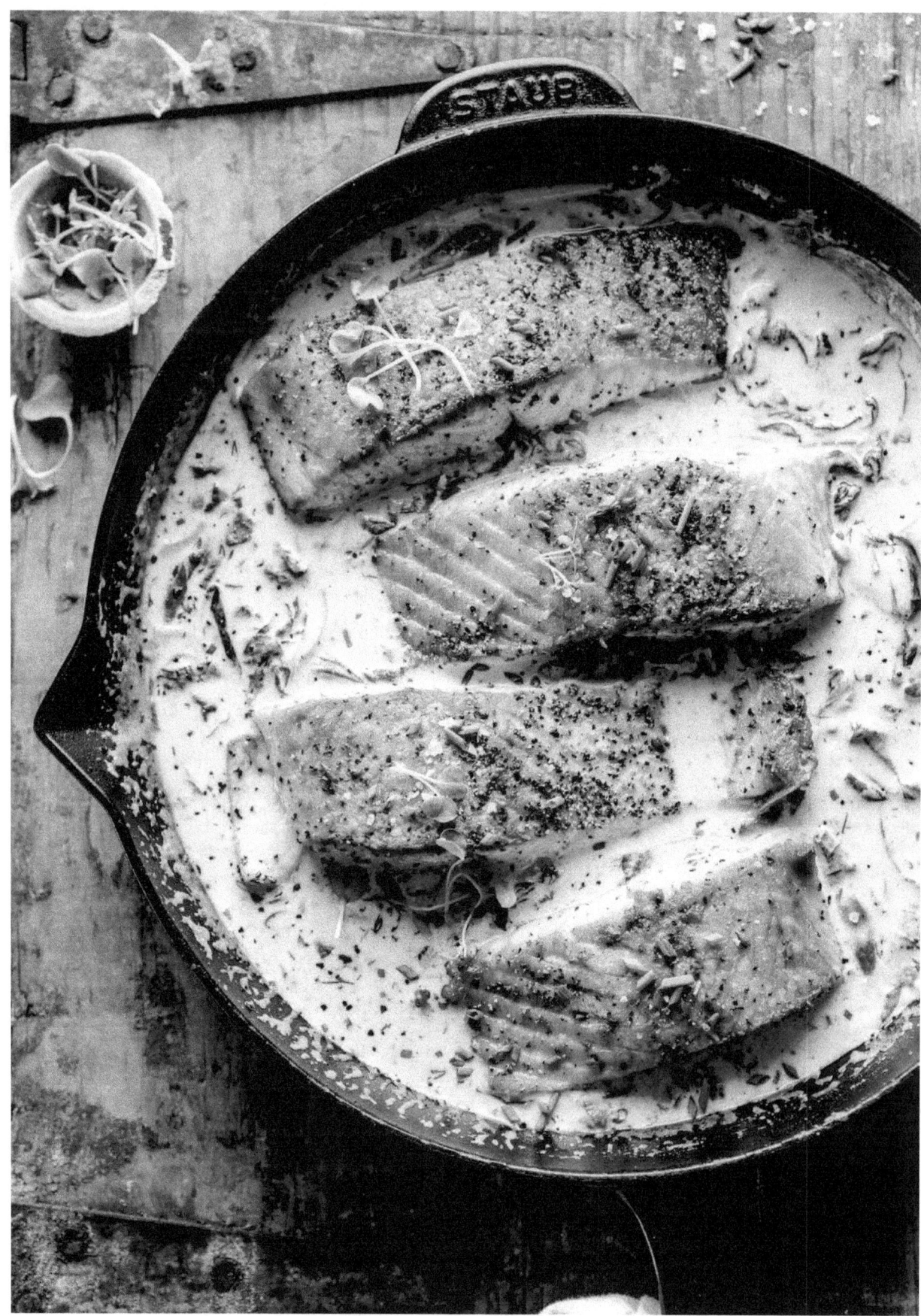

Chapter 6 Fish and Seafood

162. Anchovies and Veggies Wraps

Prep time: 10 minutes | Cook time: 0 minutes | Serves 4

2 (2-ounce / 57-g) can anchovies in olive oil, drained
1 cucumber, sliced
2 cups red cabbage, shredded
1 red onion, chopped
1 teaspoon Dijon mustard
4 tablespoons mayonnaise
¼ teaspoon ground black pepper
1 large-sized tomato, diced
12 lettuce leaves

1. In a mixing bowl, combine the anchovies with the cucumber, cabbage, onion, mustard, mayonnaise, black pepper, and tomatoes.
2. Arrange the lettuce leaves on a tray. Spoon the anchovy/vegetable mixture into the center of a lettuce leaf, taco-style.
3. Repeat until you run out of ingredients. Bon appétit!

Per Serving
calories: 191 | fat: 13g | protein: 3g | carbs: 10g net carbs: 7g | fiber: 3g

163. Haddock with Mediterranean Sauce

Prep time: 10 minutes | Cook time: 20 minutes | Serves 4

1 pound haddock fillets
1 tablespoon olive oil
Sea salt and freshly cracked black pepper, to taste
Mediterranean Sauce:
2 scallions, chopped
½ teaspoon dill weed
½ teaspoon oregano
1 teaspoon basil
¼ cup mayonnaise
¼ cup cream cheese, at room temperature

1. Start by preheating your oven to 360ºF (182ºC). Toss the haddock fillets with the olive oil, salt, and black pepper.
2. Cover with foil and bake for 20 to 25 minutes.
3. In the meantime, make the sauce by whisking all ingredients until well combined. Serve with the warm haddock fillets and enjoy!

Per Serving
calories: 260 | fat: 19g | protein: 20g | carbs: 1g net carbs: 1g | fiber: 0g

164. Tuna Fillet Salade Niçoise

Prep time: 5 minutes | Cook time: 7 minutes | Serves 2

¾ pound (340 g) tuna fillet, skinless
1 white onion, sliced
1 teaspoon Dijon mustard
8 Niçoise olives, pitted and sliced
½ teaspoon anchovy paste

1. Brush the tuna with nonstick cooking oil; season with salt and freshly cracked black pepper. Then, grill your tuna on a lightly oiled rack approximately 7 minutes, turning over once or twice.
2. Let the fish stand for 3 to 4 minutes and break into bite-sized pieces. Transfer to a nice salad bowl.
3. Toss the tuna pieces with the white onion, Dijon mustard, Niçoise olives, and anchovy paste. Serve well chilled and enjoy!

Per Serving
calories: 194 | fat: 3g | protein: 37g | carbs: 1g net carbs: 1g | fiber: 0g

165. Anchovies with Caesar Dressing

Prep time: 5 minutes | Cook time: 3 minutes | Serves 3

6 anchovies, cleaned and deboned
1 fresh garlic clove, peeled
1 teaspoon Dijon mustard
2 egg yolks
⅓ cup extra-virgin olive oil

1. Place the anchovies onto a lightly oiled grill pan; place under the grill for 2 minutes. Turn them over and cook for a further minute or so; remove from the grill.
2. Process the garlic, Dijon mustard, egg yolks, and extra-virgin olive oil in your blender. Blend until creamy and uniform.
3. Serve the warm grilled anchovies with the Caesar dressing on the side. Bon appétit!

Per Serving
calories: 449 | fat: 34g | protein: 33g | carbs: 1g net carbs: 1g | fiber: 0g

166. Seafood Chowder

Prep time: 10 minutes | Cook time: 20 minutes | Serves 4

2 tablespoons coconut oil
2 garlic cloves, pressed
1 shallot, chopped
1 cup broccoli, broken into small florets
1 bell peppers, chopped
4 cups fish broth
4 tablespoons dry sherry
6 ounces (170 g) scallops
6 ounces (170 g) shrimp, peeled and deveined
1 cup heavy cream
1 tablespoon fresh chives, chopped

1. Melt the coconut oil in a soup pot over a moderate flame. Now, cook the garlic and shallot for 3 to 4 minutes or until they have softened.
2. Stir in the broccoli florets, bell peppers, and fish broth; bring to a boil. Turn the heat to medium-low, partially cover, and let it cook for 12 minutes more.
3. Add in the dry sherry, scallops, shrimp, and heavy cream. Continue to cook an additional 7 minutes or until heated through.
4. Taste and adjust the seasonings. Serve garnished with fresh chives. Bon appétit!

Per Serving
calories: 272 | fat: 20g | protein: 17g | carbs: 7g net carbs: 6g | fiber: 1g

167. Gambas al Ajillo

Prep time: 5 minutes | Cook time: 3 minutes | Serves 5

2 tablespoons butter
2 cloves garlic, minced
2 small cayenne pepper pods
2 pounds (907 g) shrimp, peeled and deveined
¼ cup Manzanilla
Sea salt and ground black pepper, to taste

1. Melt the butter in a sauté pan over moderate heat. Add the garlic and cayenne peppers and cook for 40 seconds.
2. Add the shrimp and cook for about a minute. Pour in the Manzanilla; season with salt and black pepper.
3. Continue to cook for a minute or so, until the shrimp are cooked through. Add lemon slices to each serving if desired. Enjoy!

Per Serving
calories: 203 | fat: 6g | protein: 37g | carbs: 2g net carbs: 2g | fiber: 0g

168. Garlicky Mackerel Fillet

Prep time: 5 minutes | Cook time: 5 minutes | Serves 2

1 tablespoon olive oil
2 mackerel fillets
2 garlic cloves, minced
Sea salt and ground black pepper, to taste
½ teaspoon thyme
1 teaspoon rosemary
½ teaspoon basil

1. Heat the olive oil in a frying pan over a moderate flame and swirl to coat the bottom of the pan. Pat dry the mackerel fillets.
2. Now, brown the fish fillets for 5 minutes per side until golden and crisp, shaking the pan lightly.
3. During the last minutes, add the garlic, salt, black pepper, and herbs. Bon appétit!

Per Serving
calories: 481 | fat: 15g | protein: 80g | carbs: 1g net carbs: 1g | fiber: 0g

169. Curry White Fish Fillet

Prep time: 10 minutes | Cook time: 15 minutes | Serves 6

2 tablespoons sesame oil
1 shallot, chopped
2 bell peppers, deveined and sliced
1 teaspoon coriander, ground
1 teaspoon cumin, ground
4 tablespoons red curry paste
1 teaspoon ginger-garlic paste
1 ½ pounds (680 g) white fish fillets, skinless, boneless
½ cup tomato purée
½ cup haddi ka shorba (Indian bone broth)
1 cup coconut milk
½ teaspoon red chili powder
Kosher salt and ground black pepper, to taste

1. Heat the sesame oil in a saucepan over moderate heat; then, sauté the shallot and peppers until they have softened or about 4 minutes.
2. Now, stir in the coriander, cumin, red curry paste, and ginger-garlic paste; continue to sauté an additional 4 minutes, stirring frequently.
3. After that, fold in the fish and tomato purée; pour in the haddi ka shorba and coconut milk. Season with red chili powder, salt, and black pepper.
4. Turn the heat to simmer and let it cook for 5 minutes longer or until everything is cooked through. Enjoy!

Per Serving
calories: 349 | fat: 25g | protein: 23g | carbs: 6g net carbs: 3g | fiber: 4g

170. Sardine Burgers

Prep time: 10 minutes | Cook time: 6 minutes | Serves 3

2 (5.5-ounce / 156-g) canned sardines, drained
2 ounces (57 g) Romano cheese, preferably freshly grated
1 egg, beaten
3 tablespoons flaxseed meal
1 tablespoon dry Italian seasoning blend
1 teaspoon fresh garlic, peeled and minced
½ onion, chopped
½ teaspoon celery salt
Freshly ground black pepper, to taste
½ teaspoon smoked paprika
2 tablespoons butter

1. In a mixing dish, thoroughly combine the sardines with the cheese, egg, flaxseed meal, dry Italian seasoning blend, garlic, and onion.
2. Season with the celery salt, black pepper, and smoked paprika. Form the mixture into six equal patties.
3. Melt the butter in a frying pan over a moderate flame. Once hot, fry the fish burgers for 4 to
4. 6 minutes on each side. Serve garnished with fresh lemon slices. Bon appétit!

Per Serving
calories: 267 | fat: 21g | protein: 14g | carbs: 6g net carbs: 2g | fiber: 3g

171. Crispy Keto Creamy Fish Casserole

Prep time: 25 minutes | Cook time: 30 minutes | Serves 4

1 head broccoli, cut into florets
2 tablespoons olive oil
1 teaspoon salt
¼ teaspoon freshly ground black pepper
6 scallions, chopped
1 ounce (28 g) melted butter, for greasing the casserole dish
1 tablespoon parsley, finely chopped
1¼ cups heavy whipping cream
1 tablespoon Dijon mustard
1½ pounds (680 g) white fish, in serving-pieces
3 ounces (85 g) butter slices, under room temperature

1. Preheat the oven to 400°F (205°C).
2. Heat the olive oil in a nonstick skillet over medium heat.
3. Add the broccoli to the skillet and sauté for 5 to 7 minutes or until tender, then season the broccoli with salt and ground black pepper, add the finely chopped scallions, and sauté for 1 to 2 minutes more.
4. Prepare a casserole dish and grease it with butter to add a tasty level of flavors to the meal. Then pour the sautéed broccoli and scallions in the casserole dish, stir them well until they have a delicious butter smell.
5. In a bowl, mix finely chopped parsley with cream and Dijon mustard and pour the mixture over the casserole dish. Stir until fully incorporated. Then nestle the white fish in the casserole dish. Top them with the butter slices.
6. Cook in the preheated oven for 20 to 30 minutes, or until the fish exudes tender and takes in the flavor from the delicious butter.
7. Remove the casserole dish from the oven and serve the fish and vegetables warm.

Per Serving
calories: 611 | fat: 48.3g | total carbs: 13.2g fiber: 4.8g | protein: 34.4g

172. Asian Salmon and Veggies Salad

Prep time: 20 minutes | Cook time: 5 minutes | Serves 2

Salad:
¼ cup water
¼ cup Sauvignon Blanc
½ pound salmon fillets
1 cup Chinese cabbage, sliced
1 tomato, sliced
2 radishes, sliced
1 bell pepper, sliced
1 medium-sized white onion, sliced Salad

Dressing:
½ teaspoon fresh garlic, minced
1 fresh chili pepper, seeded and minced
½ teaspoon fresh ginger, peeled and grated
2 tablespoons fresh lime juice
1 tablespoon sesame oil
1 tablespoon tamari sauce
1 teaspoon xylitol
1 tablespoon fresh mint, roughly chopped
Sea salt and freshly ground black pepper, to taste

1. Place the water and Sauvignon Blanc in a sauté pan; bring to a simmer over moderate heat.
2. Place the salmon fillets, skin-side down in the pan and cover with the lid. Cook for 5 to 8 minutes or to your desired doneness; do not overcook the salmon; reserve.
3. Place the Chinese cabbage, tomato, radishes, bell pepper, and onion in a serving bowl.
4. Prepare the salad dressing by whisking all ingredients. Dress your salad, top with the salmon fillets and serve immediately!

Per Serving
calories: 277 | fat: 15g | protein: 24g | carbs: 5g net carbs: 4g | fiber: 1g

173. Cheesy Shrimp Stuffed Mushrooms

Prep time: 10 minutes | Cook time: 17 minutes | Serves 6

1 tablespoon butter
1 yellow onion, finely minced
1 cloves garlic, minced
Flaky salt and ground black pepper, to taste
16 ounces (454 g) fresh Bay shrimp, chopped
8 ounces (227 g) ricotta cheese, softened
6 tablespoons mayonnaise
1 ½ pounds (680 g) large-sized button mushroom cups
1 cup cheddar cheese, shredded

1. Melt the butter in a frying pan over moderate heat. Then, sauté the onion and garlic for 2 to 3 minutes or until just tender and fragrant.
2. Stir in the salt, black pepper, fresh Bay shrimp, ricotta cheese, and mayo; gently stir to combine well.
3. Bake the mushroom cups in the preheated oven at 390ºF (199ºC) until they have softened slightly.
4. Spoon the shrimp mixture into each mushroom cup. Return to the oven and bake for 8 to 11 minutes more. Top each mushroom cup with cheddar cheese.
5. Bake for a further 7 minutes or until bubbly. Bon appétit!

Per Serving

calories: 354 | fat: 24g | protein: 28g | carbs: 5g net carbs: 3g | fiber: 2g

174. Tuna Niçoise Salad

Prep time: 5 minutes | Cook time: 45 minutes | Serves 4

1 cup extra-virgin olive oil, plus more if needed
4 (3- to 4-inch) sprigs fresh rosemary
8 (3- to 4-inch) sprigs fresh thyme
2 large garlic cloves, thinly sliced
2 (2-inch) strips lemon zest
1 teaspoon salt
½ teaspoon freshly ground black pepper
1 pound (454 g) fresh tuna steaks (about 1 inch thick)

1. Select a thick pot just large enough to fit the tuna in a single layer on the bottom. The larger the pot, the more olive oil you will need to use. Combine the olive oil, rosemary, thyme, garlic, lemon zest, salt, and pepper over medium-low heat and cook until warm and fragrant, 20 to 25 minutes, lowering the heat if it begins to smoke.
2. Remove from the heat and allow to cool for 25 to 30 minutes, until warm but not hot.
3. Add the tuna to the bottom of the pan, adding additional oil if needed so that tuna is fully submerged, and return to medium-low heat. Cook for 5 to 10 minutes, or until the oil heats back up and is warm and fragrant but not smoking. Lower the heat if it gets too hot.
4. Remove the pot from the heat and let the tuna cook in warm oil 4 to 5 minutes, to your desired level of doneness. For a tuna that is rare in the center, cook for 2 to 3 minutes.
5. Remove from the oil and serve warm, drizzling 2 to 3 tablespoons seasoned oil over the tuna.
6. To store for later use, remove the tuna from the oil and place in a container with a lid. Allow tuna and oil to cool separately. When both have cooled, remove the herb stems with a slotted spoon and pour the cooking oil over the tuna. Cover and store in the refrigerator for up to 1 week. Bring to room temperature to allow the oil to liquify before serving.

Per Serving

calories: 363 | fat: 28g | protein: 27g | carbs: 1g net carbs: 1g | fiber: 0g

175. White Chowder

Prep time: 5 minutes | Cook time: 15 minutes | Serves 4

2 teaspoons butter, at room temperature
½ white onion, chopped
1 tablespoon Old Bay seasoning
¾ pound (340 g) sea bass, broken into chunks
1 cup heavy cream

1. Melt the butter in a soup pot over a moderate flame. Now, sweat the white onion until tender and translucent.
2. Then, add in the Old Bay seasoning and 3 cups of water; bring to a rapid boil. Reduce the heat to medium-low and let it simmer, covered, for 9 to 12 minutes.
3. Fold in the sea bass and heavy cream; continue to cook until everything is thoroughly heated or about 5 minutes. Serve warm and enjoy!

Per Serving

calories: 257 | fat: 18g | protein: 21g | carbs: 4g net carbs: 4g | fiber: 0g

176. Provençal Lemony Fish Stew

Prep time: 15 minutes | Cook time: 6 minutes | Serves 2

1 tablespoon olive oil
1 shallot, sliced
3 garlic cloves, minced
1 cup tomato purée
5 cups white fish stock
1 teaspoon basil
½ teaspoon rosemary
½ California bay leaf
⅓ teaspoon saffron threads, crumbled
Sea salt and freshly cracked black pepper, to taste
1 pound (454 g) grouper fish
⅓ pound (151 g) cockles, scrubbed
⅓ pound (151 g) prawns
1 tablespoon fresh lemon juice

1. Heat the olive oil in a stockpot over a moderate flame. Now, sauté the shallot for 3 minutes or until tender; add in the garlic and cook an additional 30 seconds or until aromatic.
2. Pour in the tomato purée and white fish stock; bring everything to a boil. Stir in the basil, rosemary, California bay leaf, saffron threads, salt, and black pepper.
3. Turn the heat to medium-low. Fold in the grouper and cockles; gently stir to combine and allow it to simmer for 2 to 3 minutes. Next, add in the prawns; continue to simmer for 3 minutes more or until everything is thoroughly warmed.
4. Drizzle each serving with fresh lemon juice and enjoy!

Per Serving
calories: 176 | fat: 5g | protein: 24g | carbs: 5g net carbs: 4g | fiber: 1g

177. Alaskan Cod Fillet

Prep time: 10 minutes | Cook time: 2 minutes | Serves 4

1 tablespoon coconut oil
4 Alaskan cod fillets
Salt and freshly ground black pepper, to taste
6 leaves basil, chiffonade Mustard Cream Sauce:
1 teaspoon yellow mustard
1 teaspoon paprika
¼ teaspoon ground bay leaf
3 tablespoons cream cheese
½ cup Greek-style yogurt
1 garlic clove, minced
1 teaspoon lemon zest
1 tablespoon fresh parsley, minced
Sea salt and ground black pepper, to taste

1. Heat coconut oil in a pan over medium heat. Sear the fish for 2 to 3 minutes per side. Season with salt and ground black pepper.
2. Mix all ingredients for the sauce until everything is well combined. Top the fish fillets with the sauce and serve garnished with fresh basil leaves. Bon appétit!

Per Serving
calories: 166 | fat: 8g | protein: 20g | carbs: 3g net carbs: 3g | fiber: 0g

178. Sole Fish Jambalaya

Prep time: 15 minutes | Cook time: 8 minutes | Serves 2

1 teaspoon extra virgin olive oil
1 jalapeno pepper, minced
1 small-sized leek, chopped
½ teaspoon ginger garlic paste
¼ teaspoon ground cumin
¼ teaspoon ground allspice
½ teaspoon oregano
¼ teaspoon thyme
¼ teaspoon marjoram
1 pound (454 g) sole fish fillets, cut into bite-sized strips
1 large-sized ripe tomato, pureed
½ cup water
½ cup clam juice
Kosher salt, to season
1 bay laurel
5-6 black peppercorns
1 cup spinach, torn into pieces

1. Heat the oil in a Dutch oven over a moderate flame. Then, sauté the pepper and leek until they have softened.
2. Now, stir in the ginger-garlic paste, cumin, allspice, oregano, thyme, and marjoram; continue stirring for 30 to 40 seconds more or until aromatic.
3. Add in the fish, tomatoes, water, clam juice, salt, bay laurel, and black peppercorns. Cover and decrease the temperature to medium-low.
4. Let it simmer for 4 to 6 minutes or until the liquid has reduced slightly. Stir in the spinach and let it simmer, covered, for about 2 minutes more or until it wilts.
5. Ladle into serving bowls and serve warm. Bon appétit!

Per Serving
calories: 232 | fat: 4g | protein: 38g | carbs: 6g net carbs: 4g | fiber: 2g

179. Smoked Haddock Burgers

Prep time: 10 minutes | Cook time: 6 minutes | Serves 4

2 tablespoons extra virgin olive oil
8 ounces (227 g) smoked haddock
1 egg
¼ cup Parmesan cheese, grated
1 teaspoon chili powder
1 teaspoon dried parsley flakes
¼ cup scallions, chopped
1 teaspoon fresh garlic, minced
Salt and ground black pepper, to taste
4 lemon wedges

1. Heat 1 tablespoon of oil in a pan over medium-high heat. Cook the haddock for 6 minutes or until just cooked through; discard the skin and bones and flake into small pieces.
2. Mix the smoked haddock, egg, cheese, chili powder, parsley, scallions, garlic, salt, and black pepper in a large bowl.
3. Heat the remaining tablespoon of oil and cook fish burgers until they are well cooked in the middle or about 6 minutes. Garnish each serving with a lemon wedge.

Per Serving
calories: 174 | fat: 11g | protein: 15g | carbs: 2g net carbs: 2g | fiber: 0g

180. Cajun Tilapia Fish Burgers

Prep time: 5 minutes | Cook time: 46 minutes | Serves 5

1½ pounds tilapia fish, broken into chunks
2 eggs, whisked
½ cup shallots, chopped
½ cup almond flour
1 tablespoon Cajun seasoning mix

1. Mix all of the above ingredients in a bowl. Shape the mixture into 10 patties and place in your refrigerator for about 40 minutes.
2. Cook in the preheated frying pan that is previously greased with nonstick cooking spray.
3. Cook for 3 minutes until golden brown on the bottom. Carefully flip over and cook the other side for a further 3 minutes. Remove to a paper towel-lined plate until ready to serve.
4. Serve with fresh lettuce, if desired. Bon appétit!

Per Serving
calories: 238 | fat: 11g | protein: 33g | carbs: 3g net carbs: 2g | fiber: 1g

181. Shrimp Jambalaya

Prep time: 5 minutes | Cook time: 20 minutes | Serves 4

1 shallot, chopped
1 cup ham, cut into 1/2-inch cubes
1½ cups tomatoes, crushed
1½ cups vegetable broth
¾ pound (340 g) shrimp

1. Heat up a lightly greased soup pot over a moderate flame. Now, sauté the shallots until they have softened or about 4 minutes.
2. Add in the ham, tomatoes, and vegetable broth and bring to a boil. Turn the heat to simmer, cover and continue to cook for 13 minutes longer.
3. Fold in the shrimp and continue to simmer until they are thoroughly cooked and the cooking liquid has thickened slightly, about 3 to 4 minutes.
4. Serve in individual bowls and enjoy!

Per Serving
calories: 170 | fat: 5g | protein: 26g | carbs: 6g net carbs: 5g | fiber: 1g

182. Tuna, Ham and Avocado Wraps

Prep time: 10 minutes | Cook time: 3 minutes | Serves 3

½ cup dry white wine
½ cup water
½ teaspoon mixed peppercorns
½ teaspoon dry mustard powder
½ pound Ahi tuna steak
6 slices of ham
½ Hass avocado, peeled, pitted and sliced
1 tablespoon fresh lemon juice
6 lettuce leaves

1. Add wine, water, peppercorns, and mustard powder to a skillet and bring to a boil. Add the tuna and simmer gently for 3 minutes to 5 minutes per side.
2. Discard the cooking liquid and slice tuna into bite-sized pieces. Divide the tuna pieces between slices of ham.
3. Add avocado and drizzle with fresh lemon. Roll the wraps up and place each wrap on a lettuce leaf. Serve well chilled. Bon appétit!

Per Serving
calories: 308 | fat: 20g | protein: 28g | carbs: 4g net carbs: 1g | fiber: 3g

183. Grilled Salmon Steak

Prep time: 5 minutes | Cook time: 10 minutes | Serves 4

4 (5-ounce / 142-g) salmon steaks
2 cloves garlic, pressed
4 tablespoons olive oil
1 tablespoon Taco seasoning mix
2 tablespoons fresh lemon juice

1. Place all of the above ingredients in a ceramic dish; cover and let it marinate for 40 minutes in your refrigerator.
2. Place the salmon steaks onto a lightly oiled grill pan; place under the grill for 6 minutes.
3. Turn them over and cook for a further 5 to 6 minutes, basting with the reserved marinade; remove from the grill.
4. Serve immediately and enjoy!

Per Serving
calories: 331 | fat: 21g | protein: 30g | carbs: 2g net carbs: 2g | fiber: 0g

184. Old Bay Sea Bass Fillet

Prep time: 10 minutes | Cook time: 15 minutes | Serves 6

2 tablespoons butter, at room temperature
1 leek, chopped
1 bell pepper, chopped
1 serrano pepper, chopped
2 garlic cloves, minced
2 tablespoons fresh coriander, chopped
2 vine-ripe tomatoes, pureed
4 cups fish stock
2 pounds (907 g) sea bass fillets, chopped into small chunks
1 tablespoon Old Bay seasoning
½ teaspoon sea salt, to taste
1 bay laurels

1. Melt the butter in a heavy-bottomed pot over moderate heat. Stir in the leek and peppers and sauté them for about 5 minutes or until tender.
2. Stir in the garlic and continue to sauté for 30 to 40 seconds more.
3. Add in the remaining ingredients; gently stir to combine. Turn the heat to medium-low and partially cover the pot.
4. Now, let it cook until thoroughly heated, approximately 10 minutes longer. Lastly, discard the bay laurels and serve warm. Bon appétit!

Per Serving
calories: 227 | fat: 8g | protein: 32g | carbs: 5g net carbs: 4g | fiber: 1g

185. Swedish Herring and Spinach Salad

Prep time: 10 minutes | Cook time: 0 minutes | Serves 3

6 ounces (170 g) pickled herring pieces, drained and flaked
½ cup baby spinach
2 tablespoons fresh basil leaves
2 tablespoons fresh chives, chopped
1 teaspoon garlic, minced
1 bell pepper, chopped
1 red onion, chopped
2 tablespoons key lime juice, freshly squeezed
Sea salt and ground black pepper, to taste

1. In a salad bowl, combine the herring pieces with spinach, basil leaves, chives, garlic, bell pepper, and red onion.
2. Then, drizzle key lime juice over the salad; add salt and pepper to taste and toss to combine. Smaklig maltid! Bon appétit!

Per Serving
calories: 134 | fat: 8g | protein: 10g | carbs: 5g net carbs: 4g | fiber: 1g

186. Spanish Cod à La Nage

Prep time: 5 minutes | Cook time: 15 minutes | Serves 5

2 tablespoons olive oil
1 Spanish onion, chopped
1 medium-sized zucchini, diced
1 vine-ripe tomatoes, pureed
1½ pounds (680 g) cod fish fillets

1. Heat the olive oil in a stockpot over medium-high flame. Now, cook the Spanish onion until tender and translucent.
2. Pour in the pureed tomatoes along with 2 cups of water. Bring to a boil and reduce the heat to medium-low. Let it simmer an additional 10 to 13 minutes.
3. Now, fold in the cod fish fillets. Cook, covered, an additional 5 to 6 minutes or until the codfish is just cooked through and an instant-read thermometer registers 140 ºF (60ºC).
4. Place the fish in individual bowls; ladle the fish broth over each serving, and serve hot. Enjoy!

Per Serving
calories: 177 | fat: 6g | protein: 25g | carbs: 4g net carbs: 3g | fiber: 1g

187. Thai Tuna Fillet

Prep time: 15 minutes | Cook time: 20 minutes | Serves 4

1 tablespoon peanut oil
4 tuna fillets
1 teaspoon freshly grated ginger
Kosher salt and freshly ground black pepper, to taste
1 teaspoon cayenne pepper
½ teaspoon cumin seeds
¼ teaspoon ground cinnamon

Sauce:
1 scallions, chopped
2 garlic cloves, minced
1 tablespoon fresh cilantro, chopped
1 teaspoon Sriracha sauce
4 tablespoons mayonnaise
½ cup sour cream
1 teaspoon stone-ground mustard

1. Preheat your oven to 375ºF (190ºC). Line a baking sheet with foil.
2. Place the tuna fillets onto the prepared baking sheet; now, fold up all 4 sides of the foil.
3. Add peanut oil, grated ginger, salt, black pepper, cayenne pepper, cumin, and cinnamon.
4. Fold the sides of the foil over the fish fillets, sealing the packet. Bake until cooked through, approximately 20 minutes.
5. To make the sauce, whisk together all of the sauce ingredients. Serve immediately and enjoy!

Per Serving
calories: 389 | fat: 18g | protein: 50g | carbs: 4g net carbs: 4g | fiber: 0g

188. Italian Haddock Fillet

Prep time: 5 minutes | Cook time: 10 minutes | Serves 6

2 pounds (907 g) haddock fillets
1 tablespoon Italian seasoning blend
Sea salt and freshly ground black pepper, to taste
2 tablespoons olive oil
½ cup marinara sauce

1. Season the haddock fillets and brush them on all sides with olive oil and marinara sauce.
2. Grill over medium heat for 9 to 11 minutes until golden with brown edges.
3. Use a metal spatula to gently lift the haddock fillets, place them on serving plates and serve with the remaining marinara sauce. Bon appétit!

Per Serving
calories: 226 | fat: 6g | protein: 38g | carbs: 2g net carbs: 1g | fiber: 1g

189. Mediterranean Halibut Fillet

Prep time: 5 minutes | Cook time: 30 minutes | Serves 4

1½ pounds (680 g) halibut fillets
2 tablespoons olive oil
2 tablespoons fresh lemon juice
1 tablespoon Greek seasoning blend
½ cup Kalamata olives, pitted and sliced

1. Start by preheating your oven to 380ºF (193ºC).
2. Toss the halibut fillets with the olive oil, fresh lemon juice, and Greek seasoning blend. Arrange the halibut fillets in a baking pan and cover with foil.
3. Bake approximately 30 minutes, flipping once or twice.
4. Garnish with Kalamata olives and serve warm. Bon appétit!

Per Serving
calories: 397 | fat: 32g | protein: 25g | carbs: 2g net carbs: 1g | fiber: 1g

190. Cod Patties with Creamed Horseradish

Prep time: 10 minutes | Cook time: 13 minutes | Serves 4

1 pound (454 g) cod fillets
2 eggs, beaten
1 tablespoon flax seeds meal
4 tablespoons parmesan cheese, grated
2 tablespoons olive oil

Sauce:
4 tablespoons mayonnaise
4 tablespoons Ricotta cheese
1 teaspoon creamed horseradish
2 green onions, chopped
1 tablespoon fresh basil, chopped

1. Steam the cod fillets until done and cooked through, approximately 10 minutes. Flake the fish with a fork; add in the beaten eggs, flax seeds meal, and parmesan.
2. Shape the mixture into 4 equal patties. Heat the olive oil in a nonstick skillet. Fry the fish patties over moderate heat for 3 minutes per side.
3. In the meantime, whisk the sauce ingredients until everything is well incorporated. Bon appétit!

Per Serving
calories: 346 | fat: 23g | protein: 26g | carbs: 7g net carbs: 6g | fiber: 1g

191. Red Snapper Fillet and Salad

Prep time: 10 minutes | Cook time: 18 minutes | Serves 4

1 pound (454 g) red snapper fillets
5 eggs
1 bell pepper, deseeded and sliced
1 tomato, sliced
1 cucumber, sliced
2 scallions, sliced
½ cup radishes, sliced
4 cups lettuce salad
4 tablespoons olive oil
4 tablespoons apple cider vinegar
½ cup Kalamata olives, pitted and halved

1. Steam the red snapper fillets until done and cooked through, approximately 10 minutes. Slice the fish fillets into bite-sized strips.
2. Cook the eggs in a saucepan for about 8 minutes; peel the eggs under running water and carefully slice them.
3. Place your veggies in a salad bowl; add the olive oil and vinegar and toss to combine. Top with the fish and boiled eggs. Salt to taste.
4. Garnish with Kalamata olives and serve well-chilled or at room temperature. Bon appétit!

Per Serving
calories: 300 | fat: 19g | protein: 27g | carbs: 4g net carbs: 3g | fiber: 1g

192. Lemony Shrimp and Veggie Bowl

Prep time: 10 minutes | Cook time: 4 minutes | Serves 4

2 pounds (907 g) large shrimp, peeled and deveined
1 teaspoon cayenne pepper
Sea salt and freshly ground black pepper, to taste
1 red onion, sliced
2 garlic cloves, sliced
2 Italian peppers, sliced
1 tablespoon fresh lemon juice
2 tablespoons olive oil
1 cup arugula

1. Gently pat the shrimp dry with a paper towel. Add the cayenne pepper, salt, black pepper, and toss to evenly coat.
2. Grill the shrimp over medium-high heat for 2 minutes; flip them and cook for a further 2 minutes.
3. Transfer to a bowl; add in the remaining ingredients and toss to combine. Serve immediately.

Per Serving
calories: 268 | fat: 8g | protein: 46g | carbs: 4g net carbs: 3g | fiber: 1g

193. Goan Sole Fillet Stew

Prep time: 5 minutes | Cook time: 20 minutes | Serves 3

1 tablespoon butter, at room temperature
1 shallot, chopped
1 teaspoon curry paste
1 cup tomatoes, pureed
¾ pound (340 g) sole fillets, cut into 1-inch pieces

1. Melt the butter in a stockpot over a medium-high flame. Sauté the shallot until softened.
2. Add the curry paste and pureed tomatoes along with 2 cups of water to the pot; bring to a rolling boil.
3. Immediately reduce the heat to medium-low and continue to simmer, covered, for 12 minutes longer; make sure to stir periodically.
4. Fold in the chopped sole fillets; continue to cook for a further 8 minutes or until the fish flakes easily with a fork. Enjoy!

Per Serving
calories: 191 | fat: 9g | protein: 24g | carbs: 3g net carbs: 2g | fiber: 1g

194. Cod Fillet with Summer Salad

Prep time: 10 minutes | Cook time: 10 minutes | Serves 5

4 tablespoons extra-virgin olive oil
5 cod fillets
¼ cup balsamic vinegar
1 tablespoon stone-ground mustard
Sea salt and ground black pepper, to season
½ pound (227 g) green cabbage, shredded
2 cups lettuce, cut into small pieces
1 red onion, sliced
1 garlic clove, minced
1 teaspoon red pepper flakes

1. Heat 1 tablespoon of the olive oil in a large frying pan over medium-high heat.
2. Once hot, fry the fish fillets for 5 minutes until golden brown; flip them and cook on the other side for 4 to 5 minutes more; work in batches to avoid overcrowding the pan.
3. Flake the cod fillets with two forks and reserve.
4. To make the dressing, whisk the remaining tablespoon of olive oil with the balsamic vinegar, mustard, salt, and black pepper.
5. Combine the green cabbage, lettuce, onion, and garlic in a salad bowl. Dress the salad and top with the reserved fish.
6. Garnish with red pepper flakes and serve. Enjoy!

Per Serving
calories: 276 | fat: 7g | protein: 43g | carbs: 6g net carbs: 4g | fiber: 2g

195. Cheesy Cod Fillet

Prep time: 10 minutes | Cook time: 5 minutes | Serves 3

3 cod fillets
½ cup almond meal
1 teaspoon cayenne pepper
Sea salt and ground black pepper, to season
1 teaspoon garlic powder
1 teaspoon porcini powder
½ teaspoon shallot powder
1 teaspoon dried rosemary, crushed
1 cup Romano cheese, preferably freshly grated
2 tablespoons butter

1. Pat the cod fillets dry with paper towels.
2. Add the fish, almond meal, and spices to the bag and shake to coat on all sides. Coat them with grated Romano cheese.
3. Melt the butter in a frying pan over medium-high heat.
4. Now pan-fry the fish fillets until flesh flakes easily and it is nearly opaque, about 4 to 5 minutes per side. Serve on warm plates. Bon appétit!

Per Serving
calories: 406 | fat: 30g | protein: 32g | carbs: 4g net carbs: 2g | fiber: 2g

196. Spicy Tiger Prawns

Prep time: 10 minutes | Cook time: 10 minutes | Serves 6

2 tablespoons olive oil
1 teaspoon butter
2 scallions, chopped
2 cloves garlic, pressed
2 bell peppers, chopped
2½ pounds (1.1 kg) tiger prawns, deveined
¼ teaspoon ground black pepper
1 teaspoon paprika
1 teaspoon red chili flakes
½ teaspoon mustard seeds
½ teaspoon fennel seeds
Sea salt, to taste
½ cup Marsala wine

1. Heat the olive oil and butter in a frying pan over a medium-high flame. Now, sweat the scallions, garlic, and peppers until they are crisp-tender about 2 minutes.
2. Add in the tiger prawns and cook for 1½ minutes on each side until they are opaque.
3. Stir in the remaining ingredients and continue to cook for 5 minutes more over low heat. Taste and adjust seasonings. Bon appétit!

Per Serving
calories: 219 | fat: 7g | protein: 39g | carbs: 3g net carbs: 2g | fiber: 1g

197. Baked Halibut Steaks

Prep time: 10 minutes | Cook time: 13 minutes | Serves 2

2 tablespoons olive oil
2 halibut steaks
1 red bell pepper, sliced
1 yellow onion, sliced
1 teaspoon garlic, smashed
½ teaspoon hot paprika
Sea salt cracked black pepper, to your liking
1 dried thyme sprig, leaves crushed

1. Start by preheating your oven to 390°F (199°C).
2. Then, drizzle olive oil over the halibut steaks. Place the halibut in a baking dish that is previously greased with a nonstick spray.
3. Top with the bell pepper, onion, and garlic. Sprinkle hot paprika, salt, black pepper, and dried thyme over everything.
4. Bake in the preheated oven for 13 to 15 minutes and serve immediately. Enjoy!

Per Serving
calories: 502 | fat: 19g | protein: 72g | carbs: 6g net carbs: 5g | fiber: 1g

198. Salmon Tacos with Guajillo Sauce

Prep time: 10 minutes | Cook time: 10 minutes | Serves 5

2 pounds (907 g) salmon
Flaky salt and ground black pepper, to taste
10 lettuce leaves
2 bell peppers, chopped
1 cucumber, chopped
1 avocado, pitted and peeled
1 tomato, halved
2 tablespoons extra-virgin olive oil
1 tablespoon lemon juice
4 tablespoons green onions
1 teaspoon garlic
1 guajillo chili pepper

1. Season your salmon with salt and black pepper. Brush the salmon on all sides with nonstick cooking oil.
2. Grill over medium heat for 13 minutes until golden and opaque in the middle. Flake the fish with two forks.
3. Divide the fish among the lettuce leaves; add the bell peppers and cucumber.
4. Pulse the remaining ingredients in your blender 8 to 10 times or until smooth with several small chunks of tomatoes and scallions.
5. Top each lettuce taco with the guajillo sauce and serve.

Per Serving
calories: 342 | fat: 17g | protein: 40g | carbs: 7g net carbs: 3g | fiber: 4g

199. Dijon Sea Bass Fillet

Prep time: 10 minutes | Cook time: 10 minutes | Serves 3

2 tablespoons olive oil
3 sea bass fillets
¼ teaspoon red pepper flakes, crushed
Sea salt, to taste
⅓ teaspoon mixed peppercorns, crushed
3 tablespoons butter
1 tablespoon Dijon mustard
2 cloves garlic, minced
1 tablespoon fresh lime juice

1. Heat the olive oil in a skillet over medium-high heat.
2. Pat dry the sea bass fillets with paper towels. Now pan-fry the fish fillets for about 4 minutes on each side until flesh flakes easily and it is nearly opaque.
3. Season your fish with red pepper, salt, and mixed peppercorns.
4. To make the sauce, melt the 3 tablespoons of butter in a saucepan over low heat; stir in the Dijon mustard, garlic, and lime juice. Let it simmer for 2 minutes.
5. To serve, spoon the Dijon butter sauce over the fish fillets. Bon appétit!

Per Serving
calories: 314 | fat: 23g | protein: 24g | carbs: 1g net carbs: 1g | fiber: 0g

200. Monkfish Mayonnaise Salad

Prep time: 10 minutes | Cook time: 9 minutes | Serves 5

2 pounds (57 g) monkfish
1 bell pepper, sliced
½ cup radishes, sliced
1 red onion, chopped
1 garlic clove, minced
1 tablespoon balsamic vinegar
½ cup mayonnaise
1 teaspoon stone-ground mustard
Flaky salt, to season

1. Pat the fish dry with paper towels and brush on both sides with nonstick cooking oil. Grill over medium-high heat, flipping halfway through for about 9 minutes or until opaque.
2. Flake the fish with a fork and toss with the remaining ingredients; gently toss to combine well.
3. Serve at room temperature or well-chilled. Bon appétit!

Per Serving
calories: 306 | fat: 19g | protein: 27g | carbs: 4g net carbs: 3g | fiber: 1g

201. Cod Fillet and Mustard Greens

Prep time: 10 minutes | Cook time: 13 minutes | Serves 2

1 tablespoon olive oil
1 bell pepper, seeded and sliced
1 jalapeno pepper, seeded and sliced
2 stalks green onions, sliced
1 stalk green garlic, sliced
½ cup fish broth
2 cod fish fillets
½ teaspoon paprika
Sea salt and ground black pepper, to season
1 cup mustard greens, torn into bite-sized pieces

1. Heat the olive oil in a Dutch pot over a moderate flame. Now, sauté the peppers, green onions, and garlic until just tender and aromatic.
2. Add in the broth, fish fillets, paprika, salt, black pepper, and mustard greens. Reduce the temperature to medium-low, cover, and let it cook for 11 to 13 minutes or until heated through.
3. Serve immediately garnished with lemon slices if desired. Bon appétit!

Per Serving
calories: 171 | fat: 8g | protein: 20g | carbs: 5g net carbs: 3g | fiber: 2g

202. Mahi Mahi Ceviche

Prep time: 10 minutes | Cook time: 10 minutes | Serves 4

1½ pounds mahi-mahi fish, cut into bite-sized cubes
Sea salt and ground black pepper, to taste
1 teaspoon hot paprika
2 garlic cloves, minced
4 scallions, chopped
2 Roma tomatoes, sliced
1 bell pepper, sliced
4 tablespoons olive oil
2 tablespoons fresh lemon juice

1. Season the haddock fillets with salt, black pepper, and paprika. Brush them on all sides with nonstick cooking oil.
2. Grill over medium heat for 9 to 11 minutes until golden with brown edges. Use a metal spatula to gently lift the haddock fillets.
3. Toss your fish with the remaining ingredients in a large bowl. Taste and adjust seasonings. Divide between four serving bowls and serve.

Per Serving
calories: 424 | fat: 30g | protein: 33g | carbs: 6g net carbs: 4g | fiber: 2g

203. Salmon Fillet

Prep time: 10 minutes | Cook time: 19 minutes | Serves 6

2 tablespoons peanut oil
2 bell peppers, deseeded and sliced
½ cup scallions, chopped
2 cloves garlic, minced
4 tablespoons Marsala wine
2 ripe tomatoes, pureed
2½ pounds salmon fillets
Sea salt and ground black pepper, to taste
¼ teaspoon ground bay leaf
1 teaspoon paprika

1. Heat the peanut oil in a large frying pan over a moderate flame. Now, sauté the bell peppers and scallions for 3 minutes.
2. Add in the garlic and continue to sauté for 30 seconds more or until aromatic but not until it's browned.
3. Add a splash of wine to deglaze the pan. Stir in the remaining ingredients and turn the heat to simmer.
4. Let it cook, partially covered, for 15 minutes or until the salmon is cooked through. Bon appétit!

Per Serving
calories: 347 | fat: 19g | protein: 40g | carbs: 4g net carbs: 3g | fiber: 1g

204. Tilapia Fillet

Prep time: 5 minutes | Cook time: 10 minutes | Serves 6

6 tilapia fillets, patted dry
Sea salt and ground black pepper, to taste
1 teaspoon cayenne pepper
6 tablespoons butter
1 teaspoon garlic, minced
1 tablespoon parsley, chopped
1 teaspoon fresh lime juice

1. Brush a nonstick skillet with cooking oil. Heat the skillet over medium-high heat.
2. Once the oil is heated, pan-fry the tilapia until both sides turn golden brown; gently flip them with a tong.
3. Season with salt, black pepper, and cayenne pepper.
4. Prepare the garlic butter sauce by whisking the remaining ingredients. Serve the tilapia with a dollop of garlic butter if desired. Bon appétit!

Per Serving
calories: 215 | fat: 14g | protein: 24g | carbs: 1g net carbs: 1g | fiber: 0g

205. Cod Fillet with Lemony Sesame Sauce

Prep time: 10 minutes | Cook time: 7 minutes | Serves 6

6 cod fillets, skin-on
3 tablespoons olive oil
Sea salt and ground black pepper, to season
1 lemon, freshly squeezed
½ teaspoon fresh ginger, minced
1 garlic clove, minced
1 red chili pepper, minced
3 tablespoons toasted sesame seeds
3 tablespoons toasted sesame oil

1. Prepare a grill for medium-high heat. Rub the cod fillets with olive oil; season both sides with salt and black pepper.
2. Next, place the cod fillets on the grill skin side down. Grill approximately 7 minutes until the skin is lightly charred.
3. To make the sauce, whisk the remaining ingredients until well combined; season with lots of black pepper.
4. Divide the cod fillets among serving plates. Spoon the sauce over them and enjoy!

Per Serving
calories: 341 | fat: 17g | protein: 42g | carbs: 3g net carbs: 2g | fiber: 1g

206. Shrimp and Sea Scallop

Prep time: 10 minutes | Cook time: 5 minutes | Serves 2

1 tablespoon olive oil
½ cup scallions, chopped
1 garlic clove, minced
½ pound (227 g) shrimp, deveined
½ pound (227 g) sea scallops
2 tablespoons rum
½ cup fish broth
¼ teaspoon Cajun seasoning mix
Sea salt and ground black pepper, to taste
1 tablespoon fresh parsley, chopped

1. In a sauté pan, heat the olive oil until sizzling. Now, sauté your scallions and garlic until they are just tender and fragrant.
2. Now, sear the shrimp and sea scallops for 2 to 3 minutes or until they are firm. Add a splash of rum to deglaze the pan. Now, pour in the fish broth.
3. Add in the Cajun seasoning mix, salt, and black pepper; stir and remove from heat.
4. Serve warm garnished with fresh parsley. Enjoy!

Per Serving
calories: 305 | fat: 9g | protein: 47g | carbs: 3g net carbs: 2g | fiber: 1g

207. Herbed Monkfish Fillet

Prep time: 10 minutes | Cook time: 17 minutes | Serves 6

2 tablespoons olive oil
6 monkfish fillets
Sea salt and ground black pepper, to taste
2 green onions, sliced
2 green garlic stalks, sliced
½ cup sour cream
1 teaspoon oregano
1 teaspoon basil
1 teaspoon rosemary
½ cup cheddar cheese, shredded
2 tablespoons fresh chives, chopped

1. Heat the olive oil in a frying pan over a medium-high flame. Once hot, sear the monkfish fillets for 3 minutes until golden brown; flip them and cook on the other side for 3 to 4 minutes more.
2. Season with salt and black pepper. Transfer the monkfish fillets to a lightly greased casserole dish. Add the green onions and green garlic.
3. In a mixing dish, thoroughly combine the sour cream with the oregano, basil, rosemary, and cheddar cheese.
4. Spoon the mixture into your casserole dish and bake at 360ºF (182ºC) for about 11 minutes or until golden brown on top.
5. Garnish with fresh chives and serve. Bon appétit!

Per Serving
calories: 229 | fat: 13g | protein: 26g | carbs: 2g net carbs: 2g | fiber: 0g

208. Old Bay Prawns

Prep time: 10 minutes | Cook time: 10 minutes | Serves 2

¾ pound (340 g) prawns, peeled and deveined
1 teaspoon Old Bay seasoning mix
½ teaspoon paprika
Coarse sea salt and ground black pepper, to taste
1 habanero pepper, deveined and minced
1 bell pepper, deveined and minced
1 cup pound broccoli florets
2 teaspoons olive oil
1 tablespoon fresh chives, chopped2 slices lemon, for garnish
2 dollops of sour cream, for garnish

1. Toss the prawns with the Old Bay seasoning mix, paprika, salt, and black pepper.
2. Arrange them on a parchment-lined roasting pan. Add the bell pepper and broccoli. Drizzle olive oil over everything and transfer the pan to a preheated oven.
3. Roast at 390ºF (199ºC) for 8 to 11 minutes, turning the pan halfway through the cooking time. Bake until the prawns are pink and cooked through.
4. Serve with fresh chives, lemon, and sour cream. Bon appétit!

Per Serving
calories: 269 | fat: 10g | protein: 38g | carbs: 7g net carbs: 4g | fiber: 3g

209. New Orleans Halibut and Crabmeat

Prep time: 15 minutes | Cook time: 22 minutes | Serves 6

3 teaspoons butter, at room temperature
1 pound (454 g) andouille sausage, sliced
1 red onion, chopped
2 cloves garlic, minced
1 celery stalk, chopped
1 red chili pepper, chopped
2 pounds (907 g) halibut, cut into bite-sized chunks
2 tomatoes, pureed
4 cups water
3 cubes beef bouillon
½ teaspoon Cajun seasoning blend
Flaky salt and ground black pepper, to taste
1 pound (454 g) lump crabmeat
1 teaspoon cayenne pepper
1 tablespoon fresh cilantro

1. Melt 1 teaspoon of the butter in a heavy-bottomed pot over a moderate flame. Now, brown the sausage for 2 to 3 minutes; reserve.
2. Melt the remaining 2 teaspoons of butter and add in the red onion, garlic, celery, and chili pepper; let it cook for 1 ½ minutes more.
3. Now, stir in the halibut, tomatoes, water, cubes of beef bouillon and bring to a boil. Immediately reduce the heat and let it simmer, partially covered, for 13 minutes.
4. Then, stir in the Cajun seasoning blend, salt, ground black pepper, crabmeat, and cayenne pepper; return the sausage to the pot.
5. Stir to combine well and let it cook for 5 to 6 minutes more. Ladle into individual bowls and serve garnished with fresh cilantro. Enjoy!

Per Serving
calories: 441 | fat: 28g | protein: 40g | carbs: 6g net carbs: 5g | fiber: 1g

210. Catfish Flakes and Cauliflower Casserole

Prep time: 10 minutes | Cook time: 25 minutes | Serves 4

1 tablespoon sesame oil
11 ounces (312 g) cauliflower
4 scallions
1 garlic clove, minced
1 teaspoon fresh ginger root, grated
Salt and ground black pepper, to taste
Cayenne pepper, to taste
1 sprigs dried thyme, crushed
1 sprig rosemary, crushed
24 ounces (680 g) catfish, cut into pieces
½ cup cream cheese
½ cup heavy cream
1 egg
1 ounce (28 g) butter, cold

1. Start by preheating your oven to 390ºF (199ºC). Now, lightly grease a casserole dish with a nonstick cooking spray.
2. Then, heat the oil in a pan over medium-high heat; once hot, cook the cauliflower and scallions until tender or 5 to 6 minutes. Add the garlic and ginger; continue to sauté 1 minute more.
3. Transfer the vegetables to the prepared casserole dish. Sprinkle with seasonings. Add catfish to the top.
4. In a mixing bowl, thoroughly combine the cream cheese, heavy cream, and egg. Spread this creamy mixture over the top of your casserole.
5. Top with slices of butter. Bake in the preheated oven for 18 to 22 minutes or until the fish flakes easily with a fork. Bon appétit!

Per Serving
calories: 510 | fat: 40g | protein: 31g | carbs: 6g net carbs: 4g | fiber: 2g

211. Tilapia and Shrimp Soup

Prep time: 10 minutes | Cook time: 21 minutes | Serves 5

1 tablespoon butter
4 scallions, chopped
1 cup celery, chopped
1 Italian pepper, deseeded and chopped
1 poblano pepper, deseeded and chopped
2 cups cauliflower, grated
2 Roma tomatoes, pureed
4 cups chicken broth
1 pound (454 g) tilapia, skinless and chopped into small chunks
½ pound (227 g) medium shrimp, deveined
2 tablespoons balsamic vinegar

1. Melt the butter in a heavy-bottomed pot over a moderate flame. Once hot, cook your veggies until crisp-tender or about 4 minutes, stirring periodically to ensure even cooking.
2. Add in the pureed tomatoes and chicken broth. When the soup reaches boiling, turn the heat to a simmer.
3. Add in the tilapia and let it cook, partially covered, for 12 minutes. Stir in the shrimp, partially cover, and continue to cook for 5 minutes more.
4. Afterwards, stir in the balsamic vinegar. Ladle into individual bowls and serve warm.

Per Serving
calories: 194 | fat: 6g | protein: 26g | carbs: 6g net carbs: 4g | fiber: 2g

212. Curry Tilapia

Prep time: 10 minutes | Cook time: 15 minutes | Serves 4

1 tablespoon peanut oil
3 green cardamoms
1 teaspoon cumin seeds
1 shallot, chopped
1 red chili pepper, chopped
1 red bell pepper, chopped
1 teaspoon ginger-garlic paste
1 cup tomato puree
1 cup chicken broth
1 tablespoon curry paste
1½ pounds (680 g) tilapia
1 cinnamon stick
Sea salt and ground black pepper, to taste

1. Heat the peanut oil in a saucepan over medium-heat. Now, toast the cardamoms and cumin for 2 minutes until aromatic.
2. Add in the shallot, red chili, bell pepper and continue to sauté for 2 minutes more or until just tender and translucent.
3. Add in the ginger-garlic paste and continue to sauté an additional 30 seconds. Pour the tomato puree and chicken broth into the saucepan. Bring to a boil.
4. Turn the heat to medium-low and stir in the curry paste, tilapia, cinnamon, salt, and black pepper. Let it simmer, partially covered, for 10 minutes more.
5. Flake the fish and serve in individual bowls. Enjoy!

Per Serving
calories: 209 | fat: 7g | protein: 35g | carbs: 3g net carbs: 2g | fiber: 1g

213. Cod Fillet with Parsley Pistou

Prep time: 15 minutes | Cook time: 10 minutes | Serves 4

1 cup packed roughly chopped fresh flat-leaf Italian parsley
1 to 2 small garlic cloves, minced
Zest and juice of 1 lemon
1 teaspoon salt
½ teaspoon freshly ground black pepper
1 cup extra-virgin olive oil, divided
1 pound (454 g) cod fillets, cut into 4 equal-sized pieces

1. In a food processor, combine the parsley, garlic, lemon zest and juice, salt, and pepper. Pulse to chop well.
2. While the food processor is running, slowly stream in ¾ cup olive oil until well combined. Set aside.
3. In a large skillet, heat the remaining ¼ cup olive oil over medium-high heat. Add the cod fillets, cover, and cook 4 to 5 minutes on each side, or until cooked through. Thicker fillets may require a bit more cooking time. Remove from the heat and keep warm.
4. Add the pistou to the skillet and heat over medium-low heat. Return the cooked fish to the skillet, flipping to coat in the sauce. Serve warm, covered with pistou.

Per Serving
calories: 581 | fat: 55g | protein: 21g | carbs: 3g net carbs: 2g | fiber: 1g

214. Scallops and Calamari

Prep time: 5 minutes | Cook time: 10 minutes | Serves 4

8 ounces (227 g) calamari steaks, cut into ½-inch-thick strips or rings
8 ounces (227 g) sea scallops
1½ teaspoons salt, divided
1 teaspoon freshly ground black pepper
1 teaspoon garlic powder
⅓ cup extra-virgin olive oil
2 tablespoons butter

1. Place the calamari and scallops on several layers of paper towels and pat dry. Sprinkle with 1 teaspoon salt and allow to sit for 15 minutes at room temperature. Pat dry with additional paper towels. Sprinkle with pepper and garlic powder.
2. In a deep medium skillet, heat the olive oil and butter over medium-high heat. When the oil is hot but not smoking, add the scallops and calamari in a single layer to the skillet and sprinkle with the remaining ½ teaspoon salt. Cook 2 to 4 minutes on each side, depending on the size of the scallops, until just golden but still slightly opaque in center.
3. Using a slotted spoon, remove from the skillet and transfer to a serving platter. Allow the cooking oil to cool slightly and drizzle over the seafood before serving.

Per Serving
calories: 309 | fat: 25g | protein: 18g | carbs: 3g net carbs: 3g | fiber: 0g

215. Cheesy Tilapia Omelet

Prep time: 10 minutes | Cook time: 12 minutes | Serves 4

2 tablespoons olive oil
½ cup leeks, sliced
1 pound (454 g) tilapia fillets
1 red chili pepper, deseeded and sliced
Sea salt and ground black pepper, to taste
½ teaspoon garlic powder
½ teaspoon fennel seeds
1 cup milk
4 ounces (113 g) cream cheese
8 medium-sized eggs
1 cup goat cheese, crumbled

1. Heat 1 tablespoon of the olive oil in a cast-iron skillet over moderate heat. Once hot, sweat the leeks for 4 to 5 minutes, stirring periodically.
2. Then, add in the tilapia fish and cook for 5 minutes more until flesh flakes apart easily; flake the fish using a fork and reserve.
3. Add in the chili pepper, salt, black pepper, garlic powder, and fennel seeds; stir to combine.
4. In a mixing bowl, whisk the milk, cream cheese and eggs until frothy and well combined. Heat the remaining tablespoon of olive oil. Pour the egg mixture into the skillet.
5. When the eggs are set, spoon the fish mixture over one side, add the goat cheese and fold your omelet over the filling. Heat off.
6. Cover and let stand for 2 minutes in the residual heat until the cheese has melted. Bon appétit!

Per Serving
calories: 558 | fat: 38g | protein: 46g | carbs: 7g net carbs: 7g | fiber: 0g

216. Rosemary-Lemon Snapper Fillet

Prep time: 15 minutes | Cook time: 15 minutes | Serves 4

1¼ pounds (567 g) fresh red snapper fillet, cut into two equal pieces
2 lemons, thinly sliced
6 to 8 sprigs fresh rosemary, stems removed or 1 to 2 tablespoons dried rosemary
½ cup extra-virgin olive oil
6 garlic cloves, thinly sliced
1 teaspoon salt
½ teaspoon freshly ground black pepper

1. Preheat the oven to 425°F (220°C).
2. Place two large sheets of parchment (about twice the size of each piece of fish) on the counter. Place 1 piece of fish in the center of each sheet.
3. Top the fish pieces with lemon slices and rosemary leaves.
4. In a small bowl, combine the olive oil, garlic, salt, and pepper. Drizzle the oil over each piece of fish.
5. Top each piece of fish with a second large sheet of parchment and starting on a long side, fold the paper up to about 1 inch from the fish. Repeat on the remaining sides, going in a clockwise direction. Fold in each corner once to secure.
6. Place both parchment pouches on a baking sheet and bake until the fish is cooked through, 10 to 12 minutes.

Per Serving
calories: 390 | fat: 29g | protein: 29g | carbs: 3g net carbs: 3g | fiber: 0g

217. Asian Scallop and Vegetable

Prep time: 10 minutes | Cook time: 5 minutes | Serves 4

4 teaspoons sesame oil
½ cup yellow onion, sliced
1 cup asparagus spears, sliced
½ cup celery, chopped
½ cup enoki mushrooms
1 pound (454 g) bay scallops
1 tablespoon fresh parsley, chopped
Kosher salt and ground black pepper, to taste
½ teaspoon red pepper flakes, crushed
1 tablespoon coconut aminos
2 tablespoons rice wine
½ cup dry roasted peanuts, roughly chopped

1. Heat 1 teaspoon of the sesame oil in a wok over a medium-high flame. Now, fry the onion until crisp-tender and translucent; reserve.
2. Heat another teaspoon of the sesame oil and fry the asparagus and celery for about 3 minutes until crisp-tender; reserve.
3. Then, heat another teaspoon of the sesame oil and cook the mushrooms for 2 minutes more or until they start to soften; reserve.
4. Lastly, heat the remaining teaspoon of sesame oil and cook the bay scallops just until they are opaque.
5. Return all reserved vegetables to the wok. Add in the remaining ingredients and toss to combine. Serve warm and enjoy!

Per Serving
calories: 236 | fat: 13g | protein: 27g | carbs: 6g net carbs: 4g | fiber: 2g

218. Haddock and Turkey Smoked Sausage

Prep time: 15 minutes | Cook time: 17 minutes | Serves 4

2 tablespoons butter, at room temperature
1 onion, chopped
2 cloves garlic, sliced
1 bell pepper, sliced
1 celery stalk, chopped
1 cup broccoli florets
4 ounces (113 g) turkey smoked sausage, sliced
Sea salt and ground black pepper, to taste
2 tomatoes, pureed
2 cups fish broth
1 teaspoon chili powder
¼ teaspoon ground allspice
16 ounces (454 g) haddock steak, cut into bite-sized chunks
2 tablespoons fresh coriander, minced
1 teaspoon Creole seasoning blend

1. Melt the butter in a heavy-bottomed pot over moderate heat. Now, sauté the onion, garlic, and pepper, for 2 minutes until just tender and aromatic.
2. Add in the celery, broccoli, turkey smoked sausage, salt, black pepper, pureed tomatoes, and broth. Bring to a rolling boil and immediately reduce the heat to simmer.
3. Add in the remaining ingredients, partially cover, and continue simmering for 15 minutes.
4. Ladle into soup bowls and serve immediately.

Per Serving
calories: 236 | fat: 9g | protein: 27g | carbs: 6g net carbs: 4g | fiber: 2g

219. Chepala Vepudu

Prep time: 10 minutes | Cook time: 10 minutes | Serves 3

3 carp fillets
1 teaspoon chili powder
1 teaspoon cumin powder
1 teaspoon turmeric powder
1 coriander powder
½ teaspoon garam masala
½ teaspoon flaky salt
¼ teaspoon cayenne pepper
3 tablespoons full-fat coconut milk
1 egg
2 tablespoons olive oil
6 curry leaves, for garnish

1. Pat the fish fillets with kitchen towels and add to a large resealable bag. Add the spices to the bag and shake to coat on all sides.
2. In a shallow dish, whisk the coconut milk and egg until frothy and well combined. Dip the fillets into the egg mixture.
3. Then, heat the oil in a large frying pan. Fry the fish fillets on both sides until they are cooked through and the coating becomes crispy.
4. Serve with curry leaves and enjoy!

Per Serving
calories: 443 | fat: 28g | protein: 43g | carbs: 3g net carbs: 2g | fiber: 1g

220. Goat Cheese Stuffed Squid

Prep time: 15 minutes | Cook time: 30 minutes | Serves 4

8 ounces (227 g) frozen spinach, thawed and drained (about 1½ cup)
4 ounces (113 g) crumbled goat cheese
½ cup chopped pitted olives (I like Kalamata in this recipe)
½ cup extra-virgin olive oil, divided
¼ cup chopped sun-dried tomatoes
¼ cup chopped fresh flat-leaf Italian parsley
2 garlic cloves, finely minced
¼ teaspoon freshly ground black pepper
2 pounds (907 g) baby squid, cleaned and tentacles removed

1. Preheat the oven to 350°F (180°C).
2. In a medium bowl, combine the spinach, goat cheese, olives, ¼ cup olive oil, sun-dried tomatoes, parsley, garlic, and pepper.
3. Pour 2 tablespoons olive oil in the bottom of an 8-inch square baking dish and spread to coat the bottom.
4. Stuff each cleaned squid with 2 to 3 tablespoons of the cheese mixture, depending on the size of squid, and place in the prepared baking dish.
5. Drizzle the tops with the remaining 2 tablespoons olive oil and bake until the squid are cooked through, 25 to 30 minutes. Remove from the oven and allow to cool 5 to 10 minutes before serving.

Per Serving
calories: 469 | fat: 37g | protein: 24g | carbs: 10g net carbs: 7g | fiber: 3g

221. Halászlé with Paprikash

Prep time: 15 minutes | Cook time: 10 minutes | Serves 2

1 tablespoon extra virgin olive oil
2 bell peppers, chopped
1 Hungarian wax pepper, chopped
1 garlic clove, minced
1 red onion, chopped
½ pound (227 g) tilapia, cut into bite-sized pieces
1½ cups fish broth
2 vine-ripe tomatoes, pureed
1 teaspoon sweet paprika
½ teaspoon mixed peppercorns, crushed
1 bay laurel
½ teaspoon sumac
½ teaspoon dried thyme
¼ teaspoon dried rosemary
Kosher salt, to season
½ teaspoon garlic, minced
2 tablespoons sour cream

1. Heat the extra virgin olive oil in a Dutch oven over medium-high heat. Now, sauté the peppers, garlic, and onion until tender and aromatic.
2. Now, stir in the tilapia, broth, tomatoes, and spices. Reduce the heat to medium-low. Let it simmer, covered, for 9 to 13 minutes.
3. Meanwhile, mix ½ teaspoon of minced garlic with the sour cream. Serve with the warm paprikash and enjoy!

Per Serving
calories: 252 | fat: 13g | protein: 28g | carbs: 5g net carbs: 3g | fiber: 2g

222. Mackerel Fillet and Clam

Prep time: 10 minutes | Cook time: 12 minutes | Serves 3

2 teaspoons olive oil
2 mackerel fillets, patted dry
1 shallot, finely chopped
2 cloves garlic, minced
½ cup dry white wine
9 littleneck clams, scrubbed
Flaky salt and ground black pepper, to taste
½ teaspoon cayenne pepper
½ teaspoon fennel seeds
½ teaspoon mustard seeds
1 teaspoon celery seeds
1 teaspoon coriander, minced

1. In a large skillet, heat 1 teaspoon of the olive oil until sizzling; now, cook the mackerel fillets for about 6 minutes until cooked all the way through. Make sure to shake the skillet occasionally to prevent sticking; reserve, keeping warm.
2. Heat the remaining teaspoon of olive oil and sauté the shallot and garlic for 1 to 2 minutes or until fragrant.
3. Add in the wine and remaining seasonings; cook until almost evaporated. Fold in the clams and cook for 5 to 6 minutes until they open.
4. Return the fish to the skillet and serve warm. Bon appétit!

Per Serving
calories: 379 | fat: 9g | protein: 60g | carbs: 4g net carbs: 4g | fiber: 0g

223. Stir-Fried Scallops with Cauliflower

Prep time: 10 minutes | Cook time: 6 minutes | Serves 5

1 tablespoon butter
2 medium Italian peppers, deveined and sliced
2 cups cauliflower florets
½ teaspoon fresh ginger, minced
1 teaspoon garlic, minced
2 pounds (907 g) sea scallops
½ cup dry white wine
½ teaspoon cayenne pepper
½ teaspoon oregano
½ teaspoon marjoram
½ teaspoon rosemary
Sea salt and ground black pepper, to taste
½ cup chicken broth

1. Melt the butter in a large frying pan over medium-high heat.
2. Stir in the Italian peppers, cauliflower, ginger, and garlic. Cook for about 3 minutes or until the vegetables have softened.
3. Stir in the sea scallops and continue to cook for 3 minutes. Stir to coat with the vegetable mixture.
4. Add in the remaining ingredients and let it simmer, partially covered, for a few minutes longer. Bon appétit!

Per Serving
calories: 217 | fat: 4g | protein: 24g | carbs: 5g net carbs: 4g | fiber: 1g

224. Swordfish with Greek Yogurt Sauce

Prep time: 10 minutes | Cook time: 25 minutes | Serves 6

2 tablespoons butter
4 swordfish steaks
1 teaspoon paprika
½ teaspoon ground bay leaf
½ teaspoon mustard seeds
Sea salt and ground black pepper, to season
1 yellow onion, sliced
1 teaspoon garlic, minced
1 cup Greek yogurt
4 tablespoons mayonnaise
2 tablespoons fresh basil, chopped
2 tablespoons fresh dill, chopped
1 teaspoon urfa biber chile

1. Butter the bottom and sides of your casserole dish. Toss the swordfish steaks with the seasonings. Arrange the swordfish steaks in the prepared casserole dish.
2. Scatter the onion and garlic around the swordfish steaks. Bake in the preheated oven at 390°F (199°C) for about 25 minutes.
3. Meanwhile, whisk the Greek yogurt with the remaining ingredients to make the sauce. Serve the warm fish steaks with the sauce on the side. Bon appétit!

Per Serving
calories: 346 | fat: 23g | protein: 32g | carbs: 3g net carbs: 3g | fiber: 0g

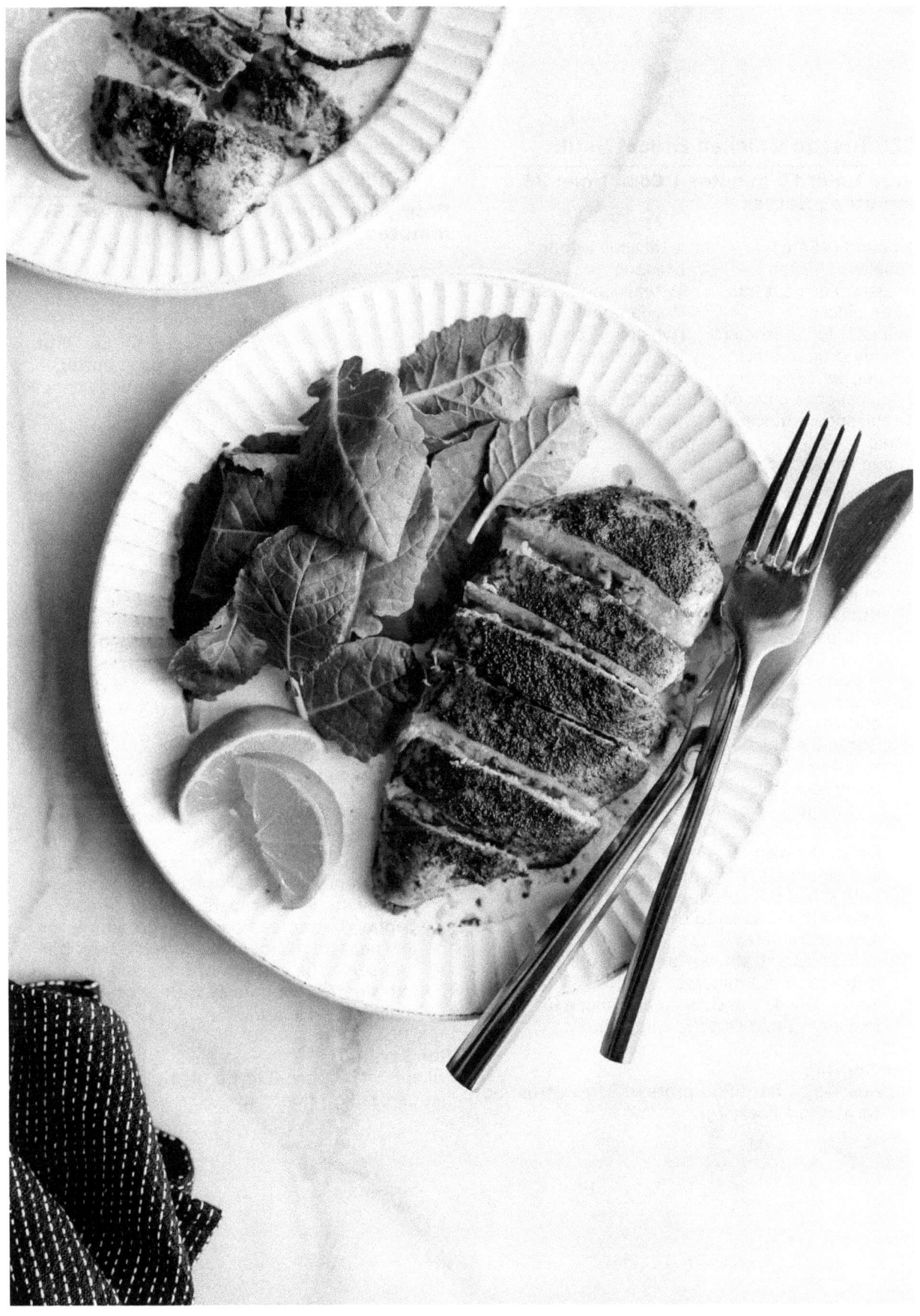

Chapter 7 Poultry

225. Tuscan Chicken Breast Sauté

Prep time: 10 minutes | Cook time: 35 minutes | Serves 4

1 pound (454 g) boneless chicken breasts, each cut into three pieces
Sea salt, for seasoning
Freshly ground black pepper, for seasoning
3 tablespoons olive oil
1 tablespoon minced garlic
¾ cup chicken stock
1 teaspoon dried oregano
½ teaspoon dried basil
½ cup heavy (whipping) cream
½ cup shredded Asiago cheese
1 cup fresh spinach
¼ cup sliced Kalamata olives

1. Prepare the chicken. Pat the chicken breasts dry and lightly season them with salt and pepper.
2. Sauté the chicken. In a large skillet over medium-high heat, warm the olive oil. Add the chicken and sauté until it is golden brown and just cooked through, about 15 minutes in total. Transfer the chicken to a plate and set it aside.
3. Make the sauce. Add the garlic to the skillet and sauté until it's softened, about 2 minutes. Stir in the chicken stock, oregano, and basil, scraping up any browned bits in the skillet. Bring to a boil, then reduce the heat to low and simmer until the sauce is reduced by about one-quarter, about 10 minutes.
4. Finish the dish. Stir in the cream and Asiago and simmer, stirring the sauce frequently, until it has thickened, about 5 minutes. Return the chicken to the skillet along with any accumulated juices. Stir in the spinach and olives and simmer until the spinach is wilted, about 2 minutes.
5. Serve. Divide the chicken and sauce between four plates and serve it immediately.

Per Serving
calories: 483 | fat: 38g | protein: 31g | carbs: 5g net carbs: 3g | fiber: 2g

226. Roasted Chicken Breasts with Capers

Prep time: 10 minutes | Cook time: 55 minutes | Serves 6

3 medium lemons, sliced
½ teaspoon salt
2 teaspoons olive oil
3 chicken breasts, halved
Salt and black pepper to season
¼ cup almond flour
1 tablespoon capers, rinsed
1¼ cup chicken broth
1 teaspoon butter
1½ tablespoon chopped fresh parsley
Parsley for garnish

1. Preheat the oven to 350ºF (180ºC) and lay a piece of parchment paper on a baking sheet.
2. Lay the lemon slices on the baking sheet, drizzle with olive oil and sprinkle with salt. Roast in the oven for 25 minutes to brown the lemon rinds.
3. Cover the chicken with plastic wrap, place them on a flat surface, and gently pound with the rolling pin to flatten to about ½-inch thickness. Remove the plastic wraps and season with salt and pepper.
4. Next, dredge the chicken in the almond flour on each side, and shake off any excess flour. Set aside.
5. Heat the olive oil in a skillet over medium heat and fry the chicken on both sides to a golden brown, for about 8 minutes in total. Pour the chicken broth in, shake the skillet, and let the broth boil and reduce to a thick consistency, about 12 minutes.
6. Lightly stir in the capers, roasted lemon, pepper, butter, and parsley, and simmer on low heat for 10 minutes. Turn the heat off and serve the chicken with the sauce hot, an extra garnish of parsley with a creamy squash mash.

Per Serving
calories: 430 | fat: 23g | protein: 33g | carbs: 7g net carbs: 3g | fiber: 4g

227. Herbed Turkey with Cucumber Salsa

Prep time: 15 minutes | Cook time: 6 minutes | Serves 4

2 spring onions, thinly sliced	1 tablespoon chopped herbs
1 pound (454 g) ground turkey	1 small chili pepper, deseeded and diced
1 egg	1 tablespoon butter
2 garlic cloves, minced	

Cucumber Salsa:

1 tablespoon apple cider vinegar	2 cucumbers, grated
1 tablespoon chopped dill	1 cup sour cream
1 garlic clove, minced	1 jalapeño pepper, minced
	1 tablespoon olive oil

1. Place all turkey ingredients, except the butter, in a bowl. Mix to combine. Make patties out of the mixture.
2. Melt the butter in a skillet over medium heat. Cook the patties for 3 minutes per side. Place all salsa ingredients in a bowl and mix to combine. Serve the patties topped with salsa.

Per Serving

calories: 350 | fat: 23g | protein: 27g | carbs: 7g net carbs: 5g | fiber: 2g

228. Spiced Chicken Breast

Prep time: 10 minutes | Cook time: 30 minutes | Serves 6

6 chicken breasts	⅔ cup olive oil
4 cloves garlic, minced	¼ cup erythritol
½ cup oregano leaves, chopped	Salt and black pepper, to taste
½ cup lemon juice	3 small chilies, minced

1. Preheat a grill to 350ºF (180ºC).
2. In a bowl, mix the garlic, oregano, lemon juice, olive oil, chilies and erythritol. Set aside.
3. While the spices incorporate in flavor, cover the chicken with plastic wraps, and use the rolling pin to pound to ½ -inch thickness. Remove the wrap, and brush the mixture on the chicken on both sides.
4. Place on the grill, cover the lid and cook for 15 minutes. Baste the chicken with more of the spice mixture, and continue cooking for 15 more minutes.

Per Serving

calories: 265 | fat: 9g | protein: 26g | carbs: 4g net carbs: 3g | fiber: 1g

229. Lemony Rosemary Chicken Thighs

Prep time: 10 minutes | Cook time: 14 minutes | Serves 4

8 chicken thighs	1 tablespoon chopped rosemary
1 teaspoon salt	¼ teaspoon black pepper
1 tablespoon lemon juice	1 garlic clove, minced
1 teaspoon lemon zest	
1 tablespoon olive oil	

1. Combine all ingredients in a bowl. Place in the fridge for one hour. Heat a skillet over medium heat. Add the chicken along with the juices and cook until crispy, about 7 minutes per side.
2. Serve immediately.

Per Serving

calories: 477 | fat: 31g | protein: 31g | carbs: 3g net carbs: 3g | fiber: 0g

230. Slow Cooked Chicken Cacciatore

Prep time: 15 minutes | Cook time: 3 to 4 hours or 6 to 8 hours | Serves 4

¼ cup good-quality olive oil	garlic
4 (4-ounce /113-g) boneless chicken breasts, each cut into three pieces	1 (28-ounce / 794-g) can sodium-free diced tomatoes
1 onion, chopped	½ cup red wine
2 celery stalks, chopped	½ cup tomato purée
1 cup sliced mushrooms	1 tablespoon dried basil
2 tablespoons minced	1 teaspoon dried oregano
	⅛ teaspoon red pepper flakes

1. Brown the chicken. In a skillet over medium-high heat, warm the olive oil. Add the chicken breasts and brown them, turning them once, about 10 minutes in total.
2. Cook in the slow cooker. Place the chicken in the slow cooker and stir in the onion, celery, mushrooms, garlic, tomatoes, red wine, tomato purée, basil, oregano, and red pepper flakes. Cook it on high for 3 to 4 hours or on low for 6 to 8 hours, until the chicken is fully cooked and tender.
3. Serve. Divide the chicken and sauce between four bowls and serve it immediately.

Per Serving

calories: 383 | fat: 26g | protein: 26g | carbs: 11g net carbs: 7g | fiber: 4g

231. Spiced Chicken Wings

Prep time: 10 minutes | Cook time: 25 minutes | Serves 4

12 chicken wings, cut in half
1 tablespoon turmeric
1 tablespoon cumin
1 tablespoon fresh ginger, grated
1 tablespoon cilantro, chopped
1 tablespoon paprika
Salt and ground black pepper, to taste
1 tablespoon olive oil
Juice of ½ lime
1 cup thyme leaves
¾ cup cilantro, chopped
1 tablespoon water
1 jalapeño pepper

1. In a bowl, stir together 1 tablespoon ginger, cumin, paprika, salt, 1 tablespoon olive oil, black pepper, and turmeric. Place in the chicken wings pieces, toss to coat, and refrigerate for 20 minutes.
2. Heat the grill, place in the marinated wings, cook for 25 minutes, turning from time to time, remove and set to a serving plate.
3. Using a blender, combine thyme, remaining ginger, salt, jalapeno pepper, black pepper, lime juice, cilantro, remaining olive oil, and water, and blend well. Drizzle the chicken wings with the sauce to serve.

Per Serving
calories: 175 | fat: 7g | protein: 21g | carbs: 7g net carbs: 4g | fiber: 3g

232. Herbed Turkey Breast

Prep time: 25 minutes | Cook time: 7 to 8 hours | Serves 6

3 tablespoons extra-virgin olive oil, divided
1½ pounds (680 g) boneless turkey breasts
Salt, for seasoning
Freshly ground black pepper, for seasoning
1 cup coconut milk
2 teaspoons minced garlic
2 teaspoons dried thyme
1 teaspoon dried oregano
1 avocado, peeled, pitted, and chopped
1 tomato, diced
½ jalapeño pepper, diced
1 tablespoon chopped cilantro

1. Lightly grease the insert of the slow cooker with 1 tablespoon of the olive oil.
2. In a large skillet over medium-high heat, heat the remaining 2 tablespoons of the olive oil.
3. Lightly season the turkey with salt and pepper. Add the turkey to the skillet and brown for about 7 minutes, turning once.
4. Transfer the turkey to the insert and add the coconut milk, garlic, thyme, and oregano.
5. Cover and cook on low for 7 to 8 hours.
6. In a small bowl, stir together the avocado, tomato, jalapeño pepper, and cilantro.
7. Serve the turkey topped with the avocado salsa.

Per Serving
calories: 347 | fat: 27g | protein: 25g | carbs: 5g net carbs: 2g | fiber: 3g

233. Cheesy Chicken and Tomato Packets

Prep time: 15 minutes | Cook time: 40 minutes | Serves 4

1 cup goat cheese
½ cup chopped oil-packed sun-dried tomatoes
1 teaspoon minced garlic
½ teaspoon dried basil
½ teaspoon dried oregano
4 (4-ounce / 113-g) boneless chicken breasts
Sea salt, for seasoning
Freshly ground black pepper, for seasoning
3 tablespoons olive oil

1. Preheat the oven. Set the oven temperature to 375ºF (190ºC).
2. Prepare the filling. In a medium bowl, stir together the goat cheese, sun-dried tomatoes, garlic, basil, and oregano until everything is well blended.
3. Stuff the chicken. Make a horizontal slice in the middle of each chicken breast to make a pocket, making sure not to cut through the sides or ends. Spoon one-quarter of the filling into each breast, folding the skin and chicken meat over the slit to form packets. Secure the packets with a toothpick. Lightly season the breasts with salt and pepper.
4. Brown the chicken. In a large oven-safe skillet over medium heat, warm the olive oil. Add the breasts and sear them, turning them once, until they are golden, about 8 minutes in total.
5. Bake the chicken. Place the skillet in the oven and bake the chicken for 30 minutes or until it's cooked through.
6. Serve. Remove the toothpicks. Divide the chicken between four plates and serve them immediately.

Per Serving
calories: 388 | fat: 29g | protein: 28g | carbs: 4g net carbs: 3g | fiber: 1g

234. Grilled Lemony Chicken Wings

Prep time: 10 minutes | Cook time: 12 minutes | Serves 4

2 pounds (907 g) chicken wings
Juice from 1 lemon
½ cup fresh parsley, chopped
2 garlic cloves, peeled and minced
1 Serrano pepper, chopped
1 tablespoon olive oil
Salt and black pepper, to taste
Lemon wedges, for serving
Ranch dip, for serving
½ teaspoon cilantro

1. In a bowl, stir together lemon juice, garlic, salt, serrano pepper, cilantro, olive oil, and black pepper. Place in the chicken wings and toss well to coat. Refrigerate for 2 hours.
2. Set a grill over high heat and add on the chicken wings; cook each side for 6 minutes.
3. Remove to a plate and serve alongside lemon wedges and ranch dip.

Per Serving
calories: 326 | fat: 12g | protein: 50g | carbs: 3g net carbs: 2g | fiber: 1g

235. Turkey and Pumpkin Ragout

Prep time: 15 minutes | Cook time: 8 hours | Serves 6

1 tablespoon extra-virgin olive oil
1 pound (454 g) boneless turkey thighs, cut into 1½-inch chunks
3 cups cubed pumpkin, cut into 1-inch chunks
1 red bell pepper, diced
½ sweet onion, cut in half and sliced
1 tablespoon minced garlic
1½ cups chicken broth
1½ cups coconut milk
2 teaspoons chopped fresh thyme
½ cup coconut cream
Salt, for seasoning
Freshly ground black pepper, for seasoning
12 slices cooked bacon, chopped, for garnish

1. Lightly grease the insert of the slow cooker with the olive oil.
2. Add the turkey, pumpkin, red bell pepper, onion, garlic, broth, coconut milk, and thyme.
3. Cover and cook on low for 8 hours.
4. Stir in the coconut cream and season with salt and pepper.
5. Serve topped with the bacon.

Per Serving
calories: 418 | fat: 34g | protein: 25g | carbs: 6g net carbs: 5g | fiber: 1g

236. Classic Jerk Chicken

Prep time: 15 minutes | Cook time: 7 to 8 hours | Serves 6

½ cup extra-virgin olive oil, divided
2 pounds (907 g) boneless chicken (breast and thighs)
1 sweet onion, quartered
4 garlic cloves
2 scallions, white and green parts, coarsely chopped
2 habanero chiles, stemmed and seeded
2 tablespoons granulated erythritol
1 tablespoon grated fresh ginger
2 teaspoons allspice
1 teaspoon dried thyme
½ teaspoon cardamom
½ teaspoon salt
2 tablespoons chopped cilantro, for garnish

1. Lightly grease the insert of the slow cooker with 1 tablespoon of the olive oil.
2. Arrange the chicken pieces in the bottom of the insert.
3. In a blender, pulse the remaining olive oil, onion, garlic, scallions, chiles, erythritol, ginger, allspice, thyme, cardamom, and salt until a thick, uniform sauce forms.
4. Pour the sauce over the chicken, turning the pieces to coat.
5. Cover and cook on low for 7 to 8 hours.
6. Serve topped with the cilantro.

Per Serving
calories: 485 | fat: 40g | protein: 27g | carbs: 5g net carbs: 4g | fiber: 1g

237. Spicy Chicken Skewers

Prep time: 10 minutes | Cook time: 6 minutes | Serves 6

2 pounds (907 g) chicken breasts, cubed
1 teaspoon sesame oil
1 tablespoon olive oil
1 cup red bell pepper pieces
1 tablespoon five spice powder
1 tablespoon granulated sweetener
1 tablespoon fish sauce

1. Combine the sesame and olive oils, fish sauce, and seasonings in a bowl. Add the chicken, and let marinate for 1 hour in the fridge.
2. Preheat the grill. Take 12 skewers and thread the chicken and bell peppers. Grill for 3 minutes per side.

Per Serving
calories: 297 | fat: 17g | protein: 32g | carbs: 2g net carbs: 1g | fiber: 1g

238. Pesto Turkey with Zucchini Spaghetti

Prep time: 10 minutes | Cook time: 32 minutes | Serves 6

2 cups sliced mushrooms
1 teaspoon olive oil
1 pound (454 g) ground turkey
1 tablespoon pesto sauce
1 cup diced onion
2 cups broccoli florets
6 cups zucchini, spiralized

1. Heat the oil in a skillet. Add zucchini and cook for 2-3 minutes, stirring continuously; set aside.
2. Add turkey to the skillet and cook until browned, about 7-8 minutes. Transfer to a plate. Add onion and cook until translucent, about 3 minutes. Add broccoli and mushrooms, and cook for 7 more minutes. Return the turkey to the skillet. Stir in the pesto sauce. Cover the pan, lower the heat, and simmer for 15 minutes. Stir in zucchini pasta and serve immediately.

Per Serving

calories: 273 | fat: 16g | protein: 19g | carbs: 7g net carbs: 4g | fiber: 3g

239. Roast Herbs Stuffed Chicken

Prep time: 10 minutes | Cook time: 1½ hours | Serves 8

5 pounds (2.3 kg) whole chicken
1 bunch oregano
1 bunch thyme
1 tablespoon marjoram
1 tablespoon parsley
1 tablespoon olive oil
2 pounds (907 g) Brussels sprouts
1 lemon
1 tablespoon butter

1. Preheat your oven to 450°F (235°C).
2. Stuff the chicken with oregano, thyme, and lemon. Roast for 15 minutes. Reduce the heat to 325°F (163°C) and cook for 40 minutes. Spread the butter over the chicken, and sprinkle parsley and marjoram. Add the brussels sprouts. Return to the oven and bake for 40 more minutes.
3. Let sit for 10 minutes before carving.

Per Serving

calories: 432 | fat: 32g | protein: 30g | carbs: 10g net carbs: 5g | fiber: 5g

240. Itanlian Chicken Cacciatore

Prep time: 15 minutes | Cook time: 8 hours | Serves 6

3 tablespoons extra-virgin olive oil, divided
2 pounds boneless chicken thighs
Salt, for seasoning
Freshly ground black pepper, for seasoning
1 (14-ounce / 397-g) can stewed tomatoes
2 cups chicken broth
1 cup quartered button mushrooms
½ sweet onion, chopped
1 tablespoon minced garlic
1 tablespoon dried oregano
1 teaspoon dried basil
pinch red pepper flakes

1. Lightly grease the insert of the slow cooker with 1 tablespoon of the olive oil.
2. Lightly season the chicken thighs with salt and pepper.
3. In a large skillet over medium-high heat, heat the remaining 2 tablespoons of the olive oil. Add the chicken thighs and brown for about 8 minutes, turning once.
4. Transfer the chicken to the insert and add the tomatoes, broth, mushrooms, onion, garlic, oregano, basil, and red pepper flakes.
5. Cover and cook on low for 8 hours.
6. Serve warm.

Per Serving

calories: 425 | fat: 32g | protein: 27g | carbs: 8g net carbs: 7g | fiber: 1g

241. Basil Turkey Meatballs

Prep time: 10 minutes | Cook time: 5 minutes | Serves 4

1 pound (454 g) ground turkey
1 tablespoon chopped sun-dried tomatoes
1 tablespoon chopped basil
½ teaspoon garlic powder
1 egg
½ teaspoon salt
¼ cup almond flour
1 tablespoon olive oil
½ cup shredded mozzarella cheese
¼ teaspoon pepper

1. Place everything, except the oil in a bowl. Mix with your hands until combined. Form into 16 balls. Heat the olive oil in a skillet over medium heat. Cook the meatballs for 4-5 minutes per each side.
2. Serve immediately.

Per Serving

calories: 310 | fat: 26g | protein: 22g | carbs: 3g net carbs: 2g | fiber: 1g

242. Hungarian Chicken Thighs

Prep time: 10 minutes | Cook time: 7 to 8 hours | Serves 4

1 tablespoon extra-virgin olive oil
2 pounds (907 g) boneless chicken thighs
½ cup chicken broth
Juice and zest of 1 lemon
2 teaspoons minced garlic
2 teaspoons paprika
¼ teaspoon salt
1 cup sour cream
1 tablespoon chopped parsley, for garnish

1. Lightly grease the insert of the slow cooker with the olive oil.
2. Place the chicken thighs in the insert.
3. In a small bowl, stir together the broth, lemon juice and zest, garlic, paprika, and salt.
4. Pour the broth mixture over the chicken.
5. Cover and cook on low for 7 to 8 hours.
6. Turn off the heat and stir in the sour cream.
7. Serve topped with the parsley.

Per Serving
calories: 404 | fat: 32g | protein: 23g | carbs: 4g net carbs: 0g | fiber: 4g

243. Braised Chicken and Veggies

Prep time: 10 minutes | Cook time: 21 minutes | Serves 4

1 tablespoon butter
1 pound (454 g) chicken thighs
Salt and black pepper, to taste
2 cloves garlic, minced
1 (14 ounce / 397-g) can whole tomatoes
1 eggplant, diced
10 fresh basil leaves, chopped, extra to garnish

1. Melt butter in a saucepan over medium heat, season the chicken with salt and black pepper and fry for 4 minutes on each side until golden brown. Remove to a plate.
2. Sauté the garlic in the butter for 2 minutes, pour in the tomatoes, and cook covered for 8 minutes. Add in the eggplant and basil. Cook for 4 minutes. Season the sauce with salt and black pepper, stir and add the chicken. Coat with sauce and simmer for 3 minutes.
3. Serve chicken with sauce on a bed of squash pasta. Garnish with extra basil.

Per Serving
calories: 330 | fat: 22g | protein: 21g | carbs: 13g net carbs: 7g | fiber: 6g

244. Cooked Chicken in Creamy Spinach Sauce

Prep time: 10 minutes | Cook time: 21 minutes | Serves 4

1 pound (454 g) chicken thighs
1 tablespoon coconut oil
1 tablespoon coconut flour
2 cups spinach, chopped
1 teaspoon oregano
1 cup heavy cream
1 cup chicken broth
1 tablespoon butter

1. Warm the coconut oil in a skillet and brown the chicken on all sides, about 6-8 minutes. Set aside.
2. Add and melt the butter and whisk in the flour over medium heat. Whisk in the heavy cream and chicken broth and bring to a boil. Stir in oregano. Add the spinach to the skillet and cook until wilted. Add the thighs in the skillet and cook for an additional 15 minutes.

Per Serving
calories: 446 | fat: 38g | protein: 18g | carbs: 3g net carbs: 2g | fiber: 1g

245. Lemony Chicken Wings

Prep time: 10 minutes | Cook time: 15 minutes | Serves 4

A pinch of garlic powder
1 teaspoon lemon zest
1 tablespoon lemon juice
½ teaspoon ground cilantro
1 tablespoon fish sauce
1 tablespoon butter
¼ teaspoon xanthan gum
1 tablespoon Swerve sweetener
20 chicken wings
Salt and black pepper, to taste

1. Combine lemon juice and zest, fish sauce, cilantro, sweetener, and garlic powder in a saucepan. Bring to a boil, cover, lower the heat, and let simmer for 10 minutes. Stir in the butter and xanthan gum. Set aside. Season the wings with some salt and pepper.
2. Preheat the grill and cook for 5 minutes per side.
3. Serve topped with the sauce.

Per Serving
calories: 365 | fat: 25g | protein: 21g | carbs: 4g net carbs: 4g | fiber: 0g

246. Creamy-Lemony Chicken Thighs

Prep time: 10 minutes | Cook time: 7 to 8 hours | Serves 6

3 tablespoons extra-virgin olive oil
2 tablespoons butter
1½ pounds (680 g) boneless chicken thighs
½ sweet onion, diced
2 teaspoons minced garlic
2 teaspoons dried oregano
½ teaspoon salt
⅛ teaspoon pepper, depending on taste
1½ cups chicken broth
Juice and zest of 1 lemon
1 tablespoon dijon mustard
1 cup heavy (whipping) cream

1. Lightly grease the insert of the slow cooker with 1 tablespoon of the olive oil.
2. In a large skillet over medium-high heat, heat the remaining 2 tablespoons of the olive oil and the butter. Add the chicken and brown for 5 minutes, turning once.
3. Transfer the chicken to the insert and add the onion, garlic, oregano, salt, and pepper.
4. In a small bowl, whisk together the broth, lemon juice and zest, and mustard. Pour the mixture over the chicken.
5. Cover and cook on low for 7 to 8 hours.
6. Remove from the heat, stir in the heavy cream, and serve.

Per Serving
calories: 400 | fat: 34g | protein: 22g | carbs: 2g net carbs: 2g | fiber: 0g

247. Dijon Chicken Thighs

Prep time: 10 minutes | Cook time: 16 minutes | Serves 4

½ cup chicken stock
1 tablespoon olive oil
½ cup chopped onion
4 chicken thighs
¼ cup heavy cream
1 tablespoon Dijon mustard
1 teaspoon thyme
1 teaspoon garlic powder

1. Heat the olive oil in a pan. Cook the chicken for about 4 minutes per side. Set aside.
2. Sauté the onion in the same pan for 3 minutes, add the stock, and simmer for 5 minutes.
3. Stir in mustard and heavy cream, along with thyme and garlic powder.
4. Pour the sauce over the chicken and serve.

Per Serving
calories: 504 | fat: 39g | protein: 33g | carbs: 4g net carbs: 3g | fiber: 1g

248. Browned Chicken and Mushrooms

Prep time: 10 minutes | Cook time: 20 minutes | Serves 6

2 cups sliced mushrooms
½ teaspoon onion powder
½ teaspoon garlic powder
¼ cup butter
1 teaspoon Dijon mustard
1 tablespoon tarragon, chopped
2 pounds (907 g) chicken thighs
Salt and black pepper, to taste

1. Season the thighs with salt, pepper, garlic, and onion powder. Melt the butter in a skillet, and cook the chicken until browned; set aside. Add mushrooms to the same fat and cook for about 5 minutes.
2. Stir in Dijon mustard and ½ cup of water. Return the chicken to the skillet. Season to taste with salt and pepper, reduce the heat and cover, and let simmer for 15 minutes. Stir in tarragon. Serve warm.

Per Serving
calories: 405 | fat: 33g | protein: 25g | carbs: 1g net carbs: 1g | fiber: 0g

249. Bacon-Wrapped Chicken with Asparagus

Prep time: 10 minutes | Cook time: 40 minutes | Serves 4

6 chicken breasts
Pink salt and black pepper to taste
8 bacon slices
1 tablespoon olive oil
1 pound (454 g) asparagus spears
1 tablespoon fresh lemon juice
Manchego cheese, for topping

1. Preheat the oven to 400ºF (205ºC).
2. Season chicken breasts with salt and black pepper, and wrap 2 bacon slices around each chicken breast. Arrange on a baking sheet that is lined with parchment paper, drizzle with oil and bake for 25-30 minutes until bacon is brown and crispy.
3. Preheat your grill to high heat.
4. Brush the asparagus spears with olive oil and season with salt. Grill for 8-10 minutes, frequently turning until slightly charred. Remove to a plate and drizzle with lemon juice. Grate over Manchego cheese so that it melts a little on contact with the hot asparagus and forms a cheesy dressing.

Per Serving
calories: 468 | fat: 38g | protein: 26g | carbs: 5g net carbs: 2g | fiber: 3g

250. Baked Cheesy Chicken and Spinach

Prep time: 10 minutes | Cook time: 35 minutes | Serves 6

6 chicken breasts, skinless and boneless
1 teaspoon mixed spice seasoning
Pink salt and black pepper to season
2 loose cups baby spinach
1 teaspoon olive oil
4 oz cream cheese, cubed
1¼ cups shredded mozzarella cheese
1 tablespoon water

1. Preheat oven to 370ºF (188ºC).
2. Season chicken with spice mix, salt, and black pepper. Pat with your hands to have the seasoning stick on the chicken. Put in the casserole dish and layer spinach over the chicken. Mix the oil with cream cheese, mozzarella, salt, and black pepper and stir in water a tablespoon at a time. Pour the mixture over the chicken and cover the pot with aluminium foil.
3. Bake for 20 minutes, remove foil and continue cooking for 15 minutes until a nice golden brown color is formed on top. Take out and allow sitting for 5 minutes. Serve warm with braised asparagus.

Per Serving

calories: 463 | fat: 18g | protein: 48g | carbs: 2g net carbs: 2g | fiber: 0g

251. Ritzy Baked Chicken with Vegetable

Prep time: 10 minutes | Cook time: 43 minutes | Serves 6

3 cups cubed leftover chicken
3 cups spinach
2 cauliflower heads, cut into florets
3 cups water
3 eggs, lightly beaten
2 cups grated sharp cheddar cheese
1 cup pork rinds, crushed
½ cup unsweetened almond milk
1 tablespoon olive oil
3 cloves garlic, minced
Salt and black pepper to taste
Cooking spray

1. Preheat the oven to 350ºF (180ºC) and grease a baking dish with cooking spray. Set aside.
2. Pour the cauli florets and water in a pot; bring to boil over medium heat. Cover and steam the cauli florets for 8 minutes. Drain them through a colander and set aside.
3. Also, combine the cheddar cheese and pork rinds in a large bowl and mix in the chicken. Set aside.
4. Heat the olive oil in a skillet and cook the garlic and spinach until the spinach has wilted, about 5 minutes. Season with salt and black pepper, and add the spinach mixture and cauli florets to the chicken bowl.
5. Top with the eggs and almond milk, mix and transfer everything to the baking dish. Layer the top of the ingredients and place the dish in the oven to bake for 30 minutes.
6. By this time the edges and top must have browned nicely, then remove the chicken from the oven, let rest for 5 minutes, and serve. Garnish with steamed and seasoned green beans.

Per Serving

calories: 472 | fat: 26g | protein: 38g | carbs: 5g net carbs: 3g | fiber: 2g

252. Chicken Paella and Chorizo

Prep time: 15 minutes | Cook time: 42 minutes | Serves 6

18 chicken drumsticks
12 ounces (340 g) chorizo, chopped
1 white onion, chopped
4 ounces (113 g) jarred Piquillo peppers, finely diced
1 tablespoon olive oil
½ cup chopped parsley
1 teaspoon smoked paprika
1 tablespoon tomato puree
½ cup white wine
1 cup chicken broth
2 cups cauli rice
1 cup chopped green beans
1 lemon, cut in wedges
Salt and pepper, to taste

1. Preheat the oven to 350ºF (180ºC).
2. Heat the olive oil in a cast iron pan over medium heat, meanwhile season the chicken with salt and black pepper, and fry in the hot oil on both sides for 10 minutes to lightly brown. After, remove onto a plate with a perforated spoon.
3. Then, add the chorizo and onion to the hot oil, and sauté for 4 minutes. Include the tomato puree, piquillo peppers, and paprika, and let simmer for 2 minutes. Add the broth, and bring the ingredients to boil for 6 minutes until slightly reduced.
4. Stir in the cauli rice, white wine, green beans, half of the parsley, and lay the chicken on top. Transfer the pan to the oven and continue cooking for 20-25 minutes. Let the paella sit to cool for 10 minutes before serving garnished with the remaining parsley and lemon wedges.

Per Serving

calories: 440 | fat: 28g | protein: 22g | carbs: 8g net carbs: 6g | fiber: 2g

253. Lemony Chicken Skewers

Prep time: 10 minutes | Cook time: 12 minutes | Serves 4

3 chicken breasts, cut into cubes
1 tablespoon olive oil, divided
2/3 jar preserved lemon, flesh removed, drained
2 cloves garlic, minced
½ cup lemon juice
Salt and black pepper to taste
1 teaspoon rosemary leaves to garnish
2 to 4 lemon wedges to garnish

1. First, thread the chicken onto skewers and set aside.
2. In a wide bowl, mix half of the oil, garlic, salt, pepper, and lemon juice, and add the chicken skewers, and lemon rind. Cover the bowl and let the chicken marinate for at least 2 hours in the refrigerator.
3. When the marinating time is almost over, preheat a grill to 350ºF (180ºC), and remove the chicken onto the grill. Cook for 6 minutes on each side.
4. Remove and serve warm garnished with rosemary leaves and lemons wedges.

Per Serving
calories: 350 | fat: 11g | protein: 34g | carbs: 6g net carbs: 4g | fiber: 2g

254. Hearty Stuffed Chicken

Prep time: 20 minutes | Cook time: 35 minutes | Serves 4

For the Chicken:
4 chicken breasts
⅓ cup baby spinach
¼ cup goat cheese
¼ cup shredded cheddar cheese
1 tablespoon butter
Salt and black pepper, to taste

For the Tomato Purée:
1 tablespoon butter
1 shallot, chopped
2 garlic cloves, chopped
½ tablespoon red wine vinegar
1 tablespoon tomato purée
14 ounces (397 g) canned crushed tomatoes
½ teaspoon salt
1 teaspoon dried basil
1 teaspoon dried oregano
Black pepper, to taste

For the Salad:
2 cucumbers, spiralized
1 tablespoon olive oil
1 tablespoon rice vinegar

1. Set oven to 400ºF (205ºC) and grease a baking dish. Set aside.
2. Place a pan over medium heat. Melt 1 tablespoon of butter and sauté spinach until it shrinks; season with salt and pepper. Transfer to a bowl containing goat cheese, stir and set aside. Cut the chicken breasts lengthwise and stuff with the cheese mixture and set into the baking dish. On top, spread the grated cheddar cheese, add 1 tablespoon of butter then set into the oven. Bake until cooked through for 20 to 30 minutes.
3. Set a pan over medium-high heat and warm 1 tablespoon of butter. Add in garlic and shallot and cook until soft. Place in herbs, tomato purée, vinegar, tomatoes, salt, and pepper. Bring the mixture to a boil. Set heat to low and simmer for 15 minutes. Arrange the cucumbers on a serving platter, season with salt, pepper, olive oil, and vinegar, Top with the chicken and pour over the sauce.

Per Serving
calories: 453 | fat: 31g | protein: 43g | carbs: 9g net carbs: 6g | fiber: 3g

255. Cheesy Spinach Stuffed Chicken

Prep time: 15 minutes | Cook time: 20 minutes | Serves 4

4 chicken breasts, boneless and skinless
½ cup mozzarella cheese
⅓ cup Parmesan cheese
6 ounces (170 g) cream cheese
2 cups spinach, chopped
A pinch of nutmeg
½ teaspoon minced garlic

Breading:
2 eggs
⅓ cup almond flour
1 tablespoon olive oil
½ teaspoon parsley
⅓ cup Parmesan cheese
A pinch of onion powder

1. Pound the chicken until it doubles in size. Mix the cream cheese, spinach, mozzarella, nutmeg, salt, black pepper, and Parmesan cheese in a bowl. Divide the mixture between the chicken breasts and spread it out evenly. Wrap the chicken in a plastic wrap. Refrigerate for 15 minutes.
2. Heat the oil in a pan and preheat the oven to 370ºF (188ºC). Beat the eggs and combine all other breading ingredients in a bowl. Dip the chicken in egg first, then in the breading mixture.
3. Cook in the pan until browned. Place on a lined baking sheet and bake for 20 minutes.

Per Serving
calories: 491 | fat: 36g | protein: 38g | carbs: 6g net carbs: 4g | fiber: 2g

256. Chicken Fingers

Prep time: 15 minutes | Cook time: 30 minutes | Serves 8

1½ pounds (680 g) chicken breasts, skinless, boneless, cubed
Salt and ground black pepper, to taste
1 egg
1 cup almond flour
¼ cup Parmesan cheese, grated
½ teaspoon garlic powder
1½ teaspoon dried parsley
½ teaspoon dried basil
1 tablespoon avocado oil
4 cups spaghetti squash, cooked
6 ounces (170 g) gruyere cheese, shredded
1½ cups tomato purée
Fresh basil, chopped, for serving

1. In a bowl, combine the almond flour with 1 teaspoon parsley, Parmesan cheese, black pepper, garlic powder, and salt. In a separate bowl, combine the egg with black pepper and salt. Dip the chicken in the egg, and then in almond flour mixture.
2. Set a pan over medium heat and warm 3 tablespoons avocado oil, add in the chicken, cook until golden, and remove to paper towels. In a bowl, combine the spaghetti squash with salt, dried basil, rest of the parsley, 1 tablespoon avocado oil, and black pepper.
3. Sprinkle this into a baking dish, top with the chicken pieces, followed by the tomato purée. Scatter shredded gruyere cheese on top, and bake for 30 minutes at 360ºF (182ºC). Remove, and sprinkle with fresh basil before serving.

Per Serving

calories: 415 | fat: 36g | protein: 28g | carbs: 7g net carbs: 5g | fiber: 2g

257. Stir-Fried Chicken, Broccoli and Cashew

Prep time: 10 minutes | Cook time: 17 minutes | Serves 4

1 chicken breasts, cut into strips
1 tablespoon olive oil
1 tablespoon coconut aminos
1 teaspoon white wine vinegar
1 teaspoon erythritol
1 teaspoon xanthan gum
1 lemon, juiced
1 cup unsalted cashew nuts
2 cups broccoli florets
1 white onion, thinly sliced
Salt and black pepper to taste

1. In a bowl, mix the coconut aminos, vinegar, lemon juice, erythritol, and xanthan gum. Set aside.
2. Heat the oil in a wok and fry the cashew for 4 minutes until golden-brown. Remove to a paper towel lined plate. Sauté the onion in the same oil for 4 minutes until soft and browned; add to the cashew nuts.
3. Add the chicken to the wok and cook for 4 minutes; include the broccoli, salt, and black pepper. Stir-fry and pour the coconut aminos mixture in. Stir and cook the sauce for 4 minutes and pour in the cashews and onion. Stir once more, cook for 1 minute, and turn the heat off.
4. Serve the chicken stir-fry with some steamed cauli rice.

Per Serving

calories: 325 | fat: 21g | protein: 22g | carbs: 6g net carbs: 4g | fiber: 2g

258. Marinated Chicken with Peanut Sauce

Prep time: 20 minutes | Cook time: 14 minutes | Serves 6

1 tablespoon wheat-free coconut aminos
1 tablespoon sugar-free fish sauce
1 tablespoon lime juice
1 teaspoon cilantro
1 teaspoon minced garlic
1 teaspoon minced ginger
1 tablespoon olive oil
1 tablespoon rice wine vinegar
1 teaspoon cayenne pepper
1 teaspoon erythritol
6 chicken thighs

Peanut sauce:
½ cup peanut butter
1 teaspoon minced garlic
1 tablespoon lime juice
1 tablespoon water
1 teaspoon minced ginger
1 tablespoon chopped jalapeño
1 tablespoon rice wine vinegar
1 tablespoon erythritol
1 tablespoon fish sauce

1. Combine all chicken ingredients in a large Ziploc bag. Seal the bag and shake to combine. Refrigerate for 1 hour. Remove from fridge about 15 minutes before cooking.
2. Preheat the grill to medium heat and cook the chicken for 7 minutes per side. Whisk together all sauce ingredients in a mixing bowl. Serve the chicken drizzled with peanut sauce.

Per Serving

calories: 492 | fat: 36g | protein: 35g | carbs: 5g net carbs: 3g | fiber: 2g

259. Chicken with Mayo-Avocado Sauce

Prep time: 10 minutes | Cook time: 12 minutes | Serves 4

For the Sauce:
1 avocado, pitted
½ cup mayonnaise
Salt to taste

For the Chicken:
1 tablespoon butter
4 chicken breasts
Pink salt and black pepper to taste
1 cup chopped cilantro leaves
½ cup chicken broth

1. Spoon the avocado, mayonnaise, and salt into a small food processor and puree until a smooth sauce is derived. Pour sauce into a jar and refrigerate while you make the chicken.
2. Melt butter in a large skillet, season chicken with salt and black pepper and fry for 4 minutes on each side to golden brown. Remove chicken to a plate.
3. Pour the broth in the same skillet and add the cilantro. Bring to simmer covered for 3 minutes and add the chicken. Cover and cook on low heat for 5 minutes until the liquid has reduced and chicken is fragrant. Dish chicken only into serving plates and spoon the mayoavocado sauce over.

Per Serving
calories: 398 | fat: 32g | protein: 24 g | carbs: 9g net carbs: 4g | fiber: 5g

260. Baked Cheesy Chicken and Zucchini

Prep time: 15 minutes | Cook time: 35 minutes | Serves 6

2 pound (907 g) chicken breasts, cubed
1 tablespoon butter
1 cup green bell peppers, sliced
1 cup yellow onions, sliced
1 zucchini, cubed
2 garlic cloves, divided
1 teaspoon Italian seasoning
½ teaspoon salt
½ teaspoon black pepper
8 ounces (227 g) cream cheese, softened
½ cup mayonnaise
1 tablespoon Worcestershire sauce (sugar-free)
2 cups cheddar cheese, shredded

1. Set oven to 370ºF (188ºC) and grease and line a baking dish.
2. Set a pan over medium heat. Place in the butter and let melt, then add in the chicken. Cook until lightly browned, about 5 minutes. Place in onions, zucchini, black pepper, garlic, bell peppers, salt, and 1 teaspoon of Italian seasoning. Cook until tender and set aside.
3. In a bowl, mix cream cheese, garlic, remaining seasoning, mayonnaise, and Worcestershire sauce. Stir in meat and sauteed vegetables. Place the mixture into the prepared baking dish, sprinkle with the shredded cheddar cheese and insert into the oven. Cook until browned for 30 minutes.
4. Serve immediately.

Per Serving
calories: 489 | fat: 37g | protein: 21g | carbs: 6g net carbs: 5g | fiber: 1g

261. Baked Chicken and Chorizo Sausages

Prep time: 20 minutes | Cook time: 45 minutes | Serves 4

½ cup mushrooms, chopped
1 pound (454 g) chorizo sausages, chopped
1 tablespoon avocado oil
4 cherry peppers, chopped
1 red bell pepper, seeded, chopped
1 onion, peeled and sliced
1 tablespoon garlic, minced
2 cups tomatoes, chopped
4 chicken thighs
Salt and black pepper, to taste
½ cup chicken stock
1 teaspoon turmeric
1 tablespoon vinegar
1 teaspoon dried oregano
Fresh parsley, chopped, for serving

1. Set a pan over medium heat and warm half of the avocado oil, stir in the chorizo sausages, and cook for 5 to 6 minutes until browned; remove to a bowl.
2. Heat the rest of the oil, place in the chicken thighs, and apply pepper and salt for seasoning. Cook each side for 3 minutes and set aside on a bowl.
3. In the same pan, add the onion, bell pepper, cherry peppers, and mushrooms, and cook for 4 minutes. Stir in the garlic and cook for 2 minutes.
4. Pour in the stock, turmeric, salt, tomatoes, pepper, vinegar, and oregano. Stir in the chorizo sausages and chicken, place everything to the oven at 400ºF (205ºC), and bake for 30 minutes. Ladle into serving bowls and garnish with chopped parsley to serve.

Per Serving
calories: 415 | fat: 33g | protein: 25g | carbs: 11g net carbs: 4g | fiber: 7g

262. Baked Chicken Skewers and Celery Fries

Prep time: 10 minutes | Cook time: 40 minutes | Serves 4

2 chicken breasts
½ teaspoon salt
¼ teaspoon ground black pepper
1 tablespoon olive oil
¼ cup chicken broth
For the Fries:
1 pound (454 g) celery root
1 tablespoon olive oil
½ teaspoon salt
¼ teaspoon ground black pepper

1. Set oven to 400°F (205°C). Grease and line a baking sheet. In a bowl, mix oil, spices and the chicken; set in the fridge for 10 minutes while covered. Peel and chop celery root to form fry shapes and place into a separate bowl. Apply oil to coat and add pepper and salt for seasoning. Arrange to the baking tray in an even layer and bake for 10 minutes.
2. Take the chicken from the refrigerator and thread onto the skewers. Place over the celery, pour in the chicken broth, then set in the oven for 30 minutes. Serve with lemon wedges.

Per Serving

calories: 579 | fat: 43g | protein: 39g | carbs: 8g net carbs: 6g | fiber: 2g

263. Chicken Garam Masala

Prep time: 15 minutes | Cook time: 26 minutes | Serves 4

1 pound (454 g) chicken breasts, sliced lengthwise
1 tablespoon butter
1 tablespoon olive oil
1 yellow bell pepper, finely chopped
1¼ cups heavy whipping cream
1 tablespoon fresh cilantro, finely chopped
Salt and pepper, to taste

For the Garam Masala:
1 teaspoon ground cumin
1 teaspoon ground coriander
1 teaspoon ground cardamom
1 teaspoon turmeric
1 teaspoon ginger
1 teaspoon paprika
1 teaspoon cayenne, ground
1 pinch ground nutmeg

1. Set your oven to 400°F (205°C). In a bowl, mix the garam masala spices. Coat the chicken with half of the masala mixture. Heat the olive oil and butter in a frying pan over medium-high heat, and brown the chicken for 3 to 5 minutes per side. Transfer to a baking dish.
2. To the remaining masala, add heavy cream and bell pepper. Season with salt and pepper and pour over chicken. Bake for 20 minutes until the mixture starts to bubble. Garnish with chopped cilantro to serve.

Per Serving

calories: 564 | fat: 50g | protein: 33g | carbs: 6g net carbs: 5g | fiber: 1g

264. Coconut-Chicken Breasts

Prep time: 15 minutes | Cook time: 7 to 8 hours | Serves 6

3 tablespoons extra-virgin olive oil, divided
1½ pounds (680 g) boneless chicken breasts
½ sweet onion, chopped
1 cup quartered baby bok choy
1 red bell pepper, diced
2 cups coconut milk
2 tablespoons almond butter
1 tablespoon red thai curry paste
1 tablespoon coconut aminos
2 teaspoons grated fresh ginger
Pinch red pepper flakes
¼ cup chopped peanuts, for garnish
2 tablespoons chopped cilantro, for garnish

1. Lightly grease the insert of the slow cooker with 1 tablespoon of the olive oil.
2. In a large skillet over medium-high heat, heat the remaining 2 tablespoons of the olive oil. Add the chicken and brown for about 7 minutes.
3. Transfer the chicken to the slow cooker and add the onion, baby bok choy, and bell pepper.
4. In a medium bowl, whisk together the coconut milk, almond butter, curry paste, coconut aminos, ginger, and red pepper flakes, until well blended.
5. Pour the sauce over the chicken and vegetables, and mix to coat.
6. Cover and cook on low for 7 to 8 hours.
7. Serve topped with the peanuts and cilantro.

Per Serving

calories: 543 | fat: 42g | protein: 35g | carbs: 10g net carbs: 5g | fiber: 5g

265. Chili Chicken Breast

Prep time: 10 minutes | Cook time: 25 minutes | Serves 4

4 chicken breasts, skinless, boneless, cubed
1 tablespoon butter
½ onion, chopped
2 cups chicken broth
8 ounces (227 g) diced tomatoes
2 ounces (57 g) tomato puree
1 tablespoon chili powder
1 tablespoon cumin
½ tablespoon garlic powder
1 Serrano pepper, minced
½ cup shredded cheddar cheese
Salt and black pepper, to taste

1. Set a large pan over medium-high heat and add the chicken. Cover with water and bring to a boil. Cook until no longer pink, for 10 minutes. Transfer the chicken to a flat surface to shred with forks.
2. In a large pot, pour in the butter and set over medium heat. Sauté onion until transparent for 5 minutes. Stir in the chicken, tomatoes, cumin, serrano pepper, garlic powder, tomato puree, broth, and chili powder. Adjust the seasoning and let the mixture boil. Reduce heat to simmer for about 10 minutes. Divide chili among bowls and top with shredded cheese to serve.

Per Serving
calories: 421 | fat: 21g | protein: 45g | carbs: 7g net carbs: 5g | fiber: 2g

266. Garlicky Sweet Chicken Skewers

Prep time: 10 minutes | Cook time: 10 minutes | Serves 4

For the Skewers:
1 tablespoon coconut aminos
1 tablespoon ginger-garlic paste
1 tablespoon Swerve
For the Dressing:
½ cup tahini
½ teaspoon garlic powder
Chili pepper to taste
1 tablespoon olive oil
3 chicken breasts, cut into cubes

Pink salt to taste
¼ cup warm water

1. In a small bowl, whisk the coconut aminos, ginger-garlic paste, Swerve, chili pepper, and olive oil.
2. Put the chicken in a zipper bag, pour the marinade over, seal and shake for an even coat. Marinate in the fridge for 2 hours.
3. Preheat a grill to 400°F and thread the chicken on skewers. Cook for 10 minutes in total with three to four turnings to be golden brown; remove to a plate. Mix the tahini, garlic powder, salt, and warm water in a bowl. Pour into serving jars.
4. Serve the chicken skewers and tahini dressing with cauli fried rice.

Per Serving
calories: 470 | fat: 25g | protein: 52g | carbs: 5g net carbs: 2g | fiber: 3g

267. Mexican Chicken Mole

Prep time: 15 minutes | Cook time: 7 to 8 hours | Serves 6

3 tablespoons extra-virgin olive oil or butter (here), divided
2 pounds (907 g) boneless chicken thighs and breasts
Salt, for seasoning
Freshly ground black pepper, for seasoning
1 sweet onion, chopped
1 tablespoon minced garlic
1 (28-ounce / 794-g) can diced tomatoes
4 dried chile peppers, soaked in water for 2 hours and chopped
3 ounces (1.4kg) dark chocolate, chopped
¼ cup natural peanut butter
1½ teaspoons ground cumin
¾ teaspoon ground cinnamon
½ teaspoon chili powder
½ cup coconut cream
2 tablespoons chopped cilantro, for garnish

1. Lightly grease the insert of the slow cooker with 1 tablespoon of the olive oil.
2. In a large skillet over medium-high heat, heat the remaining 2 tablespoons of the olive oil.
3. Lightly season the chicken with salt and pepper, add to the skillet, and brown for about 5 minutes, turning once.
4. Add the onion and garlic and sauté for an additional 3 minutes.
5. Transfer the chicken, onion, and garlic to the slow cooker, and stir in the tomatoes, chiles, chocolate, peanut butter, cumin, cinnamon, and chili powder.
6. Cover and cook on low for 7 to 8 hours.
7. Stir in the coconut cream, and serve hot, topped with the cilantro.

Per Serving
calories: 386 | fat: 30g | protein: 19g | carbs: 11g net carbs: 6g | fiber: 5g

268. Cheesy Spinach Stuffed Chicken

Prep time: 10 minutes | Cook time: 30 minutes | Serves 6

4 ounces (113 g) cream cheese
3 ounces (85 g) mozzarella slices
10 ounces (283 g) spinach
⅓ cup shredded mozzarella cheese
1 tablespoon olive oil
1 cup tomato basil sauce
3 whole chicken breasts

1. Preheat your oven to 400ºF (205ºC). Combine the cream cheese, shredded mozzarella cheese, and spinach in the microwave. Cut the chicken a couple of times horizontally and stuff with the spinach mixture. Brush with olive oil. place on a lined baking dish and bake in the oven for 25 minutes.
2. Pour the tomato basil sauce over and top with mozzarella slices. Return to the oven and cook for an additional 5 minutes.

Per Serving
calories: 338 | fat: 28g | protein: 37g | carbs: 7g net carbs: 3g | fiber: 4g

269. Paprika Chicken with Steamed Broccoli

Prep time: 10 minutes | Cook time: 15 minutes | Serves 6

1 tablespoon smoked paprika
Salt and black pepper to taste
1 teaspoon garlic powder
1 tablespoon olive oil
6 chicken breasts
1 head broccoli, cut into florets

1. Place broccoli florets onto the steamer basket over the boiling water; steam approximately 8 minutes or until crisp-tender. Set aside. Grease grill grate with cooking spray and preheat to 400ºF (205ºC).
2. Combine paprika, salt, black pepper, and garlic powder in a bowl. Brush chicken with olive oil and sprinkle spice mixture over and massage with hands.
3. Grill chicken for 7 minutes per side until well-cooked, and plate. Serve warm with steamed broccoli.

Per Serving
calories: 42 | fat: 18g | protein: 50g | carbs: 2g net carbs: 2g | fiber: 0g

270. Chicken Breast with Anchovy Tapenade

Prep time: 10 minutes | Cook time: 10 minutes | Serves 2

1 chicken breast, cut into 4 pieces
1 tablespoon coconut oil
3 garlic cloves, crushed
For the tapenade:
1 cup black olives, pitted
1 ounce (28 g) anchovy fillets, rinsed
1 garlic clove, crushed
Salt and ground black pepper, to taste
1 tablespoon olive oil
¼ cup fresh basil, chopped
1 tablespoon lemon juice

1. Using a food processor, combine the olives, salt, olive oil, basil, lemon juice, anchovy, and black pepper, blend well. Set a pan over medium heat and warm coconut oil, stir in the garlic, and sauté for 2 minutes.
2. Place in the chicken pieces and cook each side for 4 minutes. Split the chicken among plates and apply a topping of the anchovy tapenade.
3. Serve immediately.

Per Serving
calories: 155 | fat: 13g | protein: 25g | carbs: 3g net carbs: 3g | fiber: 0g

271. Bacon on Cheesy Chicken Breast

Prep time: 10 minutes | Cook time: 20 minutes | Serves 4

4 bacon strips
4 chicken breasts
3 green onions, chopped
4 ounces (113 g) ranch dressing
1 ounce coconut aminos
1 tablespoon coconut oil
4 ounces (113 g) Monterey Jack cheese, grated

1. Set a pan over high heat and warm the oil. Place in the chicken breasts, cook for 7 minutes, then flip to the other side; cook for an additional 7 minutes. Set another pan over medium heat, place in the bacon, cook until crispy, remove to paper towels, drain the grease, and crumble.
2. Add the chicken breast to a baking dish. Place the green onions, coconut aminos, cheese, and crumbled bacon on top, set in an oven, turn on the broiler, and cook for 5 minutes at high temperature. Split among serving plates and serve.

Per Serving
calories: 423 | fat: 21g | protein: 34g | carbs: 4g net carbs: 3g | fiber: 1g

272. Baked Chicken in Tomato Purée

Prep time: 15 minutes | Cook time: 1½ hours | Serves 4

8 chicken drumsticks
1½ tablespoon olive oil
1 medium white onion, diced
3 medium turnips, peeled and diced
2 green bell peppers, seeded, cut into chunks
2 cloves garlic, minced
¼ cup coconut flour
1 cup chicken broth
1 (28 ounce / 794-g) can sugar-free tomato purée
1 tablespoon dried Italian herbs
Salt and black pepper, to taste

1. Preheat oven to 400ºF (205ºC).
2. Heat the oil in a large skillet over medium heat, meanwhile season the drumsticks with salt and pepper, and fry in the oil to brown on both sides for 10 minutes. Remove to a baking dish. Sauté the onion, turnips, bell peppers, and garlic in the same oil and for 10 minutes with continuous stirring.
3. In a bowl, combine the broth, coconut flour, tomato purée, and Italian herbs together, and pour it over the vegetables in the pan. Stir and cook to thicken for 4 minutes. Pour the mixture on the chicken in the baking dish. Bake for around 1 hour. Remove from the oven and serve with steamed cauli rice.

Per Serving
calories: 515 | fat: 34g | protein: 51g | carbs: 15g net carbs: 7g | fiber: 8g

273. Bacon Fat Browned Chicken

Prep time: 15 minutes | Cook time: 7 to 8 hours | Serves 8

3 tablespoons coconut oil, divided
¼ pound (113 g) bacon, diced
2 pounds (907 g) chicken (breasts, thighs, drumsticks)
2 cups quartered button mushrooms
1 sweet onion, diced
1 tablespoon minced garlic
½ cup chicken broth
2 teaspoons chopped thyme
1 cup coconut cream

1. Lightly grease the insert of the slow cooker with 1 tablespoon of the coconut oil.
2. In a large skillet over medium-high heat, heat the remaining 2 tablespoons of the coconut oil.
3. Add the bacon and cook until it is crispy, about 5 minutes. Using a slotted spoon, transfer the bacon to a plate and set aside.
4. Add the chicken to the skillet and brown for 5 minutes, turning once.
5. Transfer the chicken and bacon to the insert and add the mushrooms, onion, garlic, broth, and thyme.
6. Cover and cook on low for 7 to 8 hours.
7. Stir in the coconut cream and serve.

Per Serving
calories: 406 | fat: 34g | protein: 22g | carbs: 5g net carbs: 3g | fiber: 2g

274. Traditional Chicken Stroganoff

Prep time: 10 minutes | Cook time: 4 hours | Serves 4

2 garlic cloves, minced
8 ounces (227 g) mushrooms, chopped
¼ teaspoon celery seeds, ground
1 cup chicken stock
1 cup sour cream
1 cup leeks, chopped
1 pound (454 g) chicken breasts
1½ teaspoon dried thyme
1 tablespoon fresh parsley, chopped
Salt and black pepper, to taste
4 zucchinis, spiralized

1. Place the chicken in a slow cooker. Place in the salt, leeks, sour cream, half of the parsley, celery seeds, garlic, black pepper, mushrooms, stock, and thyme. Cook on high for 4 hours while covered.
2. Uncover the pot and add the rest of the parsley. Heat a pan with water over medium heat, place in some salt, bring to a boil, stir in the zucchini pasta, cook for 1 minute, and drain.
3. Place in serving bowls, top with the chicken mixture, and serve.

Per Serving
calories: 365 | fat: 22g | protein: 26g | carbs: 11g net carbs: 4g | fiber: 7g

275. Garlicky Chicken Thighs

Prep time: 15 minutes | Cook time: 7 to 8 hours | Serves 4

¼ cup extra-virgin olive oil, divided
1½ pounds (680 g) boneless chicken thighs
1 teaspoon paprika
Salt, for seasoning
Freshly ground black pepper, for seasoning
1 sweet onion, chopped
4 garlic cloves, thinly sliced
½ cup chicken broth
2 tablespoons freshly squeezed lemon juice
½ cup greek yogurt

1. Lightly grease the insert of the slow cooker with 1 tablespoon of the olive oil.
2. Season the thighs with paprika, salt, and pepper.
3. In a large skillet over medium-high heat, heat the remaining olive oil. Add the chicken and brown for 5 minutes, turning once.
4. Transfer the chicken to the insert and add the onion, garlic, broth, and lemon juice.
5. Cover and cook on low for 7 to 8 hours.
6. Stir in the yogurt and serve.

Per Serving
calories: 434 | fat: 36g | protein: 22g | carbs: 5g net carbs: 4g | fiber: 1g

276. Homemade Poulet en Papillote

Prep time: 10 minutes | Cook time: 25 minutes | Serves 4

4 chicken breasts, skinless, scored
1 tablespoon white wine
1 tablespoon olive oil, plus extra for drizzling
1 tablespoon butter
3 cups mixed mushrooms, teared up
2 cups water
3 cloves garlic, minced
4 sprigs thyme, chopped
3 lemons, juiced
Salt and black pepper, to taste
1 tablespoon Dijon mustard

1. Preheat the oven to 450ºF (235ºC).
2. In a bowl, evenly mix the chicken, mushrooms, garlic, thyme, lemon juice, salt, black pepper, and mustard. Make 4 large cuts of foil, fold them in half, and then fold them in half again. Tightly fold the two open edges together to create a bag.
3. Now, share the chicken mixture into each bag, top with the white wine, olive oil, and a tablespoon of butter. Seal the last open end securely making sure not to pierce the bag. Put the bag on a baking tray and bake the chicken in the middle of the oven for 25 minutes.

Per Serving
calories: 394 | fat: 13g | protein: 25g | carbs: 6g net carbs: 5g | fiber: 1g

277. Parma Ham-Wrapped Stuffed Chicken

Prep time: 10 minutes | Cook time: 23 minutes | Serves 4

4 chicken breasts
1 tablespoon olive oil
3 cloves garlic, minced
3 shallots, finely chopped
1 tablespoon dried mixed herbs
8 slices Parma ham
8 ounces (227 g) cream cheese
2 lemons, zested
Salt, to taste

1. Preheat the oven to 350ºF (180ºC).
2. Heat the oil in a small skillet and sauté the garlic and shallots with a pinch of salt and lemon zest for 3 minutes; let it cool. After, stir the cream cheese and mixed herbs into the shallot mixture.
3. Score a pocket in each chicken breast, fill the holes with the cream cheese mixture and cover with the cut-out chicken. Wrap each breast with two Parma ham and secure the ends with a toothpick. Lay the chicken parcels on a greased baking sheet and cook in the oven for 20 minutes. Remove to rest for 4 minutes before serving with green salad and roasted tomatoes.

Per Serving
calories: 485 | fat: 35g | protein: 26g | carbs: 3g net carbs: 2g | fiber: 1g

278. oasted Chicken

Prep time: 15 minutes | Cook time: 7 to 8 hours | Serves 8

¼ cup extra-virgin olive oil, divided
1 (3-pound / 1.4-kg) whole chicken, washed and patted dry
Salt, for seasoning
Freshly ground black pepper, for seasoning
1 lemon, quartered
6 thyme sprigs
4 garlic cloves, crushed
3 bay leaves
1 sweet onion, quartered

1. Lightly grease the insert of the slow cooker with 1 tablespoon of the olive oil.
2. Rub the remaining olive oil all over the chicken and season with the salt and pepper. Stuff the lemon quarters, thyme, garlic, and bay leaves into the cavity of the chicken.
3. Place the onion quarters on the bottom of the slow cooker and place the chicken on top so it does not touch the bottom of the insert.
4. Cover and cook on low for 7 to 8 hours, or until the internal temperature reaches 165°F (74°C) on an instant-read thermometer.
5. Serve warm.

Per Serving
calories: 427 | fat: 34g | protein: 29g | carbs: 2g net carbs: 2g | fiber: 0g

279. Parmesan Chicken Wings with Yogurt Sauce

Prep time: 10 minutes | Cook time: 20 minutes | Serves 6

For the Dipping Sauce:
1 cup plain yogurt
1 teaspoon fresh lemon juice
Salt and black pepper to taste

For the Wings:
2 pounds (907 g) chicken wings
Salt and black pepper to taste
Cooking spray
½ cup melted butter
½ cup Hot sauce
¼ cup grated Parmesan cheese

1. Mix the yogurt, lemon juice, salt, and black pepper in a bowl. Chill while making the chicken.
2. Preheat oven to 400°F and season wings with salt and black pepper. Line them on a baking sheet and grease lightly with cooking spray. Bake for 20 minutes until golden brown. Mix butter, hot sauce, and Parmesan cheese in a bowl. Toss chicken in the sauce to evenly coat and plate. Serve with yogurt dipping sauce and celery strips.

Per Serving
calories: 371 | fat: 23g | protein: 36g | carbs: 3g net carbs: 3g | fiber: 0g

280. Chicken in Creamy Mushroom Sauce

Prep time: 10 minutes | Cook time: 26 minutes | Serves 4

1 tablespoon butter
4 chicken breasts, cut into chunks
Salt and black pepper to taste
1 packet white onion soup mix
2 cups chicken broth
15 baby bella mushrooms, sliced
1 cup heavy cream
1 small bunch parsley, chopped

1. Melt butter in a saucepan over medium heat, season the chicken with salt and black pepper, and brown on all sides for 6 minutes in total. Put in a plate.
2. In a bowl, stir the onion soup mix with chicken broth and add to the saucepan. Simmer for 3 minutes and add the mushrooms and chicken. Cover and simmer for another 20 minutes. Stir in heavy cream and parsley, cook on low heat for 3 minutes, and season with salt and pepper. Ladle the chicken with creamy sauce and mushrooms over beds of cauli mash. Garnish with parsley to serve.

Per Serving
calories: 448 | fat: 38g | protein: 22g | carbs: 4g net carbs: 2g | fiber: 2g

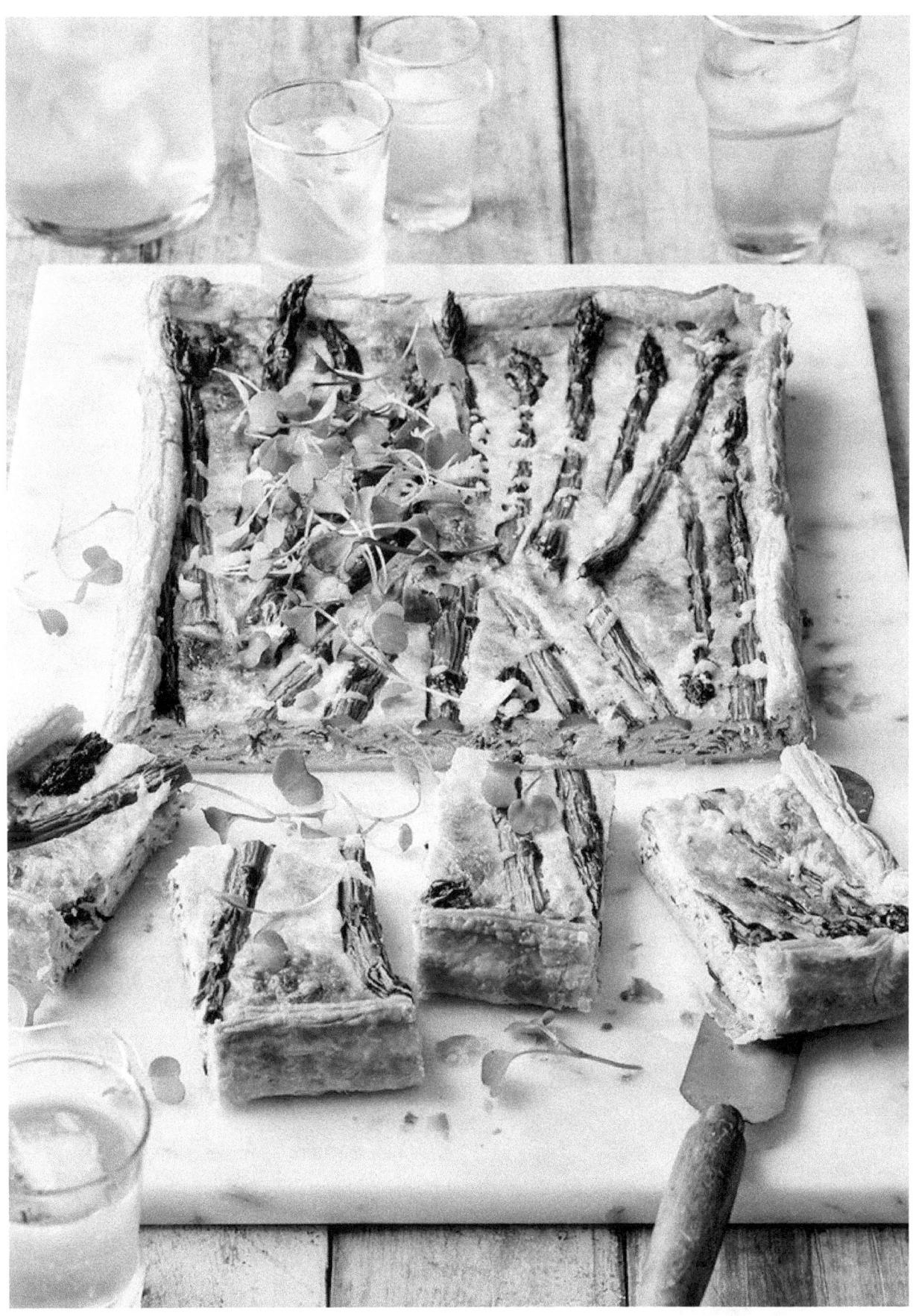

Chapter 8 Vegan and Vegetarian

281. Cauliflower and Celery Soup

Prep time: 5 minutes | Cook time: 15 minutes | Serves 4

2 green onions, chopped
½ teaspoon ginger-garlic paste
1 celery stalk, chopped
1 pound (454 g) cauliflower florets
3 cups vegetable broth

1. Heat up a lightly oiled soup pot over a medium-high flame. Now, sauté the green onions for 2 minutes, until they have softened.
2. Stir in the ginger-garlic paste, celery, cauliflower, and vegetable broth; bring to a rapid boil. Turn the heat to medium-low.
3. Continue to simmer for 13 minutes more or until heated through; heat off.
4. purée the soup in your blender until creamy and uniform. Enjoy!

Per Serving
calories: 69 | fat: 2g | protein: 6g | carbs: 7g net carbs: 4g | fiber: 3g

282. Mushroom and Bell Pepper Omelet

Prep time: 5 minutes | Cook time: 10 minutes | Serves 4

2 tablespoons olive oil
1 cup Chanterelle mushrooms, chopped
2 bell peppers, chopped
1 white onion, chopped
6 eggs

1. Heat the olive oil in a nonstick skillet over moderate heat. Now, cook the mushrooms, peppers, and onion for 5 minutes, until they have softened.
2. In a mixing bowl, whisk the eggs until frothy. Add the eggs to the skillet, reduce the heat to medium-low, and cook for approximately 5 minutes until the center starts to look dry. Do not overcook.
3. Taste and season with salt to taste. Bon appétit!

Per Serving
calories: 239 | fat: 18g | protein: 12g | carbs: 6g net carbs: 4g | fiber: 2g

283. Mushroom and Zucchini Stew

Prep time: 5 minutes | Cook time: 15 minutes | Serves 4

½ cup leeks, chopped
1 pound (454 g) brown mushrooms, chopped
1 teaspoon garlic, minced
1 medium-sized zucchini, diced
2 ripe tomatoes, puréed

1. Heat up a lightly greased soup pot over medium-high heat. Now, sauté the leeks until just tender about 3 minutes.
2. Stir in the mushrooms, garlic, and zucchini. Continue to sauté an additional 2 minutes or until tender and aromatic.
3. Add in the tomatoes and 2 cups of water. Season with Sazón spice, if desired. Reduce the temperature to simmer and continue to cook, covered, for 10 to 12 minutes more. Bon appétit!

Per Serving
calories: 108 | fat: 8g | protein: 3g | carbs: 7g net carbs: 4g | fiber: 3g

284. Double Cheese Kale Bake

Prep time: 10 minutes | Cook time: 30 to 35 minutes | Serves 4

Nonstick cooking spray
6 ounces (170 g) kale, torn into pieces
4 eggs, whisked
1 cup Cheddar cheese, grated
1 cup Romano cheese
2 tablespoons sour cream
1 garlic clove, minced
Sea salt, to taste
½ teaspoon ground black pepper, or more to taste
½ teaspoon cayenne pepper

1. Start by preheating your oven to 365ºF (185ºC). Spritz the sides and bottom of a baking pan with a nonstick cooking spray.
2. Mix all ingredients and pour the mixture into the baking pan.
3. Bake for 30 to 35 minutes or until it is thoroughly heated. Bon appétit!

Per Serving
calories: 384 | fat: 29g | protein: 25g | carbs: 6g net carbs: 4g | fiber: 2g

285. Lemony Cucumber-Avocado Salad

Prep time: 5 minutes | Cook time: 0 minutes | Serves 6

1 avocado, peeled, pitted and sliced
½ white onion, chopped
1 Lebanese cucumber, sliced
3 teaspoons fresh lemon juice
2 tablespoons extra-virgin olive oil

1. Toss all ingredients in a nice salad bowl.
2. Transfer to your refrigerator until ready to serve.
3. Serve well chilled and enjoy!

Per Serving
calories: 149 | fat: 14g | protein: 2g | carbs: 6g net carbs: 2g | fiber: 4g

286. Citrus Asparagus and Cherry Tomato Salad

Prep time: 10 minutes | Cook time: 16 minutes | Serves 3

1 pound (454 g) asparagus, trimmed
¼ teaspoon ground black pepper
Flaky salt, to season
3 tablespoons sesame seeds
1 tablespoon Dijon mustard
½ lime, freshly squeezed
3 tablespoons extra-virgin olive oil
2 garlic cloves, minced
1 tablespoon fresh tarragon, snipped
1 cup cherry tomatoes, sliced

1. Start by preheating your oven to 395°F (202°C). Spritz a roasting pan with nonstick cooking spray.
2. Roast the asparagus for about 13 minutes, turning the spears over once or twice. Sprinkle with salt, pepper, and sesame seeds; roast an additional 3 to 4 minutes.
3. To make the dressing, whisk the Dijon mustard, lime juice, olive oil, and minced garlic.
4. Chop the asparagus spears into bite-sized pieces and place them in a nice salad bowl. Add the tarragon and tomatoes to the bowl; gently toss to combine.
5. Dress your salad and serve at room temperature. Enjoy!

Per Serving
calories: 159 | fat: 12g | protein: 6g | carbs: 6g net carbs: 2g | fiber: 4g

287. Shirataki Mushroom Ramen

Prep time: 10 minutes | Cook time: 13 to 18 minutes | Serves 4

1½ tablespoons butter, melted
1 pound (454 g) brown mushrooms, chopped
1 teaspoon ginger-garlic paste
½ teaspoon ground cumin
½ teaspoon ground coriander
¼ teaspoon ground black pepper, or more to taste
Sea salt, to taste
2 tablespoons green onions, chopped
4 cups roasted vegetable broth
8 ounces (227 g) shirataki noodles

1. Melt the butter in a soup pot over moderate heat. Then, sauté the mushrooms for about 3 minutes or until they are just tender.
2. Stir in the ginger-garlic paste, cumin, coriander, black pepper, salt, and green onions. Pour in the roasted vegetable broth and bring to a boil.
3. Immediately reduce the heat to medium-low. Let it simmer for 8 to 11 minutes. Fold in the shirataki noodles and cook for 2 to 4 minutes more.
4. Serve hot and enjoy!

Per Serving
calories: 76 | fat: 5g | protein: 4g | carbs: 5g net carbs: 4g | fiber: 1g

288. Peanut Butter Crêpes with Coconut

Prep time: 5 minutes | Cook time: 4 to 5 minutes | Serves 5

4 eggs, well whisked
4 ounces (113 g) cream cheese
A pinch of salt
2 tablespoons coconut oil
3 tablespoons peanut butter
2 tablespoons toasted coconut

1. Whisk the eggs, cream cheese, and salt in a mixing bowl.
2. Heat the oil in a pancake frying pan over medium-high heat.
3. Fry each pancake for 4 to 5 minutes. Serve topped with peanut butter and coconut. Enjoy!

Per Serving
calories: 248 | fat: 22g | protein: 9g | carbs: 6g net carbs: 5g | fiber: 1g

289. Greek-Style Aubergine-Egg Casserole

Prep time: 5 minutes | Cook time: 57 minutes | Serves 5

1 pound (454 g) aubergine, cut into rounds
2 vine-ripe tomatoes, sliced
5 eggs, beaten
1 cup Greek-style yogurt
1½ cups feta cheese, grated

1. Place the aubergine on a large pan lined with paper towel; toss with 1 teaspoon of sea salt and let it stand for 25 minutes in a colander.
2. Pat your aubergine dry and transfer to a lightly oiled baking sheet. Brush them with olive oil. Bake in the preheated oven at 390ºF (199ºC) for about 40 minutes, or until they are golden brown.
3. Layer the rounds of roasted aubergine on the bottom of a lightly oiled casserole dish. Top with sliced tomatoes.
4. In a mixing dish, whisk the eggs with the yogurt. Pour the mixture over the prepared vegetables. Top with feta cheese and bake in the preheated oven at 360ºF (182ºC) for 17 minutes. Enjoy!

Per Serving

calories: 226 | fat: 14g | protein: 16g | carbs: 7g net carbs:4 g | fiber: 3g

290. Cheesy Egg-Stuffed Avocados

Prep time: 5 minutes | Cook time: 15 minutes | Serves 4

2 avocados, pitted and halved
4 eggs
Sea salt and freshly ground black pepper, to taste
1 cup Asiago cheese, grated
½ teaspoon red pepper flakes
½ teaspoon dried rosemary
1 tablespoon fresh chives, chopped

1. Crack the eggs into the avocado halves, keeping the yolks intact. Sprinkle with salt and black pepper.
2. Top with cheese, red pepper flakes, and rosemary. Arrange the stuffed avocado halves in a baking pan.
3. Bake in the preheated oven at 420ºF (216ºC) for about 15 minutes. Serve garnished with fresh chives. Enjoy!

Per Serving

calories: 300 | fat: 25g | protein: 15g | carbs: 6g net carbs: 1g | fiber: 5g

291. Mexican-Flavored Stuffed Peppers

Prep time: 5 minutes | Cook time: 40 minutes | Serves 3

3 bell peppers, halved, seeded
3 eggs, whisked
1 cup Mexican cheese blend
1 teaspoon chili powder
1 garlic clove, minced
1 teaspoon onion powder
1 ripe tomato, puréed
1 teaspoon mustard powder

1. Start by preheating your oven to 370ºF (188ºC). Spritz the bottom and sides of a baking pan with a cooking oil.
2. In a mixing bowl, thoroughly combine the eggs, cheese, chili powder, garlic, and onion powder. Divide the filling between the bell peppers.
3. Mix the tomatoes with mustard powder and transfer the mixture to the baking pan. Cover with foil and bake for 40 minutes, until the peppers are tender and the filling is thoroughly heated. Bon appétit!

Per Serving

calories: 194 | fat: 14g | protein: 13g | carbs: 4g net carbs: 3g | fiber: 1g

292. Halloumi Asparagus Frittata

Prep time: 10 minutes | Cook time: 20 minutes | Serves 4

1 tablespoon olive oil
½ red onion, sliced
4 ounces (113 g) asparagus, cut into small chunks
1 tomato, chopped
5 whole eggs, beaten
10 ounces (284 g) Halloumi cheese, crumbled
2 tablespoons green olives, pitted and sliced
1 tablespoon fresh parsley, chopped

1. Heat the oil in a skillet over medium-high heat; then, cook the onion and asparagus about 3 minutes, stirring continuously.
2. Next, add the tomato and cook for 2 minutes longer. Transfer the sautéed vegetables to a baking pan that is lightly greased with cooking oil.
3. Mix the eggs with cheese until well combined. Pour the mixture over the vegetables. Scatter sliced olives over the top. Bake in the preheated oven at 350ºF (180ºC) for 15 minutes.
4. Garnish with fresh parsley and serve immediately. Enjoy!

Per Serving

calories: 376 | fat: 29g | protein: 25g | carbs: 4g net carbs: 3g | fiber: 1g

293. Cheesy Broccoli Bake

Prep time: 5 minutes | Cook time: 27 minutes | Serves 6

6 eggs
6 ounces (170 g) sour cream
1 cup vegetable broth
¾ pound (340 g) broccoli florets
6 ounces (170 g) Swiss cheese, shredded

1. Start by preheating your oven to 360°F (182°C). Then, spritz a baking pan with nonstick cooking spray.
2. Thoroughly combine the eggs, sour cream, and vegetable broth.
3. Bring a pot with lightly salted water to a boil. Add the broccoli florets to the boiling water and cook for 2 minutes.
4. Arrange the broccoli florets on the bottom of the prepared pan. Pour the egg/cream mixture over the broccoli. Top with the shredded cheese.
5. Bake for 25 to 28 minutes, turning your pan once or twice. Bon appétit!

Per Serving
calories: 241 | fat: 16g | protein: 16g | carbs: 6g net carbs: 4g | fiber: 2g

294. Swiss Zucchini Gratin

Prep time: 10 minutes | Cook time: 10 minutes | Serves 5

10 large eggs
3 tablespoons yogurt
2 zucchinis, sliced
½ medium-sized leek, sliced
Sea salt and ground black pepper, to taste
1 teaspoon cayenne pepper
1 cup cream cheese
2 garlic cloves, minced
1 cup Swiss cheese, shredded

1. Start by preheating your oven to 360°F (182°C). Then, spritz the bottom and sides of an oven proof pan with a nonstick cooking spray. Then, mix the eggs with yogurt until well combined.
2. Overlap ½ of the zucchini and leek slices in the pan. Season with salt, black pepper, and cayenne pepper. Add cream cheese and minced garlic.
3. Add the remaining zucchini slices and leek. Add the egg mixture. Top with Swiss cheese. Bake for 40 minutes, until the top is golden brown. Bon appétit!

Per Serving
calories: 371 | fat: 32g | protein: 16g | carbs: 5g net carbs: 4g | fiber: 1g

295. Garlicky Creamed Swiss Chard

Prep time: 10 minutes | Cook time: 10 minutes | Serves 6

2 tablespoons butter
1 yellow onion, chopped
2 garlic cloves, minced
½ teaspoon kosher salt
¼ teaspoon ground black pepper
¼ teaspoon dried oregano
¼ teaspoon dried dill
1½ pounds (680 g) Swiss chard
½ cup vegetable broth
2 tablespoons dry white wine
1 cup sour cream

1. Melt the butter in a saucepan over a moderate flame. Then, sauté the onion until tender and fragrant or about 4 minutes.
2. Stir in the garlic and continue to sauté for 1 minute or until aromatic. Add in the salt, black pepper, oregano, and basil.
3. Fold in the Swiss chard in batches. Pour in vegetable broth and cook for 5 minutes or until Swiss chard wilts. Stir in the wine and sour cream. Stir to combine well and serve.

Per Serving
calories: 149 | fat: 11g | protein: 5g | carbs: 7g net carbs: 5g | fiber: 2g

296. Broccoli-Cabbage Soup

Prep time: 10 minutes | Cook time: 29 minutes | Serves 6

2 tablespoons extra-virgin olive oil
2 bell peppers, chopped
1 cup broccoli florets
1 shallot, chopped
1 teaspoon garlic, minced
1 pound (454 g) cabbage, shredded
1 cup tomato purée
5 cups vegetable broth
Sea salt and ground black pepper, to taste
½ teaspoon cayenne pepper
½ teaspoon dried dill weed
1 bay laurel

1. Heat the oil in a heavy-bottomed pot over the highest setting. Now, sauté the bell peppers, broccoli and shallot for about 4 minutes or until they have softened.
2. Add in the remaining ingredients and gently stir to combine well.
3. Turn the heat to medium-low; let it simmer, partially covered, for 25 minutes.
4. Ladle into individual bowls and serve warm. Enjoy!

Per Serving
calories: 82 | fat: 4g | protein: 2g | carbs: 6g net carbs: 3g | fiber: 3g

297. Cauliflower Chowder with Fresh Dill

Prep time: 10 minutes | Cook time: 31 minutes | Serves 4

1 tablespoon butter, softened at room temperature
½ stalk celery, chopped
1 white onion, chopped
1 teaspoon ginger-garlic paste
1 pound (454 g) cauliflower florets
Sea salt and white pepper, to taste
1 teaspoon ground sumac
4 cups roasted vegetable broth
1 cup heavy whipping cream
2 tablespoons fresh dill, chopped

1. Melt the butter in a heavy pot over medium-high heat. Then, sauté the celery and onions for 5 minutes, until just tender and fragrant.
2. Stir in the ginger-garlic paste, cauliflower, salt, white pepper, and sumac; continue to sauté for 1 minute more.
3. Pour in the vegetable broth, bringing to a rapid boil. Immediately turn the heat to medium-low. Cover part-way and continue to simmer for about 25 minutes.
4. Purée the chowder using an immersion blender or food processor until you achieve your desired smoothness. Return the chowder to the pot and fold in the heavy whipping cream.
5. Cook briefly until your chowder is all warmed through. Test and adjust seasonings as needed.
6. Garnish with fresh dill and serve warm.

Per Serving

calories: 172 | fat: 15g | protein: 3g | carbs: 7g net carbs: 4g | fiber: 3g

298. Provolone Zucchini Lasagna

Prep time: 20 minutes | Cook time: 56 minutes | Serves 2

1 large-sized zucchini, sliced lengthwise
1 tablespoon olive oil
1 red bell pepper, chopped
1 shallot, chopped
½ pound (227 g) chestnut mushrooms, chopped
2 cloves garlic, pressed
Sea salt and ground black pepper, to season
¼ teaspoon red pepper flakes
¼ teaspoon dried oregano
½ teaspoon dried dill weed
1 vine-ripe tomato, puréed
1 egg, whisked
½ cup Greek-style yogurt
½ cup Provolone cheese, grated

1. Place the zucchini slices in a bowl with a colander; add 1 teaspoon of salt and let it stand for 12 to 15 minutes; gently squeeze to discard the excess water.
2. Grill the zucchini slices for 3 minutes per side until beginning to brown; reserve.
3. Heat the olive oil in a skillet over moderate flame. Now, sauté the pepper and shallot for 3 minutes, until they have softened.
4. Next, stir in the mushrooms and garlic; continue sautéing until they are just fragrant. Add in the spices and puréed tomatoes and let it cook until heated through or about 5 minutes.
5. Pour the mushroom/tomato purée on the bottom of a lightly greased baking pan. Arrange the zucchini slices on top.
6. Mix the egg with the Greek yogurt; add the mixture to the top. Top with the grated Provolone cheese and transfer to the preheated oven.
7. Bake at 370ºF (188ºC) approximately 45 minutes until the cheese is melted and the edges are bubbling.
8. Let your lasagna stand for about 8 minutes before slicing and serving. Bon appétit!

Per Serving

calories: 284 | fat: 18g | protein: 20g | carbs: 8g net carbs: 5g | fiber: 3g

299. Creamy Broccoli and Zucchini Soup

Prep time: 10 minutes | Cook time: 25 minutes | Serves 4

3 tablespoons olive oil
2 cups broccoli florets
1 green bell pepper, chopped
1 jalapeño pepper, chopped
1 medium zucchini, cut into chunks
4 cups vegetable broth
Kosher salt and ground black pepper, to taste
½ teaspoon dried dill weed
1 bay laurel

1. Heat the olive oil in a heavy-bottomed pot over medium-high heat. Now, sauté the broccoli, peppers, and zucchini for 5 minutes, until they have softened.
2. Add in the remaining ingredients and stir to combine. Cook until the soup comes to a boil. Turn the heat to simmer.
3. Partially cover and let it simmer for a further 20 minutes or until heated through. Purée with an immersion blender and serve warm. Bon appétit!

Per Serving

calories: 111 | fat: 10g | protein: 2g | carbs: 4g net carbs: 2g | fiber: 2g

Chapter 8 Vegan and Vegetarian

300. Cheesy Veggie Fritters

Prep time: 10 minutes | Cook time: 5 to 6 minutes | Serves 5

1 pound (454 g) cauliflower florets
1 celery stalk, chopped
1 small-sized zucchini, cut into rounds
1 shallot, chopped
Sea salt and freshly ground black pepper, to taste
½ teaspoon cayenne pepper
2 garlic cloves, minced
1 cup Parmesan cheese, shredded
1 egg, beaten
½ cup almond meal
2 tablespoons sesame oil

1. Pulse the cauliflower florets and celery in a food processor until they've broken down into "rice". Then, pulse the zucchini and shallot in your food processor for 30 to 40 seconds.
2. Mix the grated vegetables with the salt, black pepper, cayenne pepper, garlic, parmesan cheese, egg, and almond meal. Shape the mixture into small patties.
3. Heat the sesame oil in a frying pan and fry the patties for 5 to 6 minutes until golden brown and thoroughly cooked. Bon appétit!

Per Serving
calories: 173 | fat: 11g | protein: 11g | carbs: 7g net carbs: 4g | fiber: 3g

301. Creamy Summer Stew with Chives

Prep time: 10 minutes | Cook time: 28 minutes | Serves 4

2 teaspoons sesame oil
2 bell peppers, seeded and chopped
1 small-sized shallot, chopped
1 summer zucchini, chopped
4 cups vegetable broth
2 vine-ripe tomatoes
4 tablespoons sour cream, well-chilled
2 tablespoons fresh chives, minced

1. Heat the sesame oil in a heavy pot over moderate flame. Sauté the bell peppers and shallot for 3 minutes, until just tender and aromatic.
2. Stir in the zucchini, broth, tomatoes, and stir to combine. Bring to a rolling boil. Immediately reduce the heat to medium-low and let it simmer for 25 minutes until everything is thoroughly cooked.
3. Ladle into individual bowls and garnish with sour cream and fresh chives. Enjoy!

Per Serving
calories: 67 | fat: 4g | protein: 2g | carbs: 6g net carbs: 4g | fiber: 2g

302. Vegetable Stir-Fry with Seeds

Prep time: 10 minutes | Cook time: 11 minutes | Serves 3

2 tablespoons sesame oil
1 yellow onion, sliced
1 red bell pepper, seeded and sliced
2 garlic cloves, minced
1 tomato, chopped
½ cup cream of mushroom soup
Sea salt and ground black pepper, to taste
½ teaspoon cayenne pepper
½ teaspoon celery seeds
½ teaspoon fennel seeds

1. Heat the sesame oil in a wok over medium-high heat. Stir fry the onion and peppers for 3 to 4 minutes.
2. Add in the garlic and continue to cook for 30 seconds more. Add in the remaining ingredients and cook for a further 8 minutes.
3. Taste, adjust seasonings and serve warm. Enjoy!

Per Serving
calories: 118 | fat: 10g | protein: 2g | carbs: 6g net carbs: 5g | fiber: 1g

303. Spinach and Zucchini Chowder

Prep time: 15 minutes | Cook time: 22 minutes | Serves 4

1 tablespoon olive oil
1 clove garlic, chopped
½ cup scallions, chopped
4 cups water
2 zucchini, sliced
1 celery stalk, chopped
2 tablespoons vegetable bouillon powder
4 ounces (113 g) baby spinach
Salt and ground black pepper, to taste
1 heaping tablespoon fresh parsley, chopped
1 tablespoon butter
1 egg, beaten

1. In a stockpot, heat the oil over medium-high heat. Now, cook the garlic and scallions until tender or about 4 minutes.
2. Add water, zucchini, celery, vegetable bouillon powder; cook for 13 minutes. Add spinach, salt, black pepper, parsley, and butter; cook for a further 5 minutes.
3. Then, stir in the egg and mix until well incorporated. Ladle into individual bowls and serve warm. Enjoy!

Per Serving
calories: 85 | fat: 6g | protein: 4g | carbs: 4g net carbs: 3g | fiber: 1g

304. Easy Roasted Asparagus with Mayo Sauce

Prep time: 10 minutes | Cook time: 9 to 11 minutes | Serves 5

1½ pounds (680 g) asparagus, trimmed
4 tablespoons olive oil
Sea salt and ground black pepper, to taste
4 tablespoons shallots, minced
½ cup mayonnaise
4 tablespoons sour cream
2 tablespoons coriander, chopped
1 teaspoon fresh garlic, minced

1. Begin by preheating your oven to 390ºF (199ºC). Brush the asparagus spears with olive oil. Add the salt, black pepper, and shallots and roast for 9 to 11 minutes in the preheated oven.
2. Meanwhile, mix the remaining ingredients to make the dipping sauce.
3. Serve the asparagus with the mayo sauce on the side and enjoy!

Per Serving
calories: 296 | fat: 28g | protein: 4g | carbs: 7g net carbs: 4g | fiber: 3g

305. Spiced Mashed Cauliflower

Prep time: 5 minutes | Cook time: 5 minutes | Serves 8

½ pound (227 g) cauliflower florets
Sea salt and ground black pepper, to taste
½ teaspoon cayenne pepper
½ teaspoon dried oregano
½ teaspoon dried basil
1 cup heavy whipping cream
5 ounces (142 g) Swiss cheese, grated

1. Steam the cauliflower for 5 minutes, until tender; pulse in your food processor until it resembles mashed potatoes.
2. Season the mashed cauliflower with salt, black pepper, cayenne pepper, oregano, and basil.
3. In a saucepan, warm the cream and stir in the cheese. Whisk until the cheese is melted.
4. Fold in the mashed cauliflower and stir again. Serve with your favorite keto veggies. Bon appétit!

Per Serving
calories: 129 | fat: 10g | protein: 6g | carbs: 3g net carbs: 2g | fiber: 1g

306. Italian Broccoli and Spinach Soup

Prep time: 15 minutes | Cook time: 30 minutes | Serves 3

4 ounces (113 g) broccoli
2 tablespoons sesame oil
1 small-sized onion, chopped
2 garlic cloves, minced
1 teaspoon cayenne pepper
Sea salt and ground black pepper, to taste
1 cup spinach leaves, torn into pieces
1 celery stalk, peeled and chopped
2 cups vegetable broth
1 cup water
1 tomato, puréed
1 jalapeño pepper, minced
1 tablespoon Italian seasonings

1. Pulse the broccoli in your food processor until rice-sized pieces are formed; work in batches; reserve.
2. Then, heat the oil in a saucepan over medium heat. Then, sauté the onion and garlic for 3 minutes, until tender and aromatic.
3. Add the broccoli and cook for 2 minutes more. Add the remaining ingredients, except the spinach.
4. Bring to a rapid boil and then, immediately reduce the heat to medium-low. Now, simmer the soup approximately 25 minutes.
5. Add spinach, turn off the heat, and cover with the lid; let it wilt. Bon appétit!

Per Serving
calories: 137 | fat: 11g | protein: 6g | carbs: 6g net carbs: 5g | fiber: 1g

307. Braised Mushrooms with Parsley

Prep time: 10 minutes | Cook time: 6 hours | Serves 8

3 tablespoons extra-virgin olive oil
1 pound (454 g) button mushrooms, wiped clean and halved
2 teaspoons minced garlic
¼ teaspoon salt
⅛ teaspoon freshly ground black pepper
2 tablespoons chopped fresh parsley

1. Place the olive oil, mushrooms, garlic, salt, and pepper in the insert of the slow cooker and toss to coat.
2. Cover and cook on low for 6 hours.
3. Serve tossed with the parsley.

Per Serving
calories: 58 | fat: 5g | protein: 2g | carbs: 2g net carbs: 1g | fiber: 1g

308. Colby Broccoli Bake

Prep time: 10 minutes | Cook time: 26 minutes | Serves 5

1 pound (454 g) broccoli florets
1 cup yellow onion, sliced
2 cloves garlic, smashed
½ cup heavy cream
1 cup vegetable broth
1 cup Colby cheese, shredded
1 teaspoon cayenne pepper
½ teaspoon dried oregano
½ teaspoon basil
½ teaspoon ground bay laurel
Sea salt and ground black pepper, to taste

1. Bring a saucepan with salted water to a boil. Parboil your broccoli for 2 to 3 minutes until crisp-tender. Throw the broccoli into a lightly oiled baking dish.
2. Add in the onion and garlic. In a mixing dish, whisk the heavy cream with the vegetable broth. Season with cayenne pepper, oregano, basil, ground bay laurel, salt, and black pepper.
3. Pour the cream mixture over the vegetables in the baking dish. Bake in the preheated oven at 390°F (199°C) for 18 minutes.
4. Top with the cheese and continue to bake an additional 6 minutes or until bubbling. Bon appétit!

Per Serving
calories: 194 | fat: 14g | protein: 9g | carbs: 7g net carbs: 4g | fiber: 3g

309. Hearty Veggie Stir-Fry

Prep time: 20 minutes | Cook time: 15 minutes | Serves 3

4 tablespoons sesame oil
½ cup shallot, chopped
2 cups white mushrooms, sliced
1 zucchini, spiralized
1 cup cauliflower rice
2 cloves garlic, minced
Kosher salt and ground black pepper, to taste
½ teaspoon turmeric powder
½ teaspoon cayenne pepper
½ teaspoon mustard seeds
2 tomatoes, puréed
3 eggs
3 ounces (85 g) Asiago cheese, shredded

1. Heat 1 tablespoon of the sesame oil in a wok over medium-high heat. Now, cook the shallot and mushrooms until just tender and fragrant or about 3 minutes; reserve.
2. In the same wok, heat another tablespoon of the sesame oil. Fry the zucchini until crisp-tender about 2 minutes or so; reserve.
3. Heat another tablespoon of the sesame oil and cook the cauliflower rice for 3 to 4 minutes or until just tender and fragrant. Return the sautéed vegetables to the wok.
4. Add in the garlic, spices and tomatoes and stir for 2 minutes more or until heated through.
5. In a nonstick skillet, heat the remaining tablespoon of sesame oil. Fry the eggs over medium-high heat until they are set or about 5 minutes.
6. Divide the vegetables between three serving plates. Top each serving with the fried egg. Garnish with Asiago cheese and serve immediately.

Per Serving
calories: 378 | fat: 32g | protein: 15g | carbs: 7g net carbs: 5g | fiber:2 g

310. Braised Mushrooms and Cabbage

Prep time: 15 minutes | Cook time: 13 minutes | Serves 3

2 tablespoons extra-virgin olive oil
½ cup onion, chopped
2 cups brown mushrooms, sliced
1 garlic clove, pressed
¾ pound (340 g) green cabbage, shredded
½ cup cream of mushroom soup
1 bay laurel
Kosher salt, to season
½ teaspoon caraway seeds
½ teaspoon ground black pepper, to taste
1 teaspoon smoked paprika
1 tablespoon apple cider vinegar

1. Heat the oil in a heavy-bottomed pot over medium-high heat. Now, sweat the onion for 3 minutes, until tender and translucent.
2. Next, stir in the mushrooms; continue to sauté until the mushrooms are caramelized or about 3 minutes. Don't crowd the mushrooms.
3. Stir in the garlic and sauté for 30 seconds longer or until aromatic. Add in the green cabbage, soup, bay laurel, salt, caraway seeds, black pepper, and paprika.
4. Continue cooking for 7 to 8 minutes more or until the cabbage leaves wilt. Ladle into three serving bowls.
5. Drizzle vinegar over each serving and serve warm. Bon appétit!

Per Serving
calories: 133 | fat: 9g | protein: 4g | carbs: 7g net carbs: 3g | fiber: 4g

311. Balsamic Zucchini Salad

Prep time: 15 minutes | Cook time: 9 minutes | Serves 5

1½ pounds (680 g) zucchini, sliced
4 tablespoons extra-virgin olive oil, divided
Sea salt and ground black pepper, to taste
½ teaspoon cayenne pepper
½ teaspoon dried dill weed
½ teaspoon dried basil
1 red onion, sliced
1 garlic clove, pressed
2 tomatoes, sliced
1 teaspoon Dijon mustard
1 tablespoon balsamic vinegar
1 tablespoon fresh lime juice
4 ounces (113 g) goat cheese, crumbled

1. Toss the zucchini with 2 tablespoons of olive oil and spices. Arrange them on a rimmed baking sheet.
2. Roast in the preheated oven at 425ºF (220ºC) until tender about 9 minutes. Toss roasted zucchini with red onion, garlic, and tomatoes.
3. Add the remaining tablespoons of olive oil, mustard, vinegar, and lime juice. Toss to combine and top with goat cheese. Enjoy!

Per Serving

calories: 186 | fat: 14g | protein: 11g | carbs: 7g net carbs: 5g | fiber: 2g

312. Creamy Cabbage and Cauliflower

Prep time: 5 minutes | Cook time: 13 minutes | Serves 4

2 tablespoons olive oil
1 white onion, chopped
½ pound (227 g) savoy cabbage, shredded
½ pound (227 g) cauliflower florets
1 bell pepper
1 cup cream of mushroom soup
1 cup heavy whipping cream
Sea salt and red pepper flakes, to taste

1. Heat the olive oil in a saucepan over a moderate flame. Now, sauté the onion for 3 minutes, until just tender and fragrant.
2. Stir in the cabbage, cauliflower, bell pepper, and cream of mushroom soup. Reduce the heat to medium-low; let it cook for 8 minutes more until the vegetables have softened.
3. Fold in the heavy whipping cream and continue to simmer for 2 to 3 minutes more. Sprinkle with salt and red pepper to taste. Serve warm.

Per Serving

calories: 256 | fat: 24g | protein: 3g | carbs: 7g net carbs: 4g | fiber: 3g

313. Peppery Omelet with Cheddar Cheese

Prep time: 10 minutes | Cook time: 8 minutes | Serves 2

2 tablespoons olive oil
1 onion, sliced
2 bell peppers, chopped
1 jalapeño pepper, chopped
4 eggs, whisked
4 tablespoons full-fat yogurt
½ teaspoon red pepper flakes
Sea salt and ground black pepper, to season
3 ounces (85 g) Cheddar cheese, shredded

1. Heat the olive oil in a frying pan over a moderate flame. Sauté the onion and peppers for 3 minutes, until tender and fragrant.
2. Then, mix the eggs with the full-fat yogurt. Now, pour the egg mixture into the frying pan. Season with red pepper, salt, and black pepper.
3. Move the pan around to spread it out evenly.
4. Continue to cook for about 5 minutes until the eggs are fully set and the surface is smooth. Top with cheese and serve immediately. Bon appétit!

Per Serving

calories: 439 | fat: 37g | protein: 23g | carbs: 4g net carbs: 4g | fiber: 0g

314. Parmesan Zoodles with Avocado Sauce

Prep time: 10 minutes | Cook time: 0 minutes | Serves 2

½ avocado, pitted and peeled
2 tablespoons sunflower seeds, hulled
1 ripe tomato, quartered
2 tablespoons water
Sea salt and ground black pepper, to taste
¼ teaspoon dried dill weed
1 medium-sized zucchini, sliced
2 tablespoons Parmesan cheese, preferably freshly grated

1. In your blender or food processor, purée the avocado, sunflower seeds, tomato, water, salt, black pepper, and dill until creamy and uniform.
2. Prepare your zoodles using a spiralizer.
3. Top the zoodles with the sauce; serve garnished with parmesan cheese. Bon appétit!

Per Serving

calories: 164 | fat: 14g | protein: 6g | carbs: 9g net carbs: 4g | fiber: 5g

315. Chinese Cabbage Stir-Fry

Prep time: 10 minutes | Cook time: 7 minutes | Serves 5

3 tablespoons sesame oil
1 shallot, sliced
2 garlic cloves, minced
1 tablespoon Shaoxing wine
Sea salt and ground black pepper, to taste
½ teaspoon chili sauce, sugar-free
¼ teaspoon rougui (Chinese cinnamon)
½ teaspoon fennel seeds
½ teaspoon Sichuan peppercorns, crushed
1½ pounds (680 g) Chinese cabbage, shredded

1. Heat the sesame oil in a wok over medium-high heat.
2. Once hot, sauté the shallot and garlic until tender and translucent or about 2 minutes. Add the Shaoxing wine to deglaze the pan.
3. Add in the remaining ingredients.
4. Cook, stirring continuously, until the cabbage leaves are wilted about 5 minutes. Serve with some extra toasted sesame seeds if desired. Enjoy!

Per Serving
calories: 108 | fat: 9g | protein: 2g | carbs: 8g net carbs: 6g | fiber: 2g

316. Balsamic Broccoli Salad

Prep time: 10 minutes | Cook time: 22 minutes | Serves 6

6 cups broccoli florets
1 red chili pepper, sliced
1 garlic clove, minced
1 shallot, sliced
½ cup mayonnaise
1 teaspoon Dijon mustard
2 tablespoons balsamic vinegar
1 tablespoon prepared horseradish
Kosher salt and ground black pepper, to taste

1. Brush the broccoli florets with nonstick cooking spray and roast at 425ºF (220ºC) for about 22 minutes until crisp-tender and little charred.
2. In a salad bowl, toss the roasted broccoli florets, chili pepper, garlic, and shallot.
3. In a small mixing dish, thoroughly combine the remaining ingredients.
4. Dress the salad and serve immediately. Bon appétit!

Per Serving
calories: 170 | fat: 14g | protein: 3g | carbs: 7g net carbs: 4g | fiber: 3g

317. Herbed Cheese Balls with Walnuts

Prep time: 5 minutes | Cook time: 0 minutes | Serves 6

4 ounces (113 g) Neufchatel cheese
4 ounces (113 g) blue cheese
Sea salt and freshly cracked black pepper, to taste
2 tablespoons fresh parsley, chopped
2 tablespoons fresh cilantro, chopped
8 tablespoons walnuts, finely chopped

1. Thoroughly combine the cheese, salt, black pepper, parsley, and cilantro in a bowl.
2. Shape into 8 balls and roll them in the chopped walnuts. Refrigerate until ready to serve. Bon appétit!

Per Serving
calories: 183 | fat: 16g | protein: 8g | carbs: 3g net carbs: 2g | fiber: 1g

318. Fried Veggies with Eggs

Prep time: 10 minutes | Cook time: 23 minutes | Serves 4

2 tablespoons olive oil
1 shallot, sliced
2 bell peppers, seeded and sliced
2 garlic cloves, minced
½ teaspoon ginger, peeled and minced
1 cup green cabbage, shredded
1 cup broccoli florets
1 cup cauliflower florets
½ cup cream of onion soup
4 eggs

1. Heat the olive oil in a large-sized frying pan over high heat. Now, fry the shallots and pepper for 3 minutes, until just tender. Add in the garlic and ginger; continue sautéing for 30 seconds more until aromatic.
2. Then, stir in the cabbage, broccoli, cauliflower, and onion soup. Turn the heat to medium-low. Continue to cook for 10 minutes or until tender and thoroughly cooked.
3. Next, make four indentations in the vegetable mixture using the back of a wooden spoon. Crack the eggs into the indentations.
4. Cover your frying pan with a lid. Cook for a further10 minutes or until the egg whites are firm but the yolks are a little runny. Serve immediately.

Per Serving
calories: 121 | fat: 7g | protein: 7g | carbs: 7g net carbs: 5g | fiber: 2g

319. Creamy Broccoli-Spinach Soup

Prep time: 15 minutes | Cook time: 10 to 13 minutes | Serves 2

1 tablespoon butter, at room temperature	1 bay laurel
½ small-sized leek, chopped	1 thyme sprig, chopped
¼ cup celery rib, chopped	1 cup spinach leaves
½ teaspoon ginger garlic paste	Kosher salt and ground black pepper, to taste
1½ cups broccoli florets	2 tablespoons cream cheese
1½ cups roasted vegetable broth	1 tablespoon tahini butter
	⅓ cup yogurt

1. In a Dutch pot, melt the butter over medium-high heat. Now, sauté the leeks and celery for 3 minutes until just tender and fragrant.
2. Add the ginger-garlic paste and continue cooking an additional 30 seconds or until aromatic.
3. Now, stir in the broccoli, broth, bay laurel, and thyme, and bring it to a rapid boil. Then, turn the heat to low and let it simmer, covered, for a further 5 to 8 minutes.
4. After that, stir in the spinach, salt, and black pepper; let it simmer for 2 minutes more or until the leaves have wilted.
5. Transfer the soup to a food processor; add the cream cheese and tahini butter; process until everything is smooth and uniform. Swirl the yogurt into the soup and serve warm. Bon appétit!

Per Serving

calories: 208 | fat: 16g | protein: 9g | carbs: 6g net carbs: 3g | fiber: 3g

320. Mediterranean Cauliflower Quiche

Prep time: 15 minutes | Cook time: 45 minutes | Serves 2

½ pound (227 g) small cauliflower florets	black pepper, to taste
½ cup vegetable broth	½ teaspoon paprika
2 scallions, chopped	½ teaspoon basil
1 teaspoon garlic, crushed	½ teaspoon oregano
½ cup almond milk	1 ounce (28 g) sour cream
2 eggs, whisked	3 ounces (85 g) Provolone cheese, freshly grated
Sea salt and ground	

1. Cook the cauliflower with the vegetable broth over medium-low flame until tender but crispy. Transfer the cauliflower florets to a lightly greased casserole dish.
2. Then, preheat your oven to 360°F (182°C). In a mixing dish, thoroughly combine the scallions, garlic, milk, eggs, salt, black pepper, paprika, basil, and oregano.
3. Pour the scallion mixture over the cauliflower florets. Mix the sour cream and Provolone cheese; add the cheese mixture to the top. Cover with foil.
4. Bake in the preheated oven for about 45 minutes, until topping is lightly golden and everything is heated through.
5. Transfer to a cooling rack for 10 minutes before serving. Bon appétit!

Per Serving

calories: 309 | fat: 21g | protein: 21g | carbs: 8g net carbs: 5g | fiber: 3g

321. Indian Tomato Soup with Raita

Prep time: 20 minutes | Cook time: 20 minutes | Serves 4

1½ tablespoons butter	seeds
1 medium-sized leek, sliced	2 garlic cloves, minced
1 red chili pepper, chopped	4 tomatoes, puréed
1 bell pepper, roughly chopped	¼ piece of a stick of cinnamon
½ teaspoon cumin	½ teaspoon mustard seeds
Raita:	2 pods cardamom
1 cup full-fat yogurt	chopped
1 cucumber, chopped	½ teaspoon powdered coriander
¼ cup fresh cilantro,	

1. Melt the butter in a heavy-bottomed pot over medium-high heat. Now, sweat the leek and peppers until just tender and fragrant.
2. Stir in the cumin seeds and garlic; continue to sauté an additional 30 seconds; just make sure they do not burn.
3. Stir in the tomatoes, cinnamon, mustard seeds, and cardamom. Bring to a rapid boil and immediately turn the heat to a simmer. Let it simmer for 20 minutes or until heated through.
4. Purée everything together with an immersion blender.
5. Meanwhile, mix all the ingredients for the Raita. Serve the warm tomato soup with the Raita on the side. Enjoy!

Per Serving

calories: 106 | fat: 6g | protein: 4g | carbs: 7g net carbs: 5g | fiber: 2g

322. Traditional Thai Tom Kha Soup

Prep time: 20 minutes | Cook time: 22 minutes | Serves 2

1 teaspoon coconut oil
1 shallot, chopped
1 clove garlic, minced
½ celery stalk, chopped
½ bell pepper, chopped
1 Bird's eye chili, divined and minced
1 cup vegetable broth
¼ teaspoon stone ground mustard
Sea salt and freshly cracked black pepper, to season
½ teaspoon ground cumin
½ teaspoon coriander seeds
2 cardamom pods
1 cup full-fat coconut milk
2 tablespoons Thai basil leaves, snipped

1. In a deep saucepan, heat the coconut oil until sizzling; now, sauté the shallot, garlic, celery, and peppers for 5 minutes, until just tender and fragrant; make sure to stir frequently.
2. Add a splash of broth to deglaze the pan. Add in the remaining broth, mustard, and spices and bring to a rolling boil.
3. Turn the heat to medium-low and let it simmer for 15 minutes or until heated through. After that, pour in the coconut milk and continue to simmer for 2 minutes more.
4. Ladle into soup bowls and serve garnished with fresh Thai basil. Enjoy!

Per Serving
calories: 273 | fat: 27g | protein: 5g | carbs: 6g net carbs: 5g | fiber: 1g

323. Italian Pepper and Mushrooms Stew

Prep time: 15 minutes | Cook time: 25 minutes | Serves 5

3 tablespoons extra-virgin olive oil
1 red onion, chopped
2 sweet Italian peppers, chopped
1 poblano pepper, chopped
1 pound (454 g) cremini mushrooms, sliced
2 garlic cloves
2 cups water
1 cup cream of mushroom soup
½ teaspoon ground cumin
½ teaspoon mustard seeds
2 vine-ripe tomatoes, puréed
2 bay laurels
Sea salt and ground black pepper, to taste

1. Heat the oil in a heavy-bottomed soup pot over medium-high heat. Once hot, sauté the onion and peppers for 3 minutes, until crisp-tender and fragrant.
2. Stir in the mushrooms and garlic and continue to sauté an additional 2 minutes.
3. Add in the remaining ingredients and turn the heat to medium-low. Cook, partially covered, for 20 minutes or until thoroughly cooked.
4. Ladle into individual bowls and serve warm. Enjoy!

Per Serving
calories: 156 | fat: 12g | protein: 5g | carbs: 6g net carbs: 4g | fiber: 2g

324. Homemade Coleslaw with Cauliflower

Prep time: 5 minutes | Cook time: 0 minutes | Serves 5

1 cup green cabbage, shredded
1 cup fresh cauliflower, chopped
4 tablespoons shallots, chopped
1 teaspoon garlic, minced
1 teaspoon lime juice
1 teaspoon white wine vinegar
⅓ cup mayonnaise
Sea salt and ground black pepper, to taste

1. Add the cabbage, cauliflower, shallots, and garlic to a salad bowl.
2. In a small mixing dish, whisk the lime juice, vinegar, mayonnaise, salt, and pepper.
3. Dress the salad and serve immediately. Bon appétit!

Per Serving
calories: 121 | fat: 9g | protein: 3g | carbs: 7g net carbs: 5g | fiber: 2g

325. Slow Cooked Spaghetti Squash

Prep time: 15 minutes | Cook time: 6 hours | Serves 8

1 small spaghetti squash, washed
½ cup vegetable stock
¼ cup butter
Salt, for seasoning
Freshly ground black pepper, for seasoning

1. Place the squash and chicken stock in the insert of the slow cooker. The squash should not touch the sides of the insert.
2. Cook on low for 6 hours.
3. Let the squash cool for 10 minutes and cut in half.
4. Scrape out the squash strands into a bowl with a fork. When finished, add the butter and toss to combine.
5. Season with salt and pepper and serve.

Per Serving
calories: 98 | fat: 5g | protein: 1g | carbs: 6g net carbs: 3g | fiber: 3g

326. Baked Stuffed Peppers with Olives

Prep time: 10 minutes | Cook time: 32 minutes | Serves 2

1 garlic clove, minced
2 scallions, chopped
3 ounces (85 g) cream cheese
3 eggs
3 ounces (85 g) Provolone cheese, grated
Sea salt and ground black pepper, to taste
½ teaspoon hot paprika
1 teaspoon coriander
3 bell peppers, seeded and sliced in half
4 Kalamata olives, pitted and sliced

1. In a mixing bowl, thoroughly combine the garlic, scallions, cream cheese, eggs, provolone cheese, salt, black pepper, paprika, and coriander.
2. Stuff the peppers and place them on a parchment lined baking sheet.
3. Bake in the preheated oven at 370°F (188°C) approximately 30 minutes until the peppers are tender. If you want your peppers nicely charred, just place them under the broiler for 2 minutes.
4. Garnish with olives and serve immediately. Bon appétit!

Per Serving
calories: 387 | fat: 30g | protein: 23g | carbs: 5g net carbs: 4g | fiber: 1g

327. Greek Roasted Cauliflower with Feta Cheese

Prep time: 5 minutes | Cook time: 40 minutes | Serves 4

1 pound (454 g) cauliflower, halved
1 medium-sized leek, cut into 2-inch pieces
2 tablespoons olive oil
1 tablespoon Greek seasoning blend
Sea salt and ground black pepper, to taste
1 cup feta cheese, crumbled

1. Begin by preheating your oven to 390°F (199°C). Toss cauliflower and leek with olive oil, Greek seasoning blend, salt, and black pepper.
2. Arrange vegetables on a parchment-lined roasting pan. Transfer to the preheated oven.
3. Roast approximately 20 minutes; turn them over and roast an additional 20 minutes. Top with feta cheese and serve immediately. Enjoy!

Per Serving
calories: 194 | fat: 15g | protein: 7g | carbs: 6g net carbs: 3g | fiber: 3g

328. Creamy Vegetable Chowder

Prep time: 15 minutes | Cook time: 36 to 38 minutes | Serves 5

1 tablespoon olive oil
½ cup shallots, chopped
1 cup celery, chopped
1 teaspoon oregano
1½ teaspoon basil
½ teaspoon rosemary
5 cups vegetable broth
1 bay laurel
2 tablespoons cilantro, chopped
Sea salt and ground black pepper, to taste
¼ cup dry white wine
1 cup heavy cream

1. Heat the olive oil in a large heavy-bottomed pot until sizzling. Then, sweat the shallot and celery until tender and aromatic.
2. Stir in the remaining ingredients, except for the heavy cream. When it comes to the boil, turn the heat to medium-low. Let it simmer, partially covered, for 30 minutes.
3. Lastly, fold in the cream. Continue to simmer an additional 6 to 8 minutes. Bon appétit!

Per Serving
calories: 131 | fat: 13g | protein: 2g | carbs: 3g net carbs: 2g | fiber: 1g

329. Double Cheese Braised Vegetables

Prep time: 15 minutes | Cook time: 6 hours | Serves 6

1 tablespoon extra-virgin olive oil
½ head cauliflower, cut into small florets
2 cups green beans, cut into 2-inch pieces
1 cup asparagus spears, cut into 2-inch pieces
½ cup sour cream
½ cup shredded Cheddar cheese
½ cup shredded Swiss cheese
3 tablespoons butter
¼ cup water
1 teaspoon ground nutmeg
Pinch freshly ground black pepper, for seasoning

1. Lightly grease the insert of the slow cooker with the olive oil.
2. Add the cauliflower, green beans, asparagus, sour cream, Cheddar cheese, Swiss cheese, butter, water, nutmeg, and pepper to the insert.
3. Cover and cook on low for 6 hours.
4. Serve warm.

Per Serving
calories: 207 | fat: 18g | protein: 8g | carbs: 5g net carbs: 3g | fiber: 2g

330. Broccoli Salad with Tahini Dressing

Prep time: 15 minutes | Cook time: 0 minutes | Serves 2

½ cup broccoli florets
1 bell pepper, seeded and sliced
1 shallot, thinly sliced
½ cup arugula
Tahini Dressing:
1 tablespoon freshly squeezed lemon juice
¼ cup tahini (sesame butter)
1 garlic clove, minced
2 ounces (57 g) Mozzarella cheese
2 tablespoons toasted sunflower seeds
½ teaspoon yellow mustard
½ teaspoon ground black pepper
Pink salt, to taste

1. Place the cabbage, pepper, shallot, and arugula in a nice salad bowl. Mix all ingredients for the dressing.
2. Now, dress your salad and top with the Mozzarella cheese and sunflower seeds.
3. Serve at room temperature or well chilled. Bon appétit!

Per Serving
calories: 323 | fat: 25g | protein: 16g | carbs: 7g net carbs: 3g | fiber: 4g

331. Spinach and Egg Salad

Prep time: 10 minutes | Cook time: 8 minutes | Serves 3

4 eggs
Sea salt and red pepper flakes, to taste
½ pound (227 g) spinach
1 roasted pepper in oil, drained and chopped
1 tomato, diced
2 scallions, sliced
¼ teaspoon dried oregano
½ teaspoon dried basil
2 tablespoons white vinegar
2 tablespoons extra-virgin olive oil

1. Cook the eggs in a saucepan for about 8 minutes; peel the eggs under running water and carefully slice them. Season the eggs with salt and red pepper.
2. Add the spinach, red pepper, tomato, scallions, oregano, and basil to a nice serving bowl.
3. Drizzle vinegar and olive oil over your vegetables. Top with the boiled eggs. Serve at room temperature or well chilled. Bon appétit!

Per Serving
calories: 156 | fat: 10g | protein: 10g | carbs: 7g net carbs: 4g | fiber: 3g

332. Garlicky Voodles with Avocado Sauce

Prep time: 5 minutes | Cook time: 6 minutes | Serves 3

1 zucchini
1 cucumber
2 bell peppers
2 tablespoons olive oil
2 garlic cloves, peeled
1 avocado, peeled and pitted
½ lemon, juiced and
zested
2 tablespoons coriander
Kosher salt and ground black pepper, to taste
½ teaspoon red pepper flakes

1. Spiralize the zucchini, cucumber, and bell peppers by using a spiralizer or a julienne peeler.
2. Heat the olive oil in a wok or a large nonstick skillet. Sauté the voodles in the hot olive oil for about 6 minutes.
3. Then, in your food processor or blender, purée the remaining ingredients until uniform and creamy. Pour the avocado sauce over the voodles and serve. Bon appétit!

Per Serving
calories: 181 | fat: 16g | protein: 2g | carbs: 7g net carbs: 3g | fiber: 4g

333. Garlicky Cauliflower-Pecan Casserole

Prep time: 15 minutes | Cook time: 6 hours | Serves 6

1 tablespoon extra-virgin olive oil
2 pounds (907 g) cauliflower florets
1 cup chopped pecans
4 garlic cloves, sliced
½ teaspoon salt
½ teaspoon freshly
ground black pepper
2 tablespoons freshly squeezed lemon juice
4 hard-boiled eggs, shredded, for garnish
1 scallion, white and green parts, chopped, for garnish

1. Lightly grease the insert of the slow cooker with the olive oil.
2. In a medium bowl, toss together the cauliflower, pecans, garlic, salt, and pepper.
3. Transfer the mixture to the insert and sprinkle the lemon juice over the top.
4. Cover and cook on low for 6 hours.
5. Garnish with hard-boiled eggs and scallion and serve.

Per Serving
calories: 219 | fat: 17g | protein: 8g | carbs: 11g net carbs: 6g | fiber: 5g

Chapter 8 Vegan and Vegetarian

334. Spicy Roasted Eggplant with Avocado

Prep time: 5 minutes | Cook time: 20 to 25 minutes | Serves 7

2 pounds (907 g) eggplant, sliced
3 teaspoons avocado oil
2 tablespoons tahini
1 teaspoon garlic paste
1 tablespoon Dijon mustard
1 tablespoon lemon juice
½ teaspoon harissa
1 avocado, pitted, peeled and mashed

1. Brush the bottom of a roasting pan with nonstick cooking oil. Arrange the eggplant slices on the prepared roasting pan. Drizzle the eggplant with 2 teaspoons of the avocado oil.
2. Transfer the pan to the preheated oven. Roast in the preheated oven at 420ºF (216ºC) for 15 to 20 minutes.
3. Meanwhile, mix the remaining ingredients, except for the avocado, until everything is well incorporated. Divide this mixture between the eggplant slices.
4. Broil approximately 5 minutes. Top with the mashed avocado and serve warm. Bon appétit!

Per Serving
calories: 94 | fat: 6g | protein: 3g | carbs: 7g net carbs: 3g | fiber: 4g

335. Button Mushroom Stroganoff

Prep time: 20 minutes | Cook time: 22 minutes | Serves 5

2 tablespoons olive oil
½ cup onion, minced
1 tablespoon butter
1½ pounds (680 g) button mushrooms, sliced
1 teaspoon garlic paste
½ teaspoon red curry paste
Sea salt and ground black pepper, to taste
1 teaspoon dried parsley flakes
½ teaspoon celery seeds
½ teaspoon mustard seeds
½ teaspoon red pepper flakes
2 tablespoons tomato purée
4 cups vegetable stock
1 cup sour cream

1. Heat the olive oil in a heavy-bottomed soup pot until sizzling. Then, sauté the onion until tender and translucent or about 4 minutes.
2. Then, melt the butter in the same pot and cook the mushrooms for 3 to 4 minutes until just tender. Add in the garlic paste, curry paste, spices, tomato purée, and stock.
3. Bring the mixture to just below boiling point. Turn the heat to simmer and let it cook for 15 minutes longer.
4. Fold in the sour cream and stir it all together. Taste, adjust the seasonings and serve warm. Enjoy!

Per Serving
calories: 166 | fat: 13g | protein: 6g | carbs: 7g net carbs: 5g | fiber: 2g

336. Mozzarella Creamed Salad with Basil

Prep time: 20 minutes | Cook time: 0 minutes | Serves 4

4 ounces (113 g) arugula
4 ounces (113 g) lettuce
4 scallions, sliced
2 green garlic stalks, sliced
½ cup celery rib, chopped
1 cucumber, sliced
1 tomato, sliced
½ cup olives, pitted and halved
½ cup mayonnaise
1 teaspoon stone-ground mustard
2 tablespoons white vinegar
Sea salt and ground black pepper, to taste
½ cup Mozzarella cheese
2 tablespoons fresh basil leaves, snipped

1. Toss the arugula, lettuce, scallions, green garlic, celery, cucumber, tomato, and olives in a large-sized bowl.
2. In a small mixing dish, whisk the mayonnaise, mustard, vinegar, salt, and black pepper. Add the mayo mixture to the vegetables and toss to combine well.
3. Top with Mozzarella and serve garnished with fresh basil. Enjoy!

Per Serving
calories: 255 | fat: 23g | protein: 7g | carbs: 7g net carbs: 4g | fiber: 3g

337. Lebanese Tabbouleh Salad

Prep time: 15 minutes | Cook time: 8 minutes | Serves 2

1 cup cauliflower florets
1 tablespoon fresh mint leaves, roughly chopped
1 tablespoon fresh parsley leaves, roughly chopped
½ white onion, thinly sliced
½ cup cherry tomatoes, halved
1 Lebanese cucumber, diced
Pink salt and freshly cracked black pepper, to taste
1 tablespoon hulled hemp seeds
1 tablespoon fresh lemon juice
2 tablespoons extra-virgin olive oil

1. Pulse the cauliflower florets in your food processor until they're broken into tiny chunks (just bigger than rice).
2. Pat dry with paper towels. Cook in a lightly greased nonstick skillet over medium heat until the cauliflower rice is turning golden or about 8 minutes; transfer to a serving bowl.
3. Add the remaining ingredients and toss to combine well.
4. Adjust the seasonings and serve. Enjoy!

Per Serving
calories: 180 | fat: 16g | protein: 3g | carbs: 7g net carbs: 4g | fiber: 3g

338. Provençal Ratatouille Casserole

Prep time: 15 minutes | Cook time: 1 hour | Serves 6

3 tablespoons extra-virgin olive oil, divided
1 tomato, sliced
2 yellow onions, sliced
3 garlic, sliced
3 bell peppers, sliced
2 medium-sized zucchinis, cut into rounds
1 medium-sized Japanese eggplant, cut into rounds
1 cup tomato purée
Sea salt and black pepper, to taste
1 tablespoon Herbes de Provence
2 tablespoons fresh cilantro, chopped

1. Start by preheating your oven to 375°F (190°C). Toss the sliced vegetables with the olive oil and brush the sides and bottom of a casserole dish with cooking spray.
2. Arrange the sliced vegetables in alternating patterns in the baking pan. Add the tomato purée, salt, black pepper, and Herbes de Provence.
3. Cover with aluminum foil. Bake in the preheated oven for 30 minutes. Remove the foil and bake for a further 30 minutes or until the tomato purée is bubbling.
4. Garnish with fresh cilantro just before serving. Enjoy!

Per Serving
calories: 104 | fat: 7g | protein: 2g | carbs: 7g net carbs: 4g | fiber: 3g

339. Gouda Cauli-Broccoli Casserole

Prep time: 15 minutes | Cook time: 6 hours | Serves 6

1 tablespoon extra-virgin olive oil
1 pound (454 g) broccoli, cut into florets
1 pound (454 g) cauliflower, cut into florets
¼ cup almond flour
2 cups coconut milk
½ teaspoon ground nutmeg
Pinch freshly ground black pepper
1½ cups shredded Gouda cheese, divided

1. Lightly grease the insert of the slow cooker with the olive oil.
2. Place the broccoli and cauliflower in the insert.
3. In a small bowl, stir together the almond flour, coconut milk, nutmeg, pepper, and 1 cup of the cheese.
4. Pour the coconut milk mixture over the vegetables and top the casserole with the remaining ½ cup of the cheese.
5. Cover and cook on low for 6 hours.
6. Serve warm.

Per Serving
calories: 377 | fat: 32g | protein: 16g | carbs: 12g net carbs: 6g | fiber: 6g

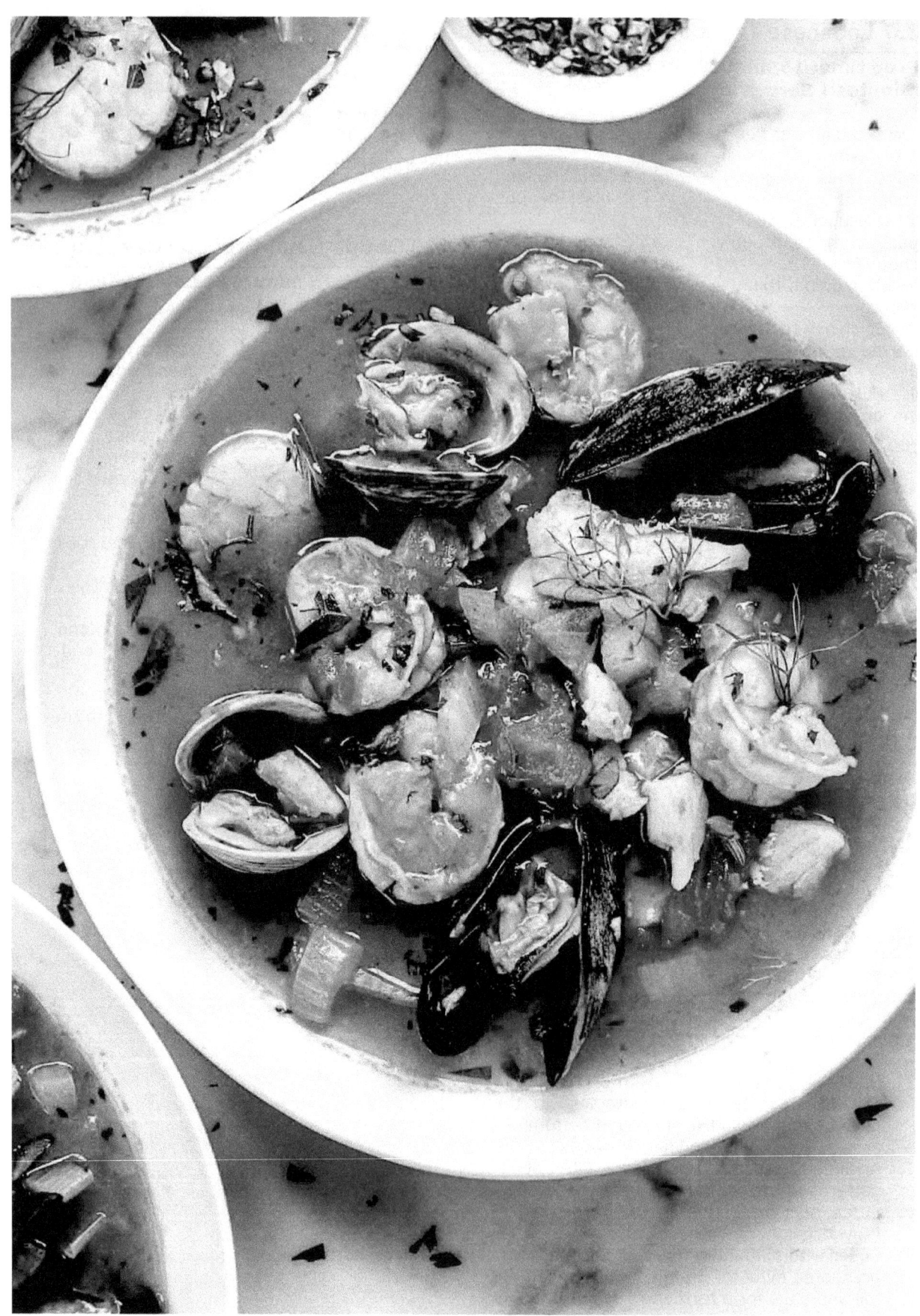

Chapter 9 Soup

340. Rich Taco Soup

Prep time: 5 minutes | Cook time: 4¼ hours | Serves 4

1 pound (454 g) ground beef
Pink Himalayan salt, to taste
Freshly ground black pepper, to taste
2 cups beef broth (I use Kettle & Fire Bone Broth)
1 (10-ounce / 283-g) can diced tomatoes (I use Rotel)
1 tablespoon taco seasoning
8 ounces (227 g) cream cheese

1. With the crock insert in place, preheat the slow cooker to low.
2. On the stove top, in a medium skillet over medium-high heat, sauté the ground beef until browned, about 8 minutes, and season with pink Himalayan salt and pepper.
3. Add the ground beef, beef broth, tomatoes, taco seasoning, and cream cheese to the slow cooker.
4. Cover and cook on low for 4 hours, stirring occasionally.
5. Ladle into four bowls and serve.

Per Serving
calories: 422 | fat: 33g | protein: 25g | carbs: 6g net carbs: 5g | fiber: 1g

341. Creamy Turkey and Celery Soup

Prep time: 15 minutes | Cook time: 4 hours | Serves 7

1 pound (454 g) turkey breast, cubed
5 cups chicken broth
1 cup cream cheese
1 stalk celery, chopped
3 cloves garlic, chopped
1 teaspoon freshly chopped rosemary
Salt and black pepper, to taste

1. Add all the ingredients minus the cream cheese to the base of a slow cooker.
2. Cook on high for 4 hours.
3. Stir in the cream cheese until well combined.

Per Serving
calories: 216 | fat: 14g | protein: 17g | carbs: 3g net carbs: 2g | fiber: 1g

342. Rich Cheesy Bacon-Cauliflower Soup

Prep time: 15 minutes | Cook time: 6 hours | Serves 6

1 tablespoon extra-virgin olive oil
4 cups chicken broth
2 cups coconut milk
2 cups chopped cooked chicken
1 cup chopped cooked bacon
2 cups chopped cauliflower
1 sweet onion, chopped
3 teaspoons minced garlic
½ cup cream cheese, cubed
2 cups shredded cheddar cheese

1. Lightly grease the insert of the slow cooker with the olive oil.
2. Place the broth, coconut milk, chicken, bacon, cauliflower, onion, and garlic in the insert.
3. Cover and cook on low for 6 hours.
4. Stir in the cream cheese and Cheddar and serve.

Per Serving
calories: 540 | fat: 44g | protein: 35g | carbs: 7g net carbs: 6g | fiber: 1g

343. Tangy Cucumber and Avocado Soup

Prep time: 10 minutes | Cook time: 0 minutes | Serves 4

4 large cucumbers, seeded, chopped
1 large avocado, peeled and pitted
Salt and black pepper to taste
2 cups water
1 tablespoon cilantro, chopped
1 tablespoon olive oil
2 limes, juiced
1 teaspoon minced garlic
2 tomatoes, chopped
1 chopped avocado for garnish

1. Pour the cucumbers, avocado halves, salt, black pepper, olive oil, lime juice, cilantro, water, and garlic in the food processor. Puree the ingredients for 2 minutes or until smooth. Pour the mixture in a bowl and top with avocado and tomatoes. Serve chilled with zero-carb bread.

Per Serving
calories: 170 | fat: 7g | protein: 4g | carbs: 10g net carbs: 4g | fiber: 6g

344. Nacho Soup

Prep time: 15 minutes | Cook time: 6 hours | Serves 8

3 tablespoons extra-virgin olive oil, divided
1 pound (454 g) ground chicken
1 sweet onion, diced
1 red bell pepper, chopped
2 teaspoons minced garlic
2 tablespoons taco seasoning
4 cups chicken broth
2 cups coconut milk
1 tomato, diced
1 jalapeño pepper, chopped
2 cups shredded cheddar cheese
½ cup sour cream, for garnish
1 scallion, white and green parts, chopped, for garnish

1. Lightly grease the insert of the slow cooker with 1 tablespoon of the olive oil.
2. In a large skillet over medium-high heat, heat the remaining 2 tablespoons of the olive oil. Add the chicken and sauté until it is cooked through, about 6 minutes.
3. Add the onion, red bell pepper, garlic, and taco seasoning, and sauté for an additional 3 minutes.
4. Transfer the chicken mixture to the insert, and stir in the broth, coconut milk, tomato, and jalapeño pepper.
5. Cover and cook on low for 6 hours.
6. Stir in the cheese.
7. Serve topped with the sour cream and scallion.

Per Serving

calories: 434 | fat: 35g | protein: 22g | carbs: 9g net carbs: 7g | fiber: 2g

345. Spiced-Pumpkin Soup

Prep time: 15 minutes | Cook time: 6 hours | Serves 6

1 tablespoon extra-virgin olive oil
4 cups chicken broth
2 cups coconut milk
1 pound pumpkin, diced
½ sweet onion, chopped
1 tablespoon grated fresh ginger
2 teaspoons minced garlic
½ teaspoon ground cinnamon
¼ teaspoon ground nutmeg
¼ teaspoon freshly ground black pepper
¼ teaspoon salt
pinch ground allspice
1 cup heavy (whipping) cream
2 cups chopped cooked chicken

1. Lightly grease the insert of the slow cooker with the olive oil.
2. Place the broth, coconut milk, pumpkin, onion, ginger, garlic, cinnamon, nutmeg, pepper, salt, and allspice in the insert.
3. Cover and cook on low for 6 hours.
4. Using an immersion blender or a regular blender, purée the soup.
5. If you removed the soup from the insert to purée, add it back to the pot, and stir in the cream and chicken.
6. Keep heating the soup on low for 15 minutes to heat the chicken through, and then serve warm.

Per Serving

calories: 389 | fat: 32g | protein: 16g | carbs: 10g net carbs: 5g | fiber: 5g

346. Saffron Coconut Shrimp Soup

Prep time: 5 minutes | Cook time: 15 minutes | Serves 4

1 tablespoon coconut oil
1 red bell pepper, chopped
2 teaspoons minced garlic
2 teaspoons grated fresh ginger
4 cups chicken stock
1 (15-ounce / 425-g) can coconut milk
1 pound shrimp, peeled, deveined, and chopped
1 cup shredded kale
Juice of 1 lime
½ cup warm water
Pinch saffron threads
Sea salt, for seasoning
2 tablespoons chopped fresh cilantro

1. Sauté the vegetables. In a large saucepan over medium heat, warm the coconut oil. Add the red pepper, garlic, and ginger and sauté until they've softened, about 5 minutes.
2. Simmer the soup. Add the chicken stock and coconut milk and bring the soup to a boil, then reduce the heat to low and stir in the shrimp, kale, and lime juice. Simmer the soup until the shrimp is cooked through, about 5 minutes.
3. Mix in the saffron. While the soup is simmering, stir the saffron and the warm water together in a small bowl and let it sit for 5 minutes. Stir the saffron mixture into the soup when the shrimp is cooked, and simmer the soup for 3 minutes more.
4. Season and serve. Season with salt. Ladle the soup into bowls, garnish it with the cilantro, and serve it hot.

Per Serving

calories: 504 | fat: 36g | protein: 32g | carbs: 15g net carbs: 12g | fiber: 3g

347. Creamy-Cheesy Cauliflower Soup

Prep time: 5 minutes | Cook time: 20 minutes | Serves 4

1 tablespoon butter
½ onion, chopped
2 cups riced/shredded cauliflower (I buy it pre-riced at Trader Joe's)
1 cup chicken broth
2 ounces (57 g) cream cheese
1 cup heavy (whipping) cream
Pink Himalayan salt
Freshly ground pepper
½ cup shredded Cheddar cheese (I use sharp Cheddar)

1. In a medium saucepan over medium heat, melt the butter. Add the onion and cook, stirring occasionally, until softened, about 5 minutes.
2. Add the cauliflower and chicken broth, and allow the mixture to come to a boil, stirring occasionally.
3. Lower the heat to medium-low and simmer until the cauliflower is soft enough to mash, about 10 minutes.
4. Add the cream cheese, and mash the mixture.
5. Add the cream and purée the mixture with an immersion blender (or you can pour the soup into the blender, blend it, and then pour it back into the pan and reheat it a bit).
6. Season the soup with pink Himalayan salt and pepper.
7. Pour the soup into four bowls, top each with the shredded Cheddar cheese, and serve.

Per Serving
calories: 372 | fat: 35g | protein: 9g | carbs: 9g net carbs: 6g | fiber: 3g

348. Colden Gazpacho Soup

Prep time: 15 minutes | Cook time: 0 minutes | Serves 6

2 small green peppers, roasted
2 large red peppers, roasted
2 medium avocados, flesh scoped out
2 garlic cloves
2 spring onions, chopped
1 cucumber, chopped
1 cup olive oil
1 tablespoon lemon juice
4 tomatoes, chopped
7 ounces (198 g) goat cheese
1 small red onion, chopped
1 tablespoon apple cider vinegar
Salt, to taste

1. Place the peppers, tomatoes, avocados, red onion, garlic, lemon juice, olive oil, vinegar, and salt, in a food processor. Pulse until your desired consistency is reached. Taste and adjust the seasoning.
2. Transfer the mixture to a pot. Stir in cucumber and spring onions. Cover and chill in the fridge at least 2 hours. Divide the soup between 6 bowls. Serve topped with goat cheese and an extra drizzle of olive oil.

Per Serving
calories: 528 | fat: 46g | protein: 8g | carbs: 7g net carbs: 4g | fiber: 3g

349. Cioppino

Prep time: 10 minutes | Cook time: 30 minutes | Serves 6

2 tablespoons olive oil
½ onion, chopped
2 celery stalks, sliced
1 red bell pepper, chopped
1 tablespoon minced garlic
2 cups fish stock
1 (15-ounce / 425-g) can coconut milk
1 cup crushed tomatoes
2 tablespoons tomato purée
1 tablespoon chopped fresh basil
2 teaspoons chopped fresh oregano
½ teaspoon sea salt
½ teaspoon freshly ground black pepper
¼ teaspoon red pepper flakes
10 ounces (283 g) salmon, cut into 1-inch pieces
½ pound (227) shrimp, peeled and deveined
12 clams or mussels, cleaned and debearded but in the shell

1. Sauté the vegetables. In a large stockpot over medium-high heat, warm the olive oil. Add the onion, celery, red bell pepper, and garlic and sauté until they've softened, about 4 minutes.
2. Make the soup base. Stir in the fish stock, coconut milk, crushed tomatoes, tomato purée, basil, oregano, salt, pepper, and red pepper flakes. Bring the soup to a boil, then reduce the heat to low and simmer the soup for 10 minutes.
3. Add the seafood. Stir in the salmon and simmer until it goes opaque, about 5 minutes. Add the shrimp and simmer until they're almost cooked through, about 3 minutes. Add the mussels and let them simmer until they open, about 3 minutes. Throw out any mussels that don't open.
4. Serve. Ladle the soup into bowls and serve it hot.

Per Serving
calories: 377 | fat: 29g | protein: 24g | carbs: 9g net carbs: 7g | fiber: 2g

350. Creamy Tomato Soup

Prep time: 10 minutes | Cook time: 14 minutes | Serves 6

1 tablespoon butter
2 large red onions, diced
½ cup raw cashew nuts, diced
2 (28-ounce / 794-g) cans tomatoes
1 teaspoon fresh thyme leaves, extra to garnish
1½ cups water
Salt and black pepper to taste
1 cup heavy cream

1. Melt butter in a pot over medium heat and sauté the onions for 4 minutes until softened.
2. Stir in the tomatoes, thyme, water, cashews, and season with salt and black pepper. Cover and bring to simmer for 10 minutes until thoroughly cooked.
3. Open, turn the heat off, and puree the ingredients with an immersion blender. Adjust to taste and stir in the heavy cream. Spoon into soup bowls and serve.

Per Serving
calories: 310 | fat: 27g | protein: 11g | carbs: 12g net carbs: 10g | fiber: 2g

351. Cheesy Cauliflower Soup

Prep time: 10 minutes | Cook time: 17 minutes | Serves 4

1 tablespoon butter
1 onion, chopped
2 head cauliflower, cut into florets
2 cups water
Salt and black pepper to taste
3 cups almond milk
1 cup shredded white cheddar cheese
3 bacon strips

1. Melt the butter in a saucepan over medium heat and sauté the onion for 3 minutes until fragrant.
2. Include the cauli florets, sauté for 3 minutes to slightly soften, add the water, and season with salt and black pepper. Bring to a boil, and then reduce the heat to low. Cover and cook for 10 minutes. Puree cauliflower with an immersion blender until the ingredients are evenly combined and stir in the almond milk and cheese until the cheese melts. Adjust taste with salt and black pepper.
3. In a non-stick skillet over high heat, fry the bacon, until crispy. Divide soup between serving bowls, top with crispy bacon, and serve hot.

Per Serving
calories: 402 | fat: 37g | protein: 8g | carbs: 9g net carbs: 6g | fiber: 3g

352. Power Green Soup

Prep time: 10 minutes | Cook time: 14 minutes | Serves 6

1 broccoli head, chopped
1 cup spinach
1 onion, chopped
2 garlic cloves, minced
½ cup watercress
5 cups veggie stock
1 cup coconut milk
1 tablespoon butter
1 bay leaf
Salt and black pepper, to taste

1. Melt the butter in a large pot over medium heat. Add onion and garlic, and cook for 3 minutes. Add broccoli and cook for an additional 5 minutes. Pour the stock over and add the bay leaf. Close the lid, bring to a boil, and reduce the heat. Simmer for about 3 minutes.
2. At the end, add spinach and watercress, and cook for 3 more minutes. Stir in the coconut cream, salt and black pepper. Discard the bay leaf, and blend the soup with a hand blender.

Per Serving
calories: 392 | fat: 37g | protein: 5g | carbs: 11g net carbs: 6g | fiber: 5g

353. Almond Soup with Sour Cream and Cilantro

Prep time: 10 minutes | Cook time: 21 minutes | Serves 4

1 tablespoon olive oil
1 cup onion, chopped
1 celery, chopped
2 cloves garlic, minced
2 turnips, peeled and chopped
4 cups vegetable broth
Salt and white pepper, to taste
¼ cup ground almonds
1 cup almond milk
1 tablespoon fresh cilantro, chopped
1 teaspoon sour cream

1. Warm oil in a pot over medium heat and sauté celery, garlic, and onion for 6 minutes. Stir in white pepper, broth, salt, and ground almonds.
2. Bring to the boil and simmer for 15 minutes.
3. Transfer soup to an immersion blender and puree. Serve garnished with sour cream and cilantro.

Per Serving
calories: 125 | fat: 7g | protein: 5g | carbs: 12g net carbs: 8g | fiber: 4g

354. Slow Cooked Faux Lasagna Soup

Prep time: 20 minutes | Cook time: 6 hours | Serves 6

3 tablespoons extra-virgin olive oil, divided
1 pound (454 g) ground beef
½ sweet onion, chopped
2 teaspoons minced garlic
4 cups beef broth
1 (28-ounce / 794-g) can diced tomatoes, undrained
1 zucchini, diced
1½ tablespoons dried basil
2 teaspoons dried oregano
4 ounces (113 g) cream cheese
1 cup shredded mozzarella

1. Lightly grease the insert of the slow cooker with 1 tablespoon of the olive oil.
2. In a large skillet over medium-high heat, heat the remaining 2 tablespoons 2. of the olive oil. Add the ground beef and sauté until it is cooked through, about 6 minutes.
3. Add the onion and garlic and sauté for an additional 3 minutes.
4. Transfer the meat mixture to the insert.
5. Stir in the broth, tomatoes, zucchini, basil, and oregano.
6. Cover and cook on low for 6 hours.
7. Stir in the cream cheese and mozzarella and serve.

Per Serving
calories: 472 | fat: 36g | protein: 30g | carbs: 9g net carbs: 6g | fiber: 3g

355. Creamy-Lemony Chicken Soup

Prep time: 10 minutes | Cook time: 30 minutes | Serves 6

½ cup grass-fed butter
½ onion, chopped
2 celery stalks, chopped
2 teaspoons minced garlic
¼ cup arrowroot
5 cups chicken stock
3 cups shredded cooked chicken
Zest and juice of 1 lemon
1 cup heavy (whipping) cream
Sea salt, for seasoning
Freshly ground black pepper, for seasoning
1 tablespoon chopped fresh oregano

1. Sauté the vegetables. In a medium stockpot over medium-high heat, melt the butter. Add the onion, celery, and garlic and sauté until they've softened, about 5 minutes.
2. Make the soup base. Add the arrowroot and whisk until it forms a paste. Whisk in the chicken stock.
3. Thicken the soup. Bring the soup to a boil, then reduce the heat to low and simmer, stirring it from time to time, until the soup thickens, about 15 minutes.
4. Add the remaining ingredients. Stir in the chicken, lemon zest, lemon juice, and cream and simmer until the chicken is heated through, about 10 minutes.
5. Season and serve. Season the soup with salt and pepper. Ladle the soup into bowls, garnish with the oregano, and serve it hot.

Per Serving
calories: 501 | fat: 36g | protein: 28g | carbs: 13g net carbs: 10g | fiber: 3g

356. Coconut Cheesy Cauliflower Soup

Prep time: 10 minutes | Cook time: 15 minutes | Serves 4

½ head cauliflower, chopped
1 tablespoon coconut oil
½ cup leeks, chopped
1 celery stalk, chopped
1 serrano pepper, finely chopped
1 teaspoon garlic puree
1½ tablespoon flax seed meal
2 cups water
1½ cups coconut milk
6 ounces (170 g) Monterey Jack cheese, shredded
Salt and black pepper, to taste
Fresh parsley, chopped

1. In a deep pan over medium heat, melt the coconut oil and sauté the serrano pepper, celery and leeks until soft, for about 5 minutes. Add in coconut milk, garlic puree, cauliflower, water and flax seed.
2. While covered partially, allow simmering for 10 minutes or until cooked through. Whizz with a immersion blender until smooth. Fold in the shredded cheese, and stir to ensure the cheese is completely melted and you have a homogenous mixture. Season with pepper and salt to taste.
3. Divide among serving bowls, decorate with parsley and serve while warm.

Per Serving
calories: 312 | fat: 16g | protein: 13g | carbs: 9g net carbs: 7g | fiber: 2g

357. Pork and Vegetable Soup

Prep time: 5 minutes | Cook time: 20 minutes | Serves 5

1½ pounds (680 g) pork stew meat, cubed	chopped
5 cups vegetable broth	2 bell peppers, chopped
½ cup scallions,	1 celery stalk, chopped

1. Spritz the bottom of a large soup pot with nonstick cooking spray. Heat up the pot over medium-high heat.
2. Now, brown the meat for 5 minutes, stirring frequently. Deglaze the skillet with a splash of vegetable broth, scraping up any brown bits stuck to the bottom. After that, stir in the remaining ingredients and bring to a rolling boil.
3. Turn the heat to simmer; cover and let it simmer for 15 minutes until everything is thoroughly warmed.
4. Ladle into individual bowls and serve hot. Bon appétit!

Per Serving

calories: 303 | fat: 18g | protein: 29g | carbs: 4g net carbs: 3g | fiber: 1g

358. Green Minestrone Soup

Prep time: 10 minutes | Cook time: 12 minutes | Serves 4

1 tablespoon butter	5 cups vegetable broth
1 tablespoon onion-garlic puree	1 cup baby spinach
2 heads broccoli, cut in florets	Salt and black pepper to taste
2 stalks celery, chopped	1 tablespoon Gruyere cheese, grated

1. Melt the butter in a saucepan over medium heat and sauté the onion-garlic puree for 3 minutes until softened. Mix in the broccoli and celery, and cook for 4 minutes until slightly tender. Pour in the broth, bring to a boil, then reduce the heat to medium-low and simmer covered for about 5 minutes.
2. Drop in the spinach to wilt, adjust the seasonings, and cook for 4 minutes. Ladle soup into serving bowls. Serve with a sprinkle of grated Gruyere cheese.

Per Serving

calories: 227 | fat: 20g | protein: 8g | carbs: 9g net carbs: 2g | fiber: 7g

359. Reuben Beef Soup

Prep time: 10 minutes | Cook time: 20 minutes | Serves 6

1 onion, diced	shredded
6 cups beef stock	1 pound (454 g) corned beef, chopped
1 teaspoon caraway seeds	1 tablespoon butter
2 celery stalks, diced	1½ cup swiss cheese, shredded
2 garlic cloves, minced	Salt and black pepper, to taste
2 cups heavy cream	
1 cup sauerkraut,	

1. Melt the butter in a large pot. Add onion and celery, and fry for 3 minutes until tender. Add garlic and cook for another minute.
2. Pour the beef stock over and stir in sauerkraut, salt, caraway seeds, and add a pinch of black pepper. Bring to a boil. Reduce the heat to low, and add the corned beef. Cook for about 15 minutes, adjust the seasoning. Stir in heavy cream and cheese and cook for 1 minute.

Per Serving

calories: 450 | fat: 37g | protein: 23g | carbs: 9g net carbs: 8g | fiber: 1g

360. Curry Green Beans and Shrimp Soup

Prep time: 10 minutes | Cook time: 10 minutes | Serves 4

1 tablespoon butter	paste
1 pound (454 g) jumbo shrimp, peeled and deveined	6 ounces (170 g) coconut milk
1 teaspoon ginger-garlic puree	Salt and chili pepper to taste
1 tablespoon red curry	1 bunch green beans, halved

1. Melt butter in a medium saucepan over medium heat. Add the shrimp, season with salt and black pepper, and cook until they are opaque, 2 to 3 minutes. Remove shrimp to a plate. Add the ginger-garlic puree and red curry paste to the butter and sauté for 2 minutes until fragrant.
2. Stir in the coconut milk; add the shrimp, salt, chili pepper, and green beans. Cook for 4 minutes. Reduce the heat to a simmer and cook an additional 3 minutes, occasionally stirring. Adjust taste with salt, fetch soup into serving bowls, and serve with cauli rice.

Per Serving

calories: 375 | fat: 35g | protein: 9g | carbs: 4g net carbs: 2g | fiber: 2g

361. Cheesy Broccoli Soup

Prep time: 10 minutes | Cook time: 14 minutes | Serves 4

¾ cup heavy cream
1 onion, diced
1 teaspoon minced garlic
4 cups chopped broccoli
4 cups veggie broth
1 tablespoon butter
3 cups grated cheddar cheese
Salt and black pepper, to taste
½ bunch fresh mint, chopped

1. Melt the butter in a large pot over medium heat. Sauté onion and garlic for 3 minutes or until tender, stirring occasionally. Season with salt and black pepper. Add the broth, broccoli and bring to a boil.
2. Reduce the heat and simmer for 10 minutes. Puree the soup with a hand blender until smooth. Add in 2 ¾ cups of the cheddar cheese and cook about 1 minute. Taste and adjust the seasoning. Stir in the heavy cream. Serve in bowls with the remaining cheddar cheese and sprinkled with fresh mint.

Per Serving
calories: 561 | fat: 52g | protein: 24g | carbs: 11g net carbs: 7g | fiber: 4g

362. Lush Vegetable Soup

Prep time: 15 minutes | Cook time: 25 minutes | Serves 4

1 teaspoon olive oil
1 onion, chopped
1 garlic clove, minced
½ celery stalk, chopped
1 cup mushrooms, sliced
½ head broccoli, chopped
1 cup spinach, torn into pieces
Salt and black pepper, to taste
2 thyme sprigs, chopped
3 cups vegetable stock
1 tomato, chopped
½ cup almond milk

1. Heat olive oil in a saucepan. Add onion, celery and garlic; sauté until translucent, stirring occasionally, about 5 minutes.
2. Place in spinach, mushrooms, salt, rosemary, tomatoes, bay leaves, black pepper, thyme, and vegetable stock. Simmer the mixture for 15 minutes while the lid is slightly open. Stir in almond milk and cook for 5 more minutes.

Per Serving
calories: 140 | fat: 6g | protein: 3g | carbs: 4g net carbs: 1g | fiber: 3g

363. Creamy Chicken Soup

Prep time: 10 minutes | Cook time: 2 minutes | Serves 4

2 cups cooked and shredded chicken
1 tablespoon butter, melted
4 cups chicken broth
1 tablespoon chopped cilantro
⅓ cup buffalo sauce
½ cup cream cheese
Salt and black pepper, to taste

1. Blend the butter, buffalo sauce, and cream cheese, in a food processor, until smooth. Transfer to a pot, add chicken broth and heat until hot but do not bring to a boil. Stir in chicken, salt, black pepper and cook until heated through.
2. When ready, remove to soup bowls and serve garnished with cilantro.

Per Serving
calories: 406 | fat: 29g | protein: 27g | carbs: 5g net carbs: 5g | fiber: 0g

364. Salsa Verde Chicken Soup

Prep time: 10 minutes | Cook time: 5 minutes | Serves 4

½ cup salsa verde
2 cups cooked and shredded chicken
2 cups chicken broth
1 cup shredded cheddar cheese
4 ounces (113 g) cream cheese
½ teaspoon chili powder
½ teaspoon ground cumin
½ teaspoon fresh cilantro, chopped
Salt and black pepper, to taste

1. Combine the cream cheese, salsa verde, and broth, in a food processor; pulse until smooth. Transfer the mixture to a pot and place over medium heat. Cook until hot, but do not bring to a boil. Add chicken, chili powder, and cumin and cook for about 3-5 minutes, or until it is heated through.
2. Stir in cheddar cheese and season with salt and pepper to taste. If it is very thick, add a few tablespoons of water and boil for 1-3 more minutes. Serve hot in bowls sprinkled with fresh cilantro.

Per Serving
calories: 346 | fat: 23g | protein: 25g | carbs: 4g net carbs: 3g | fiber: 1g

365. Creamy Cauliflower Soup with Sausage

Prep time: 10 minutes | Cook time: 35 minutes | Serves 4

1 cauliflower head, chopped
1 turnip, chopped
1 tablespoon butter
1 chorizo sausage, sliced
2 cups chicken broth
1 small onion, chopped
2 cups water
Salt and black pepper, to taste

1. Melt 1 tablespoon of the butter in a large pot over medium heat. Stir in onion and cook until soft and golden, about 3-4 minutes. Add cauliflower and turnip, and cook for another 5 minutes.
2. Pour the broth and water over. Bring to a boil, simmer covered, and cook for about 20 minutes until the vegetables are tender.
3. Remove from heat. Melt the remaining butter in a skillet. Add the chorizo sausage and cook for 5 minutes until crispy. Puree the soup with a hand blender until smooth.
4. Taste and adjust the seasonings. Serve the soup in deep bowls topped with the chorizo sausage.

Per Serving

calories: 251 | fat: 19g | protein: 10g | carbs: 8g net carbs: 6g | fiber: 2g

366. Spicy Chicken Soup

Prep time: 10 minutes | Cook time: 20 minutes | Serves 4

1 tablespoon coconut oil
1 pound (454 g) chicken thighs
¾ cup red enchilada sauce
¼ cup water
¼ cup onion, chopped
3 ounces (85 g) canned
diced green chilis
1 avocado, sliced
1 cup cheddar cheese, shredded
¼ cup pickled jalapeños, chopped
½ cup sour cream
1 tomato, diced

1. Put a large pan over medium heat. Add coconut oil and warm. Place in the chicken and cook until browned on the outside. Stir in onion, chilies, water, and enchilada sauce, then close with a lid.
2. Allow simmering for 20 minutes until the chicken is cooked through. Spoon the soup on a serving bowl and top with the sauce, cheese, sour cream, tomato, and avocado.

Per Serving

calories: 643 | fat: 44g | protein: 46g | carbs: 12g net carbs: 10g | fiber: 2g

367. Red Curry Shrimp and Bean Soup

Prep time: 10 minutes | Cook time: 11 minutes | Serves 4

1 onion, chopped
1 tablespoon red curry paste
1 tablespoon butter
1 pound jumbo shrimp, deveined
1 teaspoon ginger-garlic puree
1 cup coconut milk
Salt and chili pepper, to taste
1 bunch green beans, halved
1 tablespoon cilantro, chopped

1. Add the shrimp to melted butter in a saucepan over medium heat, season with salt and pepper, and cook until they are opaque, 2 to 3 minutes. Remove to a plate. Add in the ginger-garlic puree, onion, and red curry paste and sauté for 2 minutes until fragrant.
2. Stir in the coconut milk; add the shrimp, salt, chili pepper, and green beans. Cook for 4 minutes. Reduce the heat to a simmer and cook an additional 3 minutes, occasionally stirring. Adjust taste with salt, fetch soup into serving bowls, and serve sprinkled with cilantro.

Per Serving

calories: 351 | fat: 32g | protein: 8g | carbs: 4g net carbs: 3g | fiber: 1g

368. White Mushroom Cream Soup with Herbs

Prep time: 10 minutes | Cook time: 23 minutes | Serves 4

1 onion, chopped
½ cup crème fraiche
¼ cup butter
12 ounces (340 g) white mushrooms, chopped
1 teaspoon thyme
leaves, chopped
1 teaspoon parsley leaves, chopped
2 garlic cloves, minced
4 cups vegetable broth
Salt and black pepper, to taste

1. Add butter, onion and garlic to a pot over high heat and cook for 3 minutes. Add in mushrooms, salt and pepper, and cook for 10 minutes. Pour in broth and bring to a boil.
2. Reduce heat and simmer for 10 minutes. Puree soup with a hand blender. Stir in crème fraiche. Garnish with herbs before serving.

Per Serving

calories: 190 | fat: 15g | protein: 3g | carbs: 6g net carbs: 4g | fiber: 2g

369. Turnip and Soup with Pork Sausage

Prep time: 10 minutes | Cook time: 32 minutes | Serves 4

3 turnips, chopped
2 celery sticks, chopped
1 tablespoon butter
1 tablespoon olive oil
1 pork sausage, sliced
2 cups vegetable broth
½ cup sour cream
3 green onions, chopped
2 cups water
Salt and black pepper, to taste

1. Sauté green onions in melted butter over medium heat until soft and golden, about 3 minutes. Add celery and turnip, and cook for another 5 minutes. Pour over the vegetable broth and water over.
2. Bring to a boil, simmer covered, and cook for about 20 minutes until the vegetables are tender. Remove from heat. Puree the soup with a hand blender until smooth. Add sour cream and adjust the seasoning. Warm the olive oil in a skillet. Add the pork sausage and cook for 5 minutes. Serve the soup in deep bowls topped with pork sausage.

Per Serving
calories: 275 | fat: 23g | protein: 7 g | carbs: 10g net carbs: 6g | fiber: 4g

370. Creamy Cauliflower and Leek Soup

Prep time: 10 minutes | Cook time: 35 minutes | Serves 4

4 cups vegetable broth
2 heads cauliflower, cut into florets
1 celery stalk, chopped
1 onion, chopped
1 cup leeks, chopped
1 tablespoon butter
1 tablespoon olive oil
1 cup heavy cream
½ teaspoon red pepper flakes

1. Warm butter and olive oil in a pot set over medium heat and sauté onion, leeks, and celery for 5 minutes.
2. Stir in vegetable broth and cauliflower and bring to a boil; simmer for 30 minutes.
3. Transfer the mixture to an immersion blender and puree; add in the heavy cream and stir. Decorate with red pepper flakes to serve.

Per Serving
calories: 231 | fat: 18g | protein: 4g | carbs: 9g net carbs: 5g | fiber: 4g

371. Cheesy Broccoli and Spinach Soup

Prep time: 10 minutes | Cook time: 16 minutes | Serves 4

1 tablespoon butter
1 onion, chopped
1 garlic clove, minced
2 heads broccoli, cut in florets
2 stalks celery, chopped
4 cups vegetable broth
1 cup baby spinach
Salt and black pepper, to taste
1 tablespoon basil, chopped
Parmesan cheese, shaved to serve

1. Melt the butter in a saucepan over medium heat. Sauté the garlic and onion for 3 minutes until softened. Mix in the broccoli and celery, and cook for 4 minutes until slightly tender.
2. Pour in the broth, bring to a boil, then reduce the heat to medium-low and simmer covered for about 5 minutes.
3. Drop in the spinach to wilt, adjust the seasonings, and cook for 4 minutes. Ladle soup into serving bowls. Serve with a sprinkle of grated Parmesan cheese and chopped basil.

Per Serving
calories: 123 | fat: 11g | protein: 1g | carbs: 4g net carbs: 3g | fiber: 1g

372. Butternut Squash Soup

Prep time: 15 minutes | Cook time: 4 to 6 hours | Serves 8

1½ cups butternut squash, cubed
1 cup heavy cream
5 cups chicken broth
3 cloves garlic, chopped
2 teaspoons ground cinnamon
½ teaspoon ground nutmeg
½ teaspoon ground cloves
Salt and black pepper, to taste

1. Add all the ingredients minus the heavy cream to the base of a slow cooker.
2. Cook on high for 4 to 6 hours.
3. Warm the heavy cream, and then add to the soup.
4. Use an immersion blender and blend until smooth.

Per Serving
calories: 95 | fat: 7g | protein: 4g | carbs: 3g net carbs: 2g | fiber: 1g

373. Heavy Cream-Cheese Broccoli Soup

Prep time: 10 minutes | Cook time: 13 minutes | Serves 4

1 tablespoon olive oil
1 tablespoon peanut butter
¾ cup heavy cream
1 onion, diced
1 garlic, minced
4 cups chopped broccoli
4 cups veggie broth
2¾ cups cheddar cheese, grated
¼ cup cheddar cheese to garnish
Salt and black pepper, to taste
½ bunch fresh mint, chopped

1. Warm olive oil and peanut butter in a pot over medium heat. Sauté onion and garlic for 3 minutes, stirring occasionally. Season with salt and pepper. Add the broth and broccoli and bring to a boil.
2. Reduce the heat and simmer for 10 minutes. Puree the soup with a hand blender until smooth. Add in the cheese and cook about 1 minute. Stir in the heavy cream.
3. Serve in bowls with the reserved grated cheddar cheese and sprinkled with fresh mint.

Per Serving
calories: 508 | fat: 28g | protein: 26g | carbs: 11g net carbs: 7g | fiber: 4g

374. Creamy Tomato Soup with Basil

Prep time: 10 minutes | Cook time: 14 minutes | Serves 4

1 tablespoon olive oil
1 onion, diced
1 garlic clove, minced
¼ cup raw cashew nuts, diced
14 ounces canned tomatoes
1 teaspoon fresh basil leaves
Salt and black pepper, to taste
1 cup crème fraîche

1. Warm olive oil in a pot over medium heat and sauté the onion and garlic for 4 minutes until softened. Stir in the tomatoes, basil, 1 cup water, cashew nuts, and season with salt and black pepper.
2. Cover and bring to simmer for 10 minutes until thoroughly cooked. Puree the ingredients with an immersion blender. Adjust to taste and stir in the crème fraîche. Serve sprinkled with basil.

Per Serving
calories: 189 | fat: 14g | protein: 5g | carbs: 4g net carbs: 2g | fiber: 2g

375. Buffalo Cheese Chicken Soup

Prep time: 10 minutes | Cook time: 7 minutes | Serves 4

1 onion, chopped
2 cups cooked, shredded chicken
1 tablespoon butter
4 cups chicken broth
1 tablespoon cilantro, chopped
⅓ cup buffalo sauce
½ cup cream cheese
Salt and black pepper, to taste

1. In a skillet over medium heat, warm butter and sauté the onion until tender, about 5 minutes.
2. Add to a food processor and blend with buffalo sauce and cream cheese, until smooth.
3. Transfer to a pot, add chicken broth and heat until hot but do not bring to a boil. Stir in chicken, salt, pepper and cook until heated through. When ready, remove to soup bowls and serve garnished with cilantro.

Per Serving
calories: 487 | fat: 41g | protein: 16g | carbs: 5g net carbs: 3g | fiber: 2g

376. Cheesy Tomato and Onion Soup

Prep time: 15 minutes | Cook time: 30 minutes | Serves 6

4 cups vegetable broth
1 cup heavy cream
1 cup canned diced tomatoes
1 yellow onion, chopped
2 cloves garlic, chopped
1 cup shredded mozzarella cheese
Freshly chopped basil, for serving

1. Add all of the ingredients minus the heavy cream, cheese and fresh basil to a stockpot over medium heat. Bring to a boil, and then reduce to a simmer.
2. Simmer for 30 minutes.
3. While the soup is cooking, warm the heavy cream over low heat and add to the soup once cooked.
4. Use an immersion blender and blend until smooth.
5. Stir in the mozzarella cheese and top with fresh basil.

Per Serving
calories: 122 | fat: 9g | protein: 6g | carbs: 5g net carbs: 4g | fiber: 1g

377. Turkey and Veggies Soup

Prep time: 10 minutes | Cook time: 25 minutes | Serves 4

1 onion, chopped
1 garlic clove, minced
3 celery stalks, chopped
2 leeks, chopped
1 tablespoon butter
4 cups chicken stock
Salt and black pepper, to taste
¼ cup fresh parsley, chopped
1 large zucchini, spiralized
2 cups turkey meat, cooked and chopped

1. In a pot over medium heat, add in leeks, celery, onion, and garlic and cook for 5 minutes.
2. Place in the turkey meat, black pepper, salt, and stock, and cook for 20 minutes. Stir in the zucchini, and cook turkey soup for 5 minutes. Serve in bowls sprinkled with parsley.

Per Serving
calories: 312 | fat: 13g | protein: 16g | carbs: 9g net carbs: 4g | fiber: 5g

378. Asparagus Parmesan Soup

Prep time: 10 minutes | Cook time: 15 minutes | Serves 4

2 cups chicken broth
1 cup heavy cream
1 cup shredded Parmesan cheese
1 cup asparagus finely chopped
1 yellow onion, chopped
3 cloves garlic, chopped
1 teaspoon dried thyme
Salt and black pepper, to taste

1. Add all the ingredients minus the heavy cream and Parmesan cheese to the base of a stockpot.
2. Bring to a boil, and then simmer for 10 minutes.
3. Warm the heavy cream, and then add to the soup along with the Parmesan cheese. Stir until the cheese has melted and serve.

Per Serving
calories: 228 | fat: 17g | protein: 12g | carbs: 7g net carbs: 5g | fiber: 2g

379. Cheesy Broccoli and Bacon Soup

Prep time: 10 minutes | Cook time: 10 minutes | Serves 6

2 cups chicken broth
1 cup broccoli florets finely chopped
1 cup heavy cream
1 cup shredded cheddar cheese
½ white onion, chopped
2 cloves garlic, chopped
3 slices cooked bacon, crumbled for serving
½ teaspoon salt
¼ teaspoon black pepper

1. Add all the ingredients minus the heavy cream, cheddar cheese and bacon to a stockpot over medium heat.
2. Bring to a simmer and cook for 5 minutes.
3. Warm the cream, and then add the warm cream and cheddar cheese. Whisk until smooth.
4. Serve with crumbled bacon.

Per Serving
calories: 220 | fat: 18g | protein: 11g | carbs: 4g net carbs: 3g | fiber: 1g

380. Creamy Tomato Soup

Prep time: 10 minutes | Cook time: 40 minutes | Serves 6

3 cups canned whole, peeled tomatoes
4 cups chicken broth
1 cup heavy cream
3 cloves garlic, chopped
2 tablespoons butter
1 teaspoon freshly chopped thyme
Salt and black pepper, to taste

1. Add the butter to the bottom of a stockpot.
2. Add in all the remaining ingredients minus the heavy cream. Bring to a boil, and then simmer for 40 minutes.
3. Warm the heavy cream, and then stir into the soup.

Per Serving
calories: 144 | fat: 12g | protein: 4g | carbs: 4g net carbs: 3g | fiber: 1g

381. Spiced Pumpkin Soup

Prep time: 15 minutes | Cook time: 4 to 6 hours | Serves 8

1½ cups pumpkin, cubed
1 cup heavy cream
5 cups chicken broth
3 cloves garlic, chopped

2 teaspoons ground cinnamon
½ teaspoon ground nutmeg
½ teaspoon ground cloves
Salt and black pepper, to taste

1. Add all the ingredients minus the heavy cream to the base of a slow cooker.
2. Cook on high for 4 to 6 hours.
3. Warm the heavy cream, and then add to the soup.
4. Use an immersion blender and blend until smooth.

Per Serving

calories: 96 | fat: 7g | protein: 4g | carbs: 6g | net carbs: 4g | fiber: 2g

382. Spinach Mozzarella Soup

Prep time: 10 minutes | Cook time: 15 minutes | Serves 4

2 cups chicken broth
1 cup heavy cream
1 cup shredded mozzarella cheese
1 cup fresh spinach, chopped

3 cloves garlic, chopped
1 teaspoon onion powder
1 teaspoon dried thyme
Salt and black pepper, to taste

1. Add all the ingredients minus the heavy cream and mozzarella to the base of a stockpot.
2. Bring to a boil, and then simmer for 10 minutes.
3. Warm the heavy cream, and then add to the soup along with mozzarella. Stir until the cheese has melted.

Per Serving

calories: 151 | fat: 13g | protein: 6g | carbs: 3g | net carbs: 3g | fiber: 0g

383. Spiced Cucumber Soup

Prep time: 15 minutes | Cook time: 0 minutes | Serves 6

4 cups chicken broth
1 cup heavy cream
2 cucumbers, sliced

1 teaspoon freshly chopped rosemary
1 teaspoon freshly chopped thyme
1 pinch of Salt and black pepper, to taste

1. Add all the ingredients to a large mixing bowl and whisk well.
2. Use an immersion blender and blend until smooth.
3. Chill for 1 hour before serving.

Per Serving

calories: 111 | fat: 9g | protein: 4g | carbs: 5g | net carbs: 4g | fiber: 1g

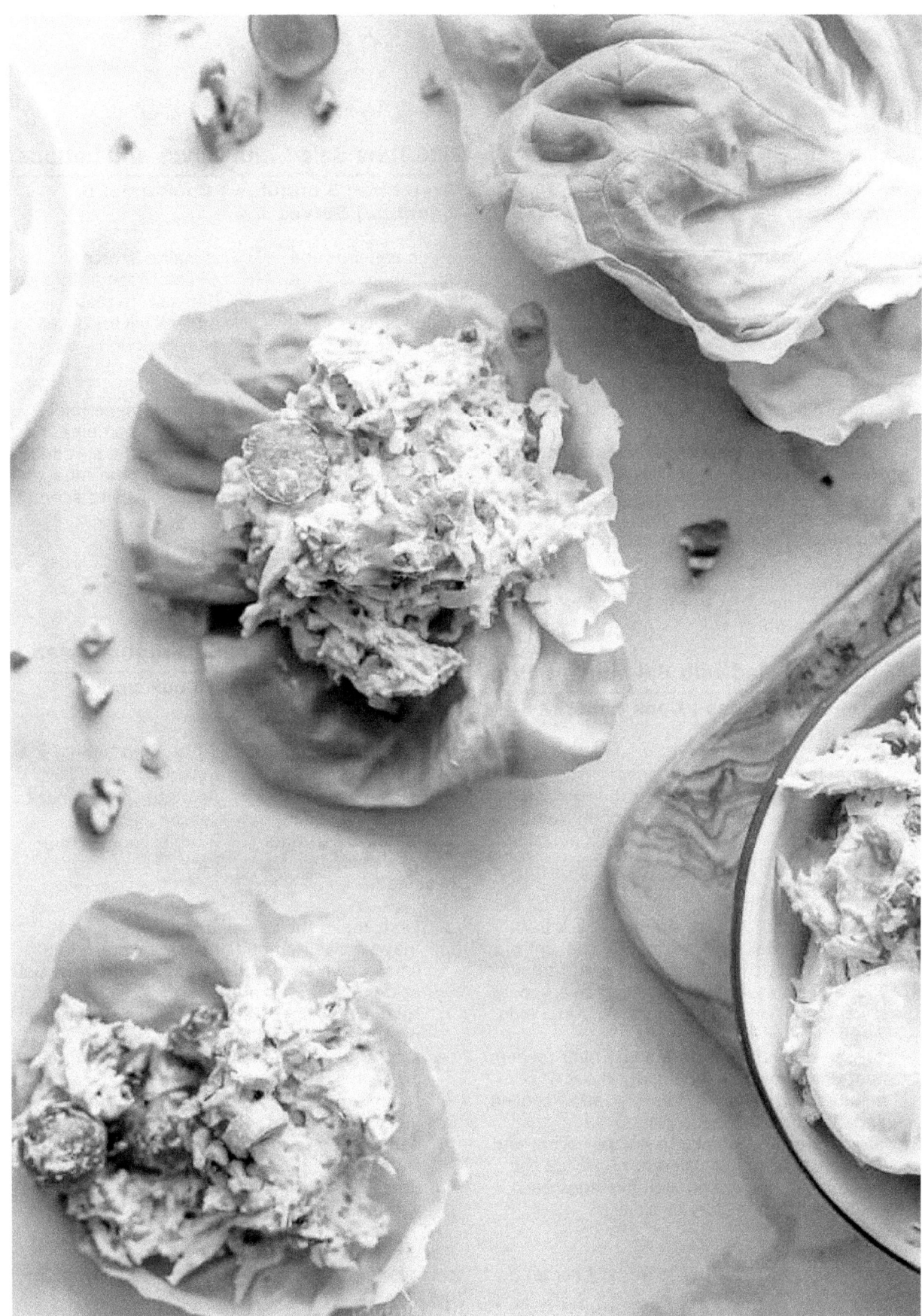

Chapter 10 Salad

384. Classic Greek Salad

Prep time: 10 minutes | Cook time: 0 minutes | Serves 4

5 tomatoes, chopped
1 large cucumber, chopped
1 green bell pepper, chopped
1 small red onion, chopped
16 kalamata olives, chopped
1 tablespoon capers
1 cup feta cheese, chopped
1 teaspoon oregano, dried
1 tablespoon olive oil
Salt to taste

1. Place tomatoes, bell pepper, cucumber, onion, feta cheese and olives in a bowl; mix to combine well. Season with salt. Combine capers, olive oil, and oregano, in a bowl. Drizzle with the dressing to serve.

Per Serving
calories: 323 | fat: 28g | protein: 9g | carbs: 12g net carbs: 8g | fiber: 4g

385. Caesar Salad with Salmon and Egg

Prep time: 5 minutes | Cook time: 27 minutes | Serves 4

2 cups water
8 eggs
2 cups torn romaine lettuce
½ cup smoked salmon, chopped
6 slices bacon
1 tablespoon Heinz low carb Caesar dressing

1. Boil the water in a pot over medium heat for 5 minutes and bring to simmer. Crack each egg into a small bowl and gently slide into the water. Poach for 2 to 3 minutes, remove with a perforated spoon, transfer to a paper towel to dry, and plate. Poach the remaining 7 eggs.
2. Put the bacon in a skillet and fry over medium heat until browned and crispy, about 6 minutes, turning once. Remove, allow cooling, and chop in small pieces.
3. Toss the lettuce, smoked salmon, bacon, and Caesar dressing in a salad bowl. Divide the salad into 4 plates, top with two eggs each, and serve immediately or chilled.

Per Serving
calories: 260 | fat: 21g | protein: 8g | carbs: 6g net carbs: 5g | fiber: 1g

386. Tuna Salad with Olives and Lettuce

Prep time: 5 minutes | Cook time: 0 minutes | Serves 2

1 cup canned tuna, drained
1 teaspoon onion flakes
1 tablespoon mayonnaise
1 cup shredded romaine lettuce
1 tablespoon lime juice
Sea salt, to taste
6 black olives, pitted and sliced

1. Combine the tuna, mayonnaise, lime juice, and salt in a small bowl; mix to combine well. In a salad platter, arrange the shredded lettuce and onion flakes. Spread the tuna mixture over; top with black olives to serve.

Per Serving
calories: 248 | fat: 20g | protein: 19g | carbs: 3g net carbs: 2g | fiber: 1g

387. Lemony Prawn and Arugula Salad

Prep time: 10 minutes | Cook time: 3 minute | Serves 4

4 cups baby arugula
½ cup garlic mayonnaise
1 tablespoon olive oil
1 pound (454 g) tiger prawns, peeled and deveined
1 teaspoon Dijon mustard
Salt and chili pepper to season
2 tablespoons lemon juice

1. First, make the dressing: add the mayonnaise, lemon juice and mustard in a small bowl. Mix until smooth and creamy. Set aside until ready to use.
2. Heat 1 tablespoon of olive oil in a skillet over medium heat, add the prawns, season with salt, and chili pepper, and fry for 3 minutes on each side until prawns are pink. Set aside to a plate.
3. Place the arugula in a serving bowl and pour half of the dressing on the salad. Toss with 2 spoons until mixed, and add the remaining dressing. Divide salad onto 4 plates and top with prawns.

Per Serving
calories: 215 | fat: 20g | protein: 8g | carbs: 3g net carbs: 2g | fiber: 1g

388. Mediterranean Tomato and Avocado Salad

Prep time: 5 minutes | Cook time: 0 minutes | Serves 4

3 tomatoes, sliced
1 large avocado, sliced
8 kalamata olives
¼ pound (113 g) buffalo mozzarella cheese, sliced
1 tablespoon pesto sauce
1 tablespoon olive oil

1. Arrange the tomato slices on a serving platter and place the avocado slices in the middle.
2. Arrange the olives around the avocado slices and drop pieces of mozzarella on the platter.
3. Drizzle the pesto sauce all over, and drizzle olive oil as well.

Per Serving
calories: 290 | fat: 25g | protein: 9g | carbs: 9g net carbs: 4g | fiber: 5g

389. Salmon Fillet and Spinach Cobb Salad

Prep time: 5 minutes | Cook time: 25 minutes | Serves 2

4 bacon slices
2 large eggs
2 (6-ounce / 170-g) salmon fillets
Pink Himalayan salt, to taste
Freshly ground black pepper, to taste
1 tablespoon butter, if needed
1 avocado, sliced
6 ounces (170-g) organic baby spinach
¼ cup crumbled blue cheese
1 tablespoon olive oil

1. In a medium skillet over medium-high heat, cook the bacon on both sides until crispy, about 8 minutes. Transfer the bacon to a paper towel–lined plate.
2. Bring a small saucepan filled with water to a boil over high heat. Put the eggs on to softboil, turn the heat down to medium-high, and cook for about 6 minutes.
3. Meanwhile, pat the salmon fillets on both sides with a paper towel to remove excess moisture. Season both sides with pink Himalayan salt and pepper.
4. With the bacon grease still in the skillet, add the salmon. If you need more grease in the pan, add some butter to the bacon grease.
5. Cook the salmon on medium-high heat for 5 minutes on each side, or until it reaches your preferred degree of doneness. (I like it medium-rare.)
6. Meanwhile, transfer the bacon to a cutting board and chop it. Peel the softboiled eggs. Season the avocado with pink Himalayan salt and pepper.
7. Divide the spinach, bacon, and avocado between two plates.
8. Carefully halve the softboiled eggs and place them on the salads. Sprinkle the blue cheese crumbles over the salads.
9. Top with the salmon, drizzle the salads with the olive oil, and serve.

Per Serving
calories: 623 | fat: 43g | protein: 54g | carbs: 12g net carbs: 5g | fiber: 7g

390. Egg and Chicken Salad in Lettuce Cups

Prep time: 10 minutes | Cook time: 18 minutes | Serves 4

2 chicken breasts, cut into pieces
1 tablespoon olive oil
Salt and black pepper to season
6 large eggs
1½ cups water
2 tomatoes, seeded, chopped
6 tablespoon Greek yogurt
1 head green lettuce, firm leaves removed for cups

1. Preheat oven to 400ºF (205ºC). Put the chicken pieces in a bowl, drizzle with olive oil, and sprinkle with salt and black pepper. Mix the ingredients until the chicken is well coated with the seasoning.
2. Put the chicken on a prepared baking sheet and spread out evenly. Slide the baking sheet in the oven and bake the chicken until cooked through and golden brown for 8 minutes, turning once.
3. Bring the eggs to boil in salted water in a pot over medium heat for 10 minutes. Run the eggs in cold water, peel, and chop into small pieces. Transfer to a salad bowl.
4. Remove the chicken from the oven when ready and add to the salad bowl. Include the tomatoes and Greek yogurt; mix evenly with a spoon. Layer two lettuce leaves each as cups and fill with two tablespoons of egg salad each. Serve with chilled blueberry juice.

Per Serving
calories: 325 | fat: 25g | protein: 21g | carbs: 7g net carbs: 4g | fiber: 3g

391. Tuna Cheese Caprese Salad

Prep time: 10 minutes | Cook time: 0 minutes | Serves 4

2 (10 ounce / 283-g) cans tuna chunks in water, drained	6 basil leaves
2 tomatoes, sliced	½ cup black olives, pitted and sliced
8 ounces (283 g) fresh mozzarella cheese, sliced	1 tablespoon extra virgin olive oil
	½ lemon, juiced

1. Place the tuna in the center of a serving platter. Arrange the cheese and tomato slices around the tuna. Alternate a slice of tomato, cheese, and a basil leaf.
2. To finish, scatter the black olives over the top, drizzle with olive oil and lemon juice and serve.

Per Serving

calories: 360 | fat: 31g | protein: 21g | carbs: 3g net carbs: 1g | fiber: 2g

392. Balsamic Brussels Sprouts Cheese Salad

Prep time: 10 minutes | Cook time: 20 minutes | Serves 6

2 pound (907 g) Brussels sprouts, halved	balsamic vinegar
1 tablespoon olive oil	¼ head red cabbage, shredded
Salt and black pepper to taste	1 tablespoon Dijon mustard
2½ tablespoon	1 cup Pecorino Romano cheese, grated

1. Preheat oven to 400ºF (205ºC) and line a baking sheet with foil. Toss the brussels sprouts with olive oil, a little salt, black pepper, and balsamic vinegar, in a bowl, and spread on the baking sheet in an even layer. Bake until tender on the inside and crispy on the outside, about 20 to 25 minutes.
2. Transfer to a salad bowl and add the red cabbage, Dijon mustard and half of the cheese. Mix until well combined. Sprinkle with the remaining cheese, share the salad onto serving plates, and serve with the salmon.

Per Serving

calories: 210 | fat: 18g | protein: 4g | carbs: 12g net carbs: 6g | fiber: 6g

393. Garlicky Chicken Salad

Prep time: 10 minutes | Cook time: 8 minutes | Serves 4

2 chicken breasts, boneless, skinless, flattened	1 teaspoon olive oil
Salt and black pepper, to taste	1½ cups mixed salad greens
1 tablespoon garlic powder	1 tablespoon red wine vinegar
	1 cup crumbled blue cheese

1. Season the chicken with salt, black pepper, and garlic powder. Heat oil in a pan over high heat and fry the chicken for 4 minutes on both sides until golden brown. Remove chicken to a cutting board and let cool before slicing.
2. Toss salad greens with red wine vinegar and share the salads into 4 plates. Divide chicken slices on top and sprinkle with blue cheese. Serve.

Per Serving

calories: 286 | fat: 23g | protein: 14g | carbs: 5g net carbs: 4g | fiber: 1g

394. Shrimp Salad with Lemony Mayonnaise

Prep time: 10 minutes | Cook time: 0 minutes | Serves 4

1 small head cauliflower, cut into florets	olives
⅓ cup diced celery	2 cups cooked large shrimp
½ cup sliced black	1 tablespoon dill, chopped
Dressing:	
½ cup mayonnaise	A pinch of black pepper
1 teaspoon apple cider vinegar	1 tablespoon lemon juice
¼ teaspoon celery seeds	1 teaspoon Swerve
	Salt to taste

1. Combine the cauliflower, celery, shrimp, and dill in a large bowl.
2. Whisk together the mayonnaise, vinegar, celery seeds, black pepper, sweetener, and lemon juice in another bowl. Season with salt to taste. Pour the dressing over and gently toss to combine; refrigerate for 1 hour. Top with olives to serve.

Per Serving

calories: 182 | fat: 15g | protein: 12g | carbs: 4g net carbs: 2g | fiber: 2g

395. Mackerel and Green Bean Salad

Prep time: 10 minutes | Cook time: 11 minutes | Serves 2

2 mackerel fillets
2 hard-boiled eggs, sliced
1 tablespoon coconut oil
2 cups green beans
1 avocado, sliced
4 cups mixed salad greens
1 tablespoon olive oil
1 tablespoon lemon juice
1 teaspoon Dijon mustard
Salt and black pepper, to taste

1. Fill a saucepan with water and add the green beans and salt. Cook over medium heat for about 3 minutes. Drain and set aside.
2. Melt the coconut oil in a pan over medium heat. Add the mackerel fillets and cook for about 4 minutes per side, or until opaque and crispy. Divide the green beans between two salad bowls. Top with mackerel, eggs, and avocado slices.
3. In a bowl, whisk together the lemon juice, olive oil, mustard, salt, and pepper, and drizzle over the salad.

Per Serving
calories: 525 | fat: 42g | protein: 27g | carbs: 22g net carbs: 8g | fiber: 14g

396. Strawberry and Spinach Salad

Prep time: 5 minutes | Cook time: 10 minutes | Serves 2

4 cups spinach
4 strawberries, sliced
½ cup flaked almonds
1½ cup grated hard goat cheese
1 tablespoon raspberry vinaigrette
Salt and black pepper, to taste

1. Preheat your oven to 400ºF (205ºC). Arrange the grated goat cheese in two circles on two pieces of parchment paper. Place in the oven and bake for 10 minutes.
2. Find two same bowls, place them upside down, and carefully put the parchment paper on top to give the cheese a bowl-like shape. Let cool that way for 15 minutes. Divide spinach among the bowls stir in salt, pepper and drizzle with vinaigrette. Top with almonds and strawberries.

Per Serving
calories: 445 | fat: 34g | protein: 33g | carbs: 7g net carbs: 5g | fiber: 2g

397. Cheesy Pork Patties Salad

Prep time: 5 minutes | Cook time: 20 minutes | Serves 4

1 pound (454 g) ground pork
Salt and black pepper to season
1 tablespoon olive oil
2 hearts romaine lettuce, torn into pieces
2 firm tomatoes, sliced
¼ red onion, sliced
3 ounces (85 g) yellow cheddar cheese, shredded

1. Season the pork with salt and black pepper, mix and make medium-sized patties out of them.
2. Heat the oil in a skillet over medium heat and fry the patties on both sides for 10 minutes until browned and cook within. Transfer to a wire rack to drain oil. When cooled, cut into quarters.
3. Mix the lettuce, tomatoes, and red onion in a salad bowl, season with a little oil, salt, and black pepper. Toss and add the pork on top.
4. Melt the cheese in the microwave for about 90 seconds. Drizzle the cheese over the salad and serve.

Per Serving
calories: 310 | fat: 23g | protein: 22g | carbs: 9g net carbs: 2g | fiber: 7g

398. Bacon, Avocado, and Veggies Salad

Prep time: 10 minutes | Cook time: 0 minutes | Serves 4

2 large avocados, 1 chopped and 1 sliced
1 spring onion, sliced
4 cooked bacon slices, crumbled
2 cups spinach
2 small lettuce heads, chopped
2 hard-boiled eggs, chopped
Vinaigrette:
1 tablespoon olive oil
1 teaspoon Dijon mustard
1 tablespoon apple cider vinegar

1. Combine the spinach, lettuce, eggs, chopped avocado, and spring onion, in a large bowl. Whisk together the vinaigrette ingredients in another bowl. Pour the dressing over, toss to combine and top with the sliced avocado and bacon.

Per Serving
calories: 350 | fat: 33g | protein: 7g | carbs: 11g net carbs: 3g | fiber: 8g

399. Cheesy Green Salad with Bacon

Prep time: 5 minutes | Cook time: 6 minutes | Serves 4

2 (8-ounce / 227-g) pack mixed salad greens
8 strips bacon
1½ cups crumbled blue cheese
1 tablespoon white wine vinegar
1 tablespoon extra virgin olive oil
Salt and black pepper to taste

1. Pour the salad greens in a salad bowl; set aside. Fry bacon strips in a skillet over medium heat for 6 minutes, until browned and crispy. Chop the bacon and scatter over the salad. Add in half of the cheese, toss and set aside.
2. In a small bowl, whisk the white wine vinegar, olive oil, salt, and black pepper until dressing is well combined. Drizzle half of the dressing over the salad, toss, and top with remaining cheese. Divide salad into four plates and serve with crusted chicken fries along with the remaining dressing.

Per Serving
calories: 205 | fat: 20g | protein: 4g | carbs: 5g net carbs: 2g | fiber: 3g

400. Shrimp, Cauliflower and Avocado Salad

Prep time: 10 minutes | Cook time: 13 minutes | Serves 6

1 cauliflower head, florets only
1 pound (454 g) medium shrimp
¼ cup plus 1 tablespoon olive oil
1 avocado, chopped
1 tablespoon chopped dill
¼ cup lemon juice
1 tablespoon lemon zest
Salt and black pepper to taste

1. Heat 1 tablespoon olive oil in a skillet and cook shrimp for 8 minutes. Microwave cauliflower for 5 minutes.
2. Place shrimp, cauliflower, and avocado in a bowl. Whisk the remaining olive oil, lemon zest, juice, dill, and salt, and pepper, in another bowl. Pour the dressing over, toss to combine and serve immediately.

Per Serving
calories: 214 | fat: 17g | protein: 15g | carbs: 9g net carbs: 5g | fiber: 4g

401. Mozzarella Bacon and Tomato Salad

Prep time: 5 minutes | Cook time: 5 minutes | Serves 2

1 large tomato, sliced
4 basil leaves
8 mozzarella cheese slices
1 teaspoon olive oil
4 bacon slices, chopped
1 teaspoon balsamic vinegar
Salt, to taste

1. Place the bacon in a skillet over medium heat and cook until crispy, about 5 minutes. Divide the tomato slices between two serving plates. Arrange the mozzarella slices over and top with the basil leaves. Add the crispy bacon on top, drizzle with olive oil and vinegar. Sprinkle with salt and serve.

Per Serving
calories: 279 | fat: 26g | protein: 21g | carbs: 3g net carbs: 2g | fiber: 1g

402. Skirt Steak, Veggies, and Pecan Salad

Prep time: 15 minutes | Cook time: 10 minutes | Serves 2

8 ounces (227 g) skirt steak
Pink Himalayan salt
Freshly ground black pepper
1 tablespoon butter
2 romaine hearts or 2 cups chopped romaine
½ cup halved grape tomatoes
¼ cup crumbled blue cheese
¼ cup pecans
1 tablespoon olive oil

1. Heat a large skillet over high heat.
2. Pat the steak dry with a paper towel, and season both sides with pink Himalayan salt and pepper.
3. Add the butter to the skillet. When it melts, put the steak in the skillet.
4. Sear the steak for about 3 minutes on each side, for medium-rare.
5. Transfer the steak to a cutting board and let it rest for at least 5 minutes.
6. Meanwhile, divide the romaine between two plates, and top with the grape tomato halves, blue cheese, and pecans. Drizzle with the olive oil.
7. Slice the skirt steak across the grain, top the salads with it, and serve.

Per Serving
calories: 451 | fat: 36g | protein: 30g | carbs: 7g net carbs: 5g | fiber: 2g

403. Spring Vegetable Salad with Cheese Balls

Prep time: 15 minutes | Cook time: 10 minutes | Serves 6

Cheese balls:
3 eggs
1 cup feta cheese, crumbled
½ cup pecorino cheese, shredded
1 cup almond flour
1 tablespoon flax meal
1 teaspoon baking powder
Salt and black pepper, to taste

Salad:
1 head iceberg lettuce, leaves separated
½ cup cucumber, thinly sliced
2 tomatoes, seeded and chopped
½ cup red onion, thinly sliced
½ cup radishes, thinly sliced
⅓ cup mayonnaise
1 teaspoon mustard
1 teaspoon paprika
1 teaspoon oregano
Salt, to taste

1. Set oven to 390°F (199°C). Line a piece of parchment paper to a baking sheet.
2. In a mixing dish, mix all ingredients for the cheese balls; form balls out of the mixture. Set the balls on the prepared baking sheet. Bake for 10 minutes until crisp. Arrange lettuce leaves on a large salad platter; add in radishes, tomatoes, cucumbers, and red onion. In a small mixing bowl, mix the mayonnaise, paprika, salt, oregano, and mustard. Sprinkle this mixture over the vegetables. Add cheese balls on top and serve.

Per Serving
calories: 234 | fat: 17g | protein: 12g | carbs: 11g net carbs: 8g | fiber: 3g

404. Baby Arugula and Walnuts Salad

Prep time: 10 minutes | Cook time: 0 minutes | Serves 4

4 tablespoons extra-virgin olive oil
Zest and juice of 2 lemon (2 to 3 tablespoons)
1 tablespoon red wine vinegar
½ teaspoon salt
¼ teaspoon freshly ground black pepper
8 cups baby arugula
1 cup coarsely chopped walnuts
1 cup crumbled goat cheese
½ cup pomegranate seeds

1. In a small bowl, whisk together the olive oil, zest and juice, vinegar, salt, and pepper and set aside.
2. To assemble the salad for serving, in a large bowl, combine the arugula, walnuts, goat cheese, and pomegranate seeds. Drizzle with the dressing and toss to coat.

Per Serving
calories: 444 | fat: 40g | protein: 10g | carbs: 11g net carbs: 8g | fiber: 3g

405. Ritzy Chicken Salad with Tzatziki Sauce

Prep time: 15 minutes | Cook time: 20 minutes | Serves 2

Chicken:
3 tablespoons extra virgin olive oil, divided
Juice of ½ lemon
1 tablespoon organic apple cider vinegar
½ teaspoon garlic powder
1 pound (454 g) boneless, skinless chicken thighs

Tzatziki Sauce:
1 cup full-fat organic Greek yogurt
1 tablespoon extra virgin olive oil
½ cup deseeded and grated Persian cucumber
2 garlic cloves, minced
Juice of 1 lemon
¼ teaspoon sea salt

Salad:
3 to 4 cups baby spinach leaves
½ cup cherry tomatoes, sliced
½ red onion, sliced
¼ cup full-fat feta, crumbled
¼ cup Kalamata olives, sliced

1. In a small bowl, mix together 2 tablespoons olive oil, lemon juice, cider vinegar, and garlic powder. Put the chicken thighs in a large bowl and pour the marinade over them. Put the chicken in the refrigerator to marinate for 30 minutes.
2. While the chicken marinates, mix together the tzatziki ingredients in a small bowl and set aside.
3. Heat the remaining 1 tablespoon olive oil in a large skillet over medium heat. Add the chicken, cooking the thighs on each side for 8 to 10 minutes, or until cooked through and the internal temperature reaches 165°F (74°C).
4. Remove the chicken from the skillet and slice each thigh into four or five pieces.
5. Combine the salad ingredients and serve in two bowls, topped with the chicken and tzatziki sauce.

Per Serving
calories: 899 | fat: 68g | protein: 61g | carbs: 19g net carbs: 16g | fiber: 3g

406. Tuscan Kale Salad with Lemony Anchovies

Prep time: 15 minutes | Cook time: 0 minutes | Serves 4

1 large bunch lacinato or dinosaur kale
¼ cup toasted pine nuts
1 cup shaved or coarsely shredded fresh Parmesan cheese
¼ cup extra-virgin olive oil
8 anchovy fillets, roughly chopped
2 to 3 tablespoons freshly squeezed lemon juice (from 1 large lemon)
2 teaspoons red pepper flakes (optional)

1. Remove the rough center stems from the kale leaves and roughly tear each leaf into about 4-by-1-inch strips. Place the torn kale in a large bowl and add the pine nuts and cheese.
2. In a small bowl, whisk together the olive oil, anchovies, lemon juice, and red pepper flakes (if using). Drizzle over the salad and toss to coat well. Let sit at room temperature 30 minutes before serving, tossing again just prior to serving.

Per Serving
calories: 337 | fat: 25g | protein: 16g | carbs: 12g net carbs: 10g | fiber: 2g

407. Caesar Salad with Chicken and Cheese

Prep time: 10 minutes | Cook time: 11 minutes | Serves 4

4 boneless, skinless chicken thighs
¼ cup lemon juice
2 garlic cloves, minced
1 tablespoon olive oil
½ cup Caesar salad dressing, sugar-free
12 bok choy leaves
3 Parmesan crisps
Parmesan cheese, grated for garnishing

1. Mix chicken, lemon juice, 1 tablespoon olive oil and garlic in a ziploc bag. Seal the bag, shake well, and refrigerate for 1 hour.
2. Preheat the grill to medium and grill the chicken for 4 minutes per side. Cut bok choy lengthwise, and brush with the remaining oil. Grill the bok choy for about 3 minutes.
3. Place on a bowl. Top with chicken and Parmesan; drizzle the dressing over. Top with Parmesan crisps to serve.

Per Serving
calories: 529 | fat: 39g | protein: 33g | carbs: 6g net carbs: 5g | fiber: 1g

408. Tangy Squid and Veggies Salad

Prep time: 15 minutes | Cook time: 5 minutes | Serves 4

4 medium squid tubes, cut into strips
½ cup mint leaves
2 medium cucumbers, halved and cut in strips
½ cup coriander leaves, reserve the stems
½ red onion, finely sliced
Salt and black pepper, to taste
1 teaspoon fish sauce
1 red chili, roughly chopped
1 clove garlic
2 limes, juiced
1 tablespoon chopped coriander
1 teaspoon olive oil

1. In a salad bowl, mix mint leaves, cucumber strips, coriander leaves, and red onion. Season with salt, black pepper and some olive oil; set aside. In the mortar, pound the coriander stems, and red chili to form a paste using the pestle. Add the fish sauce and lime juice, and mix with the pestle.
2. Heat a skillet over high heat on a stovetop and sear the squid on both sides to lightly brown, about 5 minutes. Pour the squid on the salad and drizzle with the chili dressing. Toss the ingredients with two spoons, garnish with coriander, and serve the salad as a single dish or with some more seafood.

Per Serving
calories: 318 | fat: 23g | protein: 25g | carbs: 3g net carbs: 2g | fiber: 1g

409. Mustard Eggs Salad

Prep time: 10 minutes | Cook time: 10 minutes | Serves 8

10 eggs
¾ cup mayonnaise
1 teaspoon sriracha sauce
1 tablespoon mustard
½ cup scallions
½ stalk celery, minced
½ teaspoon fresh lemon juice
½ teaspoon sea salt
½ teaspoon black pepper
1 head romaine lettuce, torn into pieces

1. Add the eggs in a pan and cover with enough water and boil. Get them from the heat and allow to set for 10 minutes while covered. Chop the eggs and add to a salad bowl. Stir in the remaining ingredients until everything is well combined. Refrigerate until ready to serve.

Per Serving
calories: 174 | fat: 13g | protein: 7g | carbs: 10g net carbs: 8g | fiber: 2g

410. Skirt Steak and Pickled Peppers Salad

Prep time: 10 minutes | Cook time: 10 minutes | Serves 4

1 pound (454 g) skirt steak, sliced
Salt and black pepper to season
1 teaspoon olive oil
1½ cups mixed salad greens
3 chopped pickled peppers
1 tablespoon red wine vinaigrette
½ cup crumbled queso fresco

1. Brush the steak slices with olive oil and season with salt and black pepper on both sides. Heat pan over high heat and cook the steaks on each side for about 5-6 minutes. Remove to a bow.
2. Mix the salad greens, pickled peppers, and vinaigrette in a salad bowl. Add the beef and sprinkle with queso fresco.

Per Serving
calories: 315 | fat: 26g | protein: 18g | carbs: 3g net carbs: 2g | fiber: 1g

411. Lush Greek Salad

Prep time: 10 minutes | Cook time: 0 minutes | Serves 4

2 large English cucumbers
4 Roma tomatoes, quartered
1 green bell pepper, cut into 1- to 1½-inch chunks
¼ small red onion, thinly sliced
4 ounces pitted Kalamata olives
¼ cup extra-virgin olive oil
2 tablespoons freshly squeezed lemon juice
1 tablespoon red wine vinegar
1 tablespoon chopped fresh oregano or 1 teaspoon dried oregano
¼ teaspoon freshly ground black pepper
4 ounces (113 g) crumbled traditional feta cheese

1. Cut the cucumbers in half lengthwise and then into ½-inch-thick half-moons. Place in a large bowl.
2. Add the quartered tomatoes, bell pepper, red onion, and olives.
3. In a small bowl, whisk together the olive oil, lemon juice, vinegar, oregano, and pepper. Drizzle over the vegetables and toss to coat.
4. Divide between salad plates and top each with 1 ounce of feta.

Per Serving
calories: 278 | fat: 22g | protein: 8g | carbs: 12g net carbs: 8g | fiber: 4g

412. Dijon Broccoli Slaw Salad

Prep time: 10 minutes | Cook time: 0 minutes | Serves 6

1 tablespoon granulated Swerve
1 tablespoon Dijon mustard
1 tablespoon olive oil
4 cups broccoli slaw
⅓ cup mayonnaise, sugar-free
1 teaspoon celery seeds
1½ tablespoon apple cider vinegar
Salt and black pepper, to taste

1. Whisk together all ingredients except the broccoli slaw. Place broccoli slaw in a large salad bowl. Pour the dressing over. Mix with your hands to combine well.

Per Serving
calories: 110 | fat: 10g | protein: 3g | carbs: 5g net carbs: 2g | fiber: 3g

413. Tangy Shrimp Ceviche Salad

Prep time: 15 minutes | Cook time: 0 minutes | Serves 4

1 pound fresh shrimp, peeled and deveined
1 small red or yellow bell pepper, cut into ½-inch chunks
½ English cucumber, peeled and cut into ½-inch chunks
½ small red onion, cut into thin slivers
¼ cup chopped fresh cilantro or flat-leaf Italian parsley
⅓ cup freshly squeezed lime juice
2 tablespoons freshly squeezed lemon juice
2 tablespoons freshly squeezed lemon juice
½ cup extra-virgin olive oil
1 teaspoon salt
½ teaspoon freshly ground black pepper
2 ripe avocados, peeled, pitted, and cut into ½-inch chunks

1. Cut the shrimp in half lengthwise. In a large glass bowl, combine the shrimp, bell pepper, cucumber, onion, and cilantro.
2. In a small bowl, whisk together the lime, lemon, and clementine juices, olive oil, salt, and pepper. Pour the mixture over the shrimp and veggies and toss to coat. Cover and refrigerate for at least 2 hours, or up to 8 hours. Give the mixture a toss every 30 minutes for the first 2 hours to make sure all the shrimp "cook" in the juices.
3. Add the cut avocado just before serving and toss to combine.

Per Serving
calories: 497 | fat: 40g | protein: 25g | carbs: 14g net carbs: 8g | fiber: 6g

414. Dijon Cauliflower Salad

Prep time: 10 minutes | Cook time: 10 minutes | Serves 6

1 large cauliflower
Sea salt and freshly ground black pepper, to taste
3 hard-boiled eggs, diced
¾ cup avocado oil mayonnaise
2 tablespoons Dijon mustard
¼ cup dill pickle, diced
3 celery stalks, diced
1 tablespoon apple cider vinegar
1 teaspoon garlic powder

1. Remove the stem and cut the cauliflower into florets.
2. Put 1 to 2 inches water in a large pot, add a pinch of salt, and bring to a boil. Add the cauliflower, reduce the heat to low, and cover the pot. Steam the cauliflower for 10 minutes, or until fork-tender.
3. Drain the cauliflower and let it cool for 15 minutes.
4. Mix the remaining ingredients in a large bowl. When cooled, add the cauliflower and mix together.
5. Cover and refrigerate for 1 to 2 hours, until chilled. Serve cold.

Per Serving

calories: 305 | fat: 30g | protein: 6g | carbs: 4g
net carbs: 3g | fiber: 1g

415. Classic Caprese Salad

Prep time: 10 minutes | Cook time: 0 minutes | Serves 8

8 ounces (227 g) fresh mozzarella cheese
4 tomatoes
¼ cup balsamic vinegar
¼ cup extra virgin olive oil
1 cup fresh basil
1 teaspoon sea salt
½ teaspoon freshly ground black pepper

1. Cut the mozzarella and tomatoes into ¼-inch-thick slices and arrange in an alternating pattern on a plate.
2. In a small bowl, mix the balsamic vinegar and olive oil. Drizzle on top of the mozzarella and tomatoes.
3. Stack the fresh basil and roll it into a tight log. Carefully cut into thin julienne slices, and toss over the salad.
4. Sprinkle the salt and pepper on top and enjoy.

Per Serving

calories: 148 | fat: 11g | protein: 9g | carbs: 4g
net carbs: 3g | fiber: 1g

416. Cheesy Bacon Salad with Walnuts

Prep time: 5 minutes | Cook time: 10 minutes | Serves 4

½ pound bacon, diced
1 (8-ounce) log fresh goat cheese
½ cup pork dust (or pork rinds crushed into a powder)
3 tablespoons plus 2 teaspoons coconut vinegar or red wine vinegar
3 tablespoons avocado oil, MCT oil, or extra-virgin olive oil
1 teaspoon Dijon mustard
½ teaspoon fine sea salt
¼ teaspoon ground black pepper
2 drops stevia glycerite (optional)
4 cups leafy greens
½ avocado, sliced (optional)
½ cup raw walnuts, for garnish (optional; omit for nut-free)

1. Sauté the diced bacon in a skillet over medium heat until crisp, about 5 minutes. Using a slotted spoon, remove the bacon to a bowl, leaving the drippings in the pan.
2. Meanwhile, cut the goat cheese log into 8 medallions that are about ¼ inch thick.
3. Place the pork dust in a shallow bowl. Gently roll each goat cheese medallion in the pork dust to cover the medallions.
4. In batches, fry the medallions in the hot skillet with the bacon drippings over medium heat for 1 minute or until golden brown, then flip and fry for another minute. Remove the medallions from the skillet and set aside on a plate.
5. Add the vinegar, oil, mustard, salt, pepper, and stevia, if using, to the skillet and stir well to combine. Stir in the cooked bacon.
6. Plate the greens and avocado slices, if using, on a serving platter and top with the fried goat cheese medallions. Drizzle the bacon vinaigrette over the greens and garnish with walnuts and freshly ground pepper, if desired.

Per Serving

calories: 766 | fat: 67g | protein: 36g | carbs: 8g
net carbs: 4g | fiber: 4g

417. Turkey and Walnuts Salad

Prep time: 10 minutes | Cook time: 0 minutes | Serves 4

1 pound (454 g) turkey breast, cooked
3 green onions, sliced
2 celery stalks, diced
½ cup chopped walnuts
½ cup avocado oil mayonnaise
1 teaspoon fresh lemon juice
¼ teaspoon sea salt
¼ teaspoon freshly ground black pepper
Mixed greens

1. Chop the turkey breast into small pieces.
2. In a large bowl, combine the turkey, onions, celery, walnuts, mayonnaise, lemon juice, salt, and pepper, and mix well.
3. Serve on a bed of mixed greens.

Per Serving

calories: 351 | fat: 23g | protein: 32g | carbs: 5g net carbs: 3g | fiber: 2g

418. Dijon Egg Salad

Prep time: 5 minutes | Cook time: 0 minutes | Serves 4

6 hard boiled eggs, finely chopped
1 celery stalk, diced
½ cup cashews, finely diced
¼ cup olive oil mayonnaise
1 tablespoon Dijon mustard
1½ teaspoons curry powder
¼ teaspoon salt
¼ teaspoon freshly ground black pepper
8 butter lettuce leaves

1. In a medium mixing bowl, combine the eggs with the celery and cashews.
2. Add the mayonnaise, mustard, curry powder, salt, and pepper, and stir until thoroughly combined.
3. Divide the salad into four equal servings and serve on top of the butter lettuce leaves.

Per Serving

calories: 600 | fat: 50g | protein: 23g | carbs: 15g net carbs: 13g | fiber: 2g

419. Vinegary Cucumber Salad

Prep time: 5 minutes | Cook time: 0 minutes | Serves 2

1 large hothouse or English cucumber
¼ red onion, finely sliced
2 tablespoons organic apple cider vinegar
2 tablespoons extra virgin olive oil
5 drops liquid stevia
1 teaspoon sea salt

1. Slice the cucumber and place in a medium bowl. Add the red onion.
2. In a small bowl, mix the apple cider vinegar, olive oil, stevia, and salt together. Pour over the cucumbers and onion.
3. Stir together well to combine and refrigerate for 30 minutes. Serve chilled.

Per Serving

calories: 151 | fat: 14g | protein: 1g | carbs: 7g net carbs: 6g | fiber: 1g

420. Homemade Albacore Tuna Salad

Prep time: 5 minutes | Cook time: 0 minutes | Serves 4

2 (5-ounce / 142-g) cans albacore tuna packed in water, drained
¼ cup avocado oil mayonnaise
2 teaspoons Dijon mustard
3 teaspoons dried dill
2 teaspoons lime juice
½ cup diced bell pepper

1. In a small bowl, combine the tuna, mayonnaise, mustard, dill, lime juice, and bell pepper.
2. Serve on a bed of mixed greens.

Per Serving

calories: 294 | fat: 21g | protein: 13g | carbs: 19g net carbs: 12g | fiber: 7g

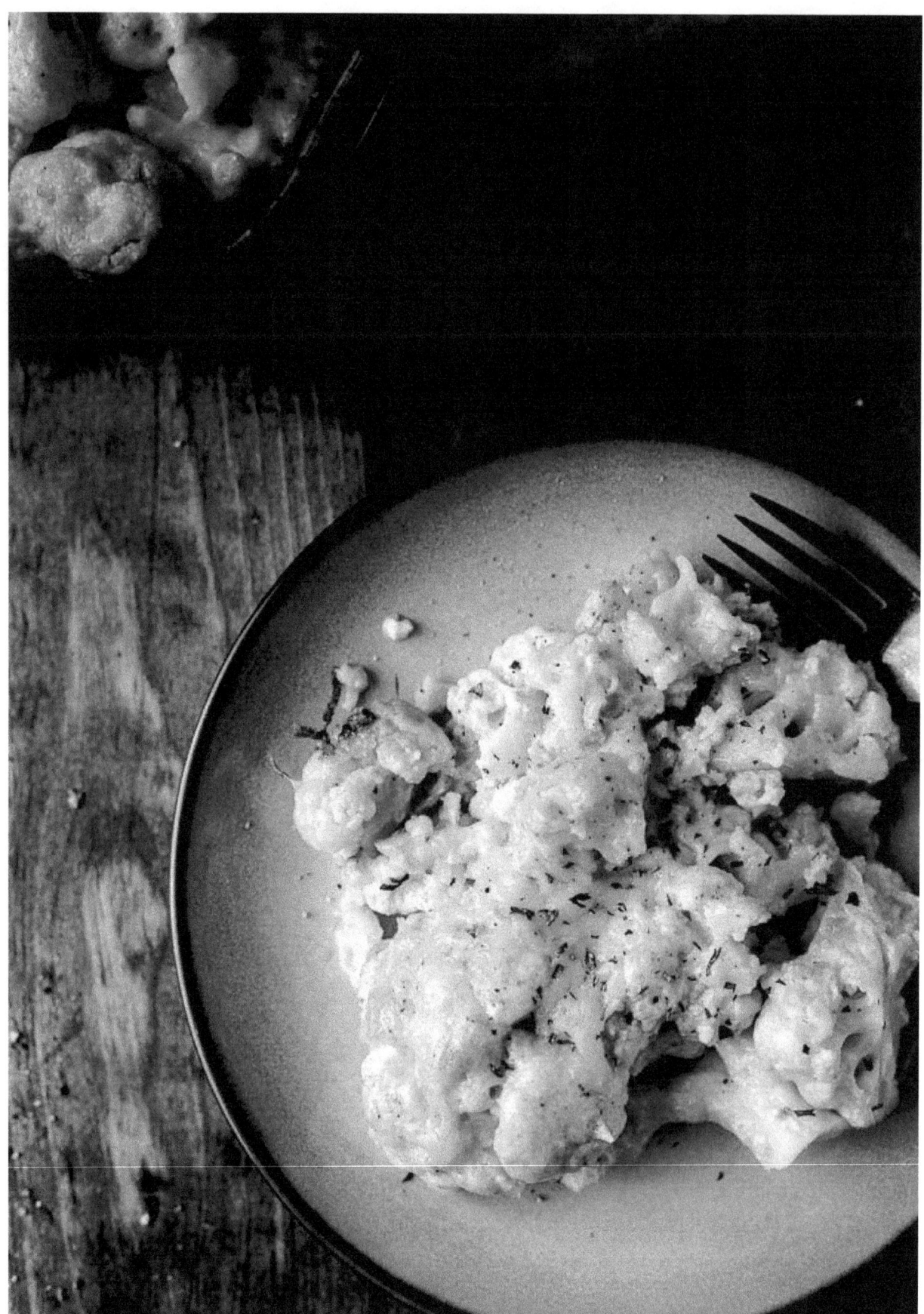

Chapter 11 Side Dishes

421. Roasted Cauliflower with Serrano Ham

Prep time: 5 minutes | Cook time: 20 minutes | Serves 6

1 head cauliflower, cut into 1-inch slices
2 tablespoons olive oil
Salt and chili pepper, to taste
1 teaspoon garlic powder
10 slices Serrano ham, chopped
¼ cup pine nuts, chopped
1 teaspoon capers
1 teaspoon parsley

1. Preheat oven to 450°F and line a baking sheet with foil. Brush the cauli steaks with olive oil and season with chili pepper, garlic, and salt. Spread the cauli slices on the baking sheet.
2. Roast in the oven for 10 minutes until tender and lightly browned. Remove the sheet and sprinkle the ham and pine nuts all over the cauli. Bake for another 10 minutes until the ham is crispy and a nutty aroma is perceived. Take out, sprinkle with capers and parsley and serve.

Per Serving
calories: 180 | fat: 13g | protein: 11g | carbs: 8g net carbs: 5g | fiber: 3g

422. Chicken-Stuffed Cucumber Bites

Prep time: 5 minutes | Cook time: 0 minutes | Serves 6

2 cucumbers, sliced with a 3-inch thickness
2 cups small dices leftover chicken
1. ¼ jalapeño pepper, seeded and minced
5.
6. Cut mid-level holes in cucumber slices with a knife and set aside. Combine chicken, jalapeño pepper, mustard, mayonnaise, salt, and black pepper to be evenly mixed. Fill cucumber holes with chicken mixture and serve.

2. 1 tablespoon Dijon mustard
3. ⅓ cup mayonnaise
4. Salt and black pepper, to taste

Per Serving
calories: 115 | fat: 14g | protein: 14g | carbs: 5g net carbs: 4g | fiber: 1g

423. Roasted Brussels Sprouts with Balsamic Glaze

Prep time: 5 minutes | Cook time: 30 minutes | Serves 4

3 tablespoons balsamic vinegar
1 tablespoon erythritol
½ tablespoon olive oil
Salt and black pepper, to taste
1 pound (454 g) Brussels sprouts, halved
5 slices prosciutto, chopped

1. Preheat oven to 400°F and line a baking sheet with parchment paper. Mix balsamic vinegar, erythritol, olive oil, salt, and black pepper and combine with the Brussels sprouts in a bowl.
2. Spread the mixture on the baking sheet and roast for 30 minutes until tender on the inside and crispy on the outside. Toss with prosciutto, share among 4 plates, and serve with chicken breasts.

Per Serving
calories: 143 | fat: 5g | protein: 10g | carbs: 16g net carbs: 11g | fiber: 5g

424. Cheddar Buffalo Chicken Bake

Prep time: 5 minutes | Cook time: 28 minutes | Serves 6

2 tablespoons olive oil
8 ounces (227 g) cream cheese
1 pound (454 g) ground chicken
1 cup buffalo sauce
1 cup ranch dressing
3 cups grated yellow Cheddar cheese

1. Preheat oven to 350°F. Lightly grease a baking sheet with a cooking spray. Warm the oil in a skillet over medium heat and brown the chicken for 5 minutes, take off the heat, and set aside.
2. Spread cream cheese at the bottom of the baking sheet, top with chicken, pour buffalo sauce over, add ranch dressing, and sprinkle with Cheddar cheese. Bake for 23 minutes until cheese has melted and golden brown on top. Remove and serve with veggie sticks.

Per Serving
calories: 618 | fat: 49g | protein: 33g | carbs: 14g net carbs: 12g | fiber: 2g

425. Chicken Breast Fritters with Dill Dip

Prep time: 10 minutes | Cook time: 8 minutes | Serves 4

1 pound (454 g) chicken breasts, thinly sliced	4 tablespoons dill, chopped
1¼ cup mayonnaise	3 tablespoons olive oil
¼ cup coconut flour	1 cup sour cream
2 eggs	1 teaspoon garlic powder
Salt and black pepper, to taste	1 tablespoon parsley, chopped
1 cup Mozzarella cheese, grated	1 onion, finely chopped

1. In a bowl, mix 1 cup of the mayonnaise, 3 tablespoons of dill, sour cream, garlic powder, onion, and salt. Cover the bowl with plastic wrap and refrigerate for 30 minutes.
2. Mix the chicken, remaining mayonnaise, coconut flour, eggs, salt, black pepper, Mozzarella, and remaining dill, in a bowl. Cover the bowl with plastic wrap and refrigerate it for 2 hours. After the marinating time is over, remove from the fridge.
3. Place a skillet over medium fire and heat the olive oil. Fetch 2 tablespoons of chicken mixture into the skillet, use the back of a spatula to flatten the top. Cook for 4 minutes, flip, and fry for 4 more.
4. Remove onto a wire rack and repeat the cooking process until the batter is finished, adding more oil as needed. Garnish the fritters with parsley and serve with dill dip.

Per Serving

calories: 671 | fat: 42g | protein: 45g | carbs: 15g net carbs: 13g | fiber: 2g

426. Simple Buttery Broccoli

Prep time: 5 minutes | Cook time: 3 minutes | Serves 6

1 broccoli head, florets only	pepper, to taste
Kosher salt and black	¼ cup butter

1. Place the broccoli in a pot filled with salted water and bring to a boil. Cook for about 3 minutes until crisp-tender. Drain the broccoli and transfer to a plate.
2. Melt the butter in a microwave. Drizzle the butter over and season with some salt and black pepper.

Per Serving

calories: 102 | fat: 8g | protein: 3g | carbs: 7g net carbs: 4g | fiber: 3g

427. Classic Devilled Eggs with Sriracha Mayo

Prep time: 5 minutes | Cook time: 10 minutes | Serves 4

8 large eggs	mayonnaise
3 cups water	Salt, to taste
3 tablespoons sriracha sauce	¼ teaspoon smoked paprika
4 tablespoons	

1. Bring eggs to boil in salted water in a pot over high heat, and then reduce the heat to simmer for 10 minutes. Transfer eggs to an ice water bath, let cool completely and peel the shells.
2. Slice the eggs in half height wise and empty the yolks into a bowl. Smash with a fork and mix in sriracha sauce, mayonnaise, and half of the paprika until smooth. Spoon filling into a piping bag with a round nozzle and fill the egg whites to be slightly above the brim.
3. Garnish with remaining paprika and serve.

Per Serving

calories: 180 | fat: 12g | protein: 13g | carbs: 4g net carbs: 4g | fiber: 0g

428. Cheesy Cauli Bake with Mayo

Prep time: 5 minutes | Cook time: 25 minutes | Serves 6

2 heads cauliflower, cut into florets	flakes
¼ cup melted butter	½ cup mayonnaise
Salt and black pepper to taste	¼ teaspoon Dijon mustard
1 pinch red pepper	3 tablespoons grated pecorino cheese

1. Preheat oven to 400ºF (205ºC) and grease a baking dish with cooking spray.
2. Combine the cauli florets, butter, salt, black pepper, and red pepper flakes in a bowl until well mixed. Mix the mayonnaise and Dijon mustard in a bowl, and set aside until ready to serve.
3. Arrange cauliflower florets on the prepared baking dish. Sprinkle with grated pecorino cheese and bake for 25 minutes until the cheese has melted and golden brown on the top.
4. Remove, let sit for 3 minutes to cool, and serve with the mayo sauce.

Per Serving

calories: 171 | fat: 13g | protein: 5g | carbs: 13g net carbs: 9g | fiber: 4g

429. Mashed Cauliflower with Bacon and Chives

Prep time: 5 minutes | Cook time: 16 minutes | Serves 6

6 slices bacon
3 heads cauliflower, leaves removed
2 cups water
2 tablespoons melted butter
½ cup coconut milk
Salt and black pepper, to taste
¼ cup grated yellow Cheddar cheese
2 tablespoons chopped chives

1. Preheat oven to 350°F. Fry bacon in a heated skillet over medium heat for 5 minutes until crispy. Remove to a paper towel-lined plate, allow to cool, and crumble. Set aside and keep bacon fat. Boil cauli heads in water in a pot over high heat for 7 minutes, until tender. Drain and put in a bowl.
2. Include butter, coconut milk, salt, black pepper, and purée using a hand blender until smooth and creamy. Lightly grease a casserole dish with the bacon fat and spread the mash on it.
3. Sprinkle with Cheddar cheese and place under the broiler for 4 minutes on high until the cheese melts. Remove and top with bacon and chopped chives. Serve with pan-seared scallops.

Per Serving
calories: 206 | fat: 17g | protein: 8g | carbs: 8g net carbs: 5g | fiber: 3g

430. Baked Zucchini Sticks with Garlic Aioli

Prep time: 5 minutes | Cook time: 15 minutes | Serves 4

¼ cup pork rind crumbs
1 teaspoon sweet paprika
¼ cup shredded Parmesan cheese
Salt and chili pepper, to taste
3 fresh eggs
2 zucchinis, cut into strips
Aioli:
½ cup mayonnaise
1 garlic clove, minced
Juice and zest from ½ lemon

1. Preheat oven to 425°F and line a baking sheet with foil. Grease with cooking spray and set aside.
2. Mix the pork rinds, paprika, Parmesan cheese, salt, and chili pepper in a bowl. Beat the eggs in another bowl.
3. Coat zucchini strips in eggs, then in Parmesan mixture, and arrange on the baking sheet. Grease lightly with cooking spray and bake for 15 minutes to be crispy.
4. To make the aioli, combine in a bowl mayonnaise, lemon juice, and garlic, and gently stir until everything is well incorporated. Add the lemon zest, adjust the seasoning and stir again. Cover and place in the refrigerator until ready to serve.
5. Serve the zucchini strips with garlic aioli for dipping.

Per Serving
calories: 186 | fat: 11g | protein: 8g | carbs: 7g net carbs: 5g | fiber: 2g

431. Crispy Chorizo with Parsley

Prep time: 5 minutes | Cook time: 15 minutes | Serves 6

7 ounces (198 g) Spanish chorizo, sliced
4 ounces (113 g) cream cheese
¼ cup chopped parsley

1. Preheat oven to 325°F (163°C). Line a baking dish with waxed paper. Bake chorizo for 15 minutes until crispy. Remove and let cool. Arrange on a serving platter. Top with cream cheese. Serve sprinkled with parsley.

Per Serving
calories: 207 | fat: 18g | protein: 9g | carbs: 1g net carbs: 1g | fiber: 0g

432. Simple Boiled Stuffed Eggs

Prep time: 5 minutes | Cook time: 10 minutes | Serves 6

6 eggs
1 tablespoon Sriracha
⅓ cup mayonnaise
Salt, to taste

1. Place the eggs in a saucepan and cover with salted water. Bring to a boil over medium heat. Boil for 10 minutes. Place the eggs in an ice bath and let cool for 10 minutes.
2. Peel and slice in half lengthwise. Scoop out the yolks to a bowl; mash with a fork. Whisk together the Sriracha, mayonnaise, mashed yolks, and salt, in a bowl. Spoon this mixture into egg whites.

Per Serving
calories: 92 | fat: 6g | protein: 6g | carbs: 3g net carbs: 3g | fiber: 0g

433. Garlicky Roasted Vegetable Mix

Prep time: 10 minutes | Cook time: 15 to 20 minutes | Serves 4

1 butternut squash, cut into chunks
¼ pound (113 g) shallots, peeled
¼ pound (113 g) Brussels sprouts
1 sprig rosemary, chopped
1 sprig thyme, chopped
4 cloves garlic, peeled only
3 tablespoons olive oil
Salt and black pepper, to taste

1. Preheat the oven to 450ºF (235ºC).
2. Pour the butternut squash, shallots, garlic cloves, and Brussels sprouts in a bowl. Season with salt, black pepper, olive oil, and toss. Pour the mixture on a baking sheet and sprinkle with the chopped thyme and rosemary. Roast the vegetables for 15–20 minutes.
3. Once ready, remove and spoon into a serving bowl. Serve with oven roasted chicken thighs.

Per Serving
calories: 159 | fat: 10g | protein: 3g | carbs: 14g net carbs: 10g | fiber: 4g

434. Avocado Crostini Nori with Walnuts

Prep time: 5 minutes | Cook time: 2 minutes | Serves 4

8 slices low carb bread (baguette)
4 nori sheets
1 cup mashed avocado
⅓ teaspoon salt
1 teaspoon lemon juice
1½ tablespoons coconut oil
⅓ cup chopped raw walnuts
1 tablespoon chia seeds

1. In a bowl, flake the nori sheets into the smallest possible pieces.
2. In another bowl, mix the avocado, salt, and lemon juice, and stir in half of the nori flakes. Set aside.
3. Place the bread slices on a baking sheet and toast in a broiler on medium heat for 2 minutes, making sure not to burn. Remove the crostini after and brush with coconut oil on both sides. Top each crostini with the avocado mixture and garnish with the chia seeds, chopped walnuts, Serve.

Per Serving
calories: 317 | fat: 18g | protein: 9g | carbs: 10g net carbs: 3g | fiber: 7g

435. Baked Spinach Cheese Balls

Prep time: 10 minutes | Cook time: 10 to 12 minutes | Serves 8

⅓ cup crumbled ricotta cheese
¼ teaspoon nutmeg
¼ teaspoon pepper
3 tablespoons heavy cream
1 teaspoon garlic powder
1 tablespoon onion powder
2 tablespoons butter, melted
⅓ cup Parmesan cheese, shredded
2 eggs
1 cup spinach
1 cup almond flour

1. Place all ingredients in a food processor. Process until smooth. Place in the freezer for about 10 minutes.
2. Make balls out of the mixture and arrange them on a lined baking sheet. Bake in the oven at 350ºF for about 10-12 minutes.

Per Serving
calories: 149 | fat: 9g | protein: 6g | carbs: 3g net carbs: 1g | fiber: 2g

436. Pecorino Mushroom Burgers

Prep time: 15 minutes | Cook time: 13 minutes | Serves 4

2 tablespoons butter, softened
2 tablespoons olive oil
2 garlic cloves, minced
2 cups portobello mushrooms, chopped
4 tablespoons blanched almond flour
4 tablespoons ground flax seeds
4 tablespoons hemp seeds
4 tablespoons sunflower seeds
1 tablespoon Cajun seasoning
1 teaspoon mustard
2 eggs, whisked
½ cup Pecorino cheese, shredded

1. Set a pan over medium heat and warm the olive oil. Add in mushrooms and garlic and sauté until there is no more water in mushrooms. Remove to a plate and let cool for a few minutes.
2. In a bowl, place Pecorino cheese, almond flour, hemp seeds, mustard, eggs, sunflower seeds, flax seeds, mushrooms, and Cajun seasoning. Create 4 burgers from the mixture.
3. To the same pan, add and warm the butter; fry the burgers for 7 minutes. Flip them over with a wide spatula and cook for 6 more minutes. Serve with guacamole.

Per Serving
calories: 368 | fat: 30g | protein: 14g | carbs: 15g net carbs: 11g | fiber: 4g

437. Feta Zucchini and Pepper Gratin

Prep time: 5 minutes | Cook time: 30 to 40 minutes | Serves 6

2 pounds (907 g) zucchinis, sliced
2 red bell peppers, seeded and sliced
Salt and black pepper, to taste
1½ cups crumbled feta cheese
2 tablespoons butter, melted
½ cup heavy whipping cream

1. Preheat oven to 370ºF. Place the sliced zucchinis in a colander over the sink, sprinkle with salt and let sit for 20 minutes. Transfer to paper towels to drain the excess liquid.
2. Grease a baking dish with cooking spray and make a layer of zucchini and bell peppers overlapping one another. Season with pepper, and sprinkle with feta cheese. Repeat the layering process a second time.
3. Combine the butter and whipping cream in a bowl, stir to mix completely, and pour over the vegetables. Bake for 30-40 minutes or until golden brown on top.

Per Serving
calories: 211 | fat: 16g | protein: 10g | carbs: 9g net carbs: 6g | fiber: 3g

438. Prosciutto-Wrapped Piquillo Peppers

Prep time: 15 minutes | Cook time: 0 minutes | Serves 8

8 canned roasted piquillo peppers
1 tablespoon olive oil
3 slices prosciutto, cut into thin slices
1 tablespoon balsamic vinegar
Filling:
8 ounces (227 g) goat cheese
3 tablespoons heavy cream
3 tablespoons chopped parsley
½ teaspoon minced garlic
1 tablespoon olive oil
1 tablespoon chopped mint

1. Mix all filling ingredients in a bowl. Place in a freezer bag, press down and squeeze, and cut off the bottom. Drain and deseed the peppers. Squeeze about 2 tablespoons of the filling into each pepper.
2. Wrap a prosciutto slice onto each pepper. Secure with toothpicks. Arrange them on a serving platter. Sprinkle the olive oil and vinegar over.

Per Serving
calories: 216 | fat: 17g | protein: 11g | carbs: 6g net carbs: 5g | fiber: 1g

439. Colby Bacon-Wrapped Jalapeño Peppers

Prep time: 5 minutes | Cook time: 25 minutes | Serves 6

12 jalapeño peppers
¼ cup shredded Colby cheese
6 ounces (170 g) cream cheese, softened
6 slices bacon, halved

1. Cut the jalapeño peppers in half, and then remove the membrane and seeds. Combine cheeses and stuff into the pepper halves. Wrap each pepper with a bacon strip and secure with toothpicks.
2. Place the filled peppers on a baking sheet lined with a piece of foil. Bake at 350ºF for 25 minutes until bacon has browned, and crispy and cheese is golden brown on the top. Remove to a paper towel lined plate to absorb grease, arrange on a serving plate, and serve warm.

Per Serving
calories: 219 | fat: 20g | protein: 7g | carbs: 3g net carbs: 2g | fiber: 1g

440. Ricotta Spinach Gnocchi

Prep time: 5 minutes | Cook time: 7 minutes | Serves 4

1 cup ricotta cheese
1 cup Parmesan cheese, grated
¼ teaspoon nutmeg powder
1 egg, cracked into a bowl
Salt and black pepper, to taste
3 cups chopped spinach
1½ cups almond flour
2½ cups water
2 tablespoons butter

1. To a bowl, add the ricotta cheese, half of the Parmesan cheese, egg, nutmeg powder, salt, spinach, almond flour, and black pepper. Mix well. Make gnocchi of the mixture using 2 tablespoons and set aside.
2. Bring the water to a boil over high heat on a stovetop, about 5 minutes. Place one gnocchi onto the water, if it breaks apart; add some more flour to the other gnocchi to firm it up.
3. Put the remaining gnocchi in the water to poach and rise to the top, about 2 minutes. Remove the gnocchi with a perforated spoon to a serving plate. Melt the butter in a microwave and pour over the gnocchi. Sprinkle with the remaining Parmesan cheese and serve with green salad.

Per Serving
calories: 238 | fat: 16g | protein: 18g | carbs: 9g net carbs: 4g | fiber: 5g

441. Mascarpone Turkey Pastrami Pinwheels

Prep time: 5 minutes | Cook time: 0 minutes | Serves 4

Cooking spray
8 ounces (227 g) mascarpone cheese
10 ounces (284 g) turkey pastrami, sliced
10 canned pepperoncini peppers, sliced and drained

1. Lay a 12 x 12 plastic wrap on a flat surface and arrange the pastrami all over slightly overlapping each other. Spread the cheese on top of the salami layers and arrange the pepperoncini on top.
2. Hold two opposite ends of the plastic wrap and roll the pastrami. Twist both ends to tighten and refrigerate for 2 hours. Unwrap the salami roll and slice into 2-inch pinwheels. Serve.

Per Serving
calories: 549 | fat: 49g | protein: 29g | carbs: 10g net carbs: 7g | fiber: 3g

442. Scrambled Eggs with Swiss Chard Pesto

Prep time: 10 minutes | Cook time: 3 minutes | Serves 4

3 tablespoons butter
8 eggs, beaten
¼ cup almond milk
Salt and black pepper, to taste
Swiss Chard Pesto:
2 cups Swiss chard
1 cup Parmesan cheese, grated
2 garlic cloves, minced
½ cup olive oil
2 tablespoons lime juice
½ cup walnuts, chopped

1. Set a pan over medium heat and warm butter. Mix eggs, black pepper, salt, and almond milk. Cook the egg mixture while stirring gently, until eggs are set but still tender and moist, for 3 minutes.
2. In your blender, place all the ingredients for the pesto, excluding the olive oil. Pulse until roughly blended. While the machine is still running, slowly add in the olive oil until the desired consistency is attained. Serve alongside warm scrambled eggs.

Per Serving
calories: 626 | fat: 58g | protein: 20g | carbs: 8g net carbs: 7g | fiber: 1g

443. Parmesan Cauliflower Fritters

Prep time: 5 minutes | Cook time: 6 minutes | Serves 4

1 pound (454 g) grated cauliflower
½ cup Parmesan cheese, grated
3 ounces (85 g) chopped onion
½ teaspoon baking powder
½ cup almond flour
2 eggs
½ teaspoon lemon juice
2 tablespoons olive oil
⅓ teaspoon salt

1. Sprinkle the salt over the cauliflower in a bowl, and let it stand for 10 minutes. Add in the other ingredients. Mix with your hands to combine. Place a skillet over medium heat, and heat olive oil.
2. Shape fritters out of the cauliflower mixture. Fry in batches, for about 3 minutes per side.

Per Serving
calories: 231 | fat: 13g | protein: 11g | carbs: 10g net carbs: 6g | fiber: 4g

444. Garlicky Roasted Broccoli

Prep time: 5 minutes | Cook time: 20 to 30 minutes | Serves 6

¼ cup olive oil
1 teaspoon lemon zest
1 tablespoon lemon juice
6 cloves garlic, minced
½ teaspoon sea salt
¼ teaspoon black pepper
1 pound (454 g) broccoli florets

1. Preheat the oven to 400ºF (205ºC). Grease a 20 × 14-inch baking sheet or two 10 × 14-inch pans.
2. In a large bowl, whisk together the oil, lemon zest, lemon juice, garlic, sea salt, and black pepper. (You can tilt the bowl to the side to help when whisking this small amount in a large bowl.)
3. Add the broccoli florets and toss to coat.
4. Arrange the broccoli florets in a single layer on the baking sheet so that each piece is touching the baking sheet.
5. Roast for 20 to 30 minutes, until the edges of the florets are browned.

Per Serving
calories: 109 | fat: 9g | protein: 2g | carbs: 5g net carbs: 3g | fiber: 2g

445. Grilled Prosciutto-Chicken Wraps

Prep time: 5 minutes | Cook time: 6 minutes | Serves 8

¼ teaspoon garlic powder
8 ounces (227 g) Provolone cheese
8 raw chicken tenders
Salt and black pepper, to taste
8 prosciutto slices

1. Pound the chicken until half an inch thick. Season with salt, black pepper, and garlic powder. Cut the provolone cheese into 8 strips. Place a slice of prosciutto on a flat surface. Place one chicken tender on top. Top with a provolone strip.
2. Roll the chicken and secure with previously soaked skewers. Grill the wraps for 3 minutes per side.

Per Serving
calories: 271 | fat: 13g | protein: 35g | carbs: 2g net carbs: 1g | fiber: 1g

446. Buttered Mushrooms with Sage

Prep time: 5 minutes | Cook time: 14 to 19 minutes | Serves 8

5 tablespoons butter, divided
¼ teaspoon ground sage
2 cloves garlic, minced
1 pound (454 g) baby portobello mushrooms,
cut into quarters
½ teaspoon sea salt
⅛ teaspoon black pepper
8 medium fresh sage leaves

1. In a large sauté pan, melt 4 tablespoons of the butter over medium heat. Add the dried sage and heat for 2 to 3 minutes, stirring occasionally, until the butter starts to turn golden.
2. Add the garlic and heat for another 2 to 3 minutes, until the butter is dark golden brown and smells nutty. Watch the pan closely, because the butter can go from browned to burned quickly.
3. Add the mushrooms. Sprinkle with sea salt and black pepper. Cover and cook for 7 to 10 minutes, lifting the lid to stir occasionally, until the mushrooms are soft and most of the moisture evaporates. Uncover and stir-fry for another 3 minutes to evaporate any remaining excess moisture. Remove the mushrooms from the pan and cover to keep warm.
4. Melt the remaining 1 tablespoon butter in the pan. Add the fresh sage leaves in a single layer. Fry for just a few seconds, until crispy.
5. Use the crispy sage leaves for topping the mushrooms—whole for garnish or crumbled for flavor.

Per Serving
calories: 154 | fat: 14g | protein: 2g | carbs: 4g net carbs: 3g | fiber: 1g

447. Tuna-Mayo Topped Dill Pickles

Prep time: 5 minutes | Cook time: 0 minutes | Serves 12

18 ounces (510 g) canned and drained tuna
6 large dill pickles
¼ teaspoon garlic powder
⅓ cup sugar-free mayonnaise
1 tablespoon onion flakes

1. Combine the mayonnaise, tuna, onion flakes, and garlic powder in a bowl. Cut the pickles in half lengthwise. Top each half with tuna mixture. Place in the fridge for 30 minutes before serving.

Per Serving
calories: 59 | fat: 2g | protein: 9g | carbs: 3g net carbs: 2g | fiber: 1g

448. Parmesan Creamed Spinach

Prep time: 5 minutes | Cook time: 5 minutes | Serves 4

1 tablespoon unsalted butter
1 clove garlic, minced
9 ounces (255 g) fresh spinach, chopped
2 ounces (57 g) cream cheese
½ cup grated Parmesan cheese
2 tablespoons heavy whipping cream
Salt and pepper, to taste

1. In a large pot over medium heat, combine the butter and garlic. Sauté, stirring frequently, for 3 to 4 minutes, until fragrant.
2. Add the spinach and cream cheese and use a spatula to combine.
3. Stir in the Parmesan cheese and cream. Bring to a simmer and cook, stirring, for about 1 minute to reduce a bit.
4. Remove from the heat and season with salt and pepper to taste before serving.

Per Serving
calories: 172 | fat: 14g | protein: 7g | carbs: 4g net carbs: 3g | fiber: 1g

449. Mozzarella Prosciutto Wraps with Basil

Prep time: 5 minutes | Cook time: 0 minutes | Serves 6

6 thin prosciutto slices	balls
18 basil leaves	2 tablespoons extra-virgin olive oil
18 ciliegine Mozzarella	

1. Cut the prosciutto slices into three strips each. Place basil leaves at the end of each strip. Top with a ciliegine Mozzarella ball. Wrap the Mozzarella in prosciutto. Secure with toothpicks. Arrange on a platter, drizzle with olive oil, and serve.

Per Serving

calories: 211 | fat: 16g | protein: 14g | carbs: 2g net carbs: 1g | fiber: 1g

450. Fried Cauliflower Rice with Peppers

Prep time: 10 minutes | Cook time: 14 minutes | Serves 6

1 head cauliflower	divided
2 tablespoons butter, divided	¼ teaspoon black pepper
½ medium orange bell pepper, finely diced	2 tablespoons coconut aminos
½ medium green bell pepper, finely diced	1 teaspoon toasted sesame oil
3 cloves garlic, minced	3 green onions, chopped
2 large eggs	
1¼ teaspoons sea salt,	

1. Remove the cauliflower leaves and stems. (Cut off as much of the stems as you can.) Push the cauliflower florets into a running food processor with a grating attachment, to make cauliflower rice. Alternatively, rice the cauliflower using a box grater.
2. In a large sauté pan, heat 1 tablespoon of the butter over medium heat. Add the bell peppers and sauté for about 5 minutes, until the peppers are soft. Add the garlic and sauté for about 1 minute, until fragrant.
3. Meanwhile, whisk the eggs with ¼ teaspoon sea salt and a pinch of black pepper.
4. Push the veggies to one side of the skillet. (If the pan is dry, you can melt in more butter.) Add the whisked eggs to the other side and cook for 3 minutes, until barely scrambled.
5. Push everything to the side again and add the remaining 1 tablespoon butter to the pan. Once it melts, increase the heat to medium-high, immediately add the cauliflower rice, and stir everything together. Season with 1 teaspoon sea salt and ¼ teaspoon black pepper, or to taste. Stir-fry for about 5 minutes, until the cauliflower is soft but not mushy.
6. Remove from the heat. Stir in the coconut aminos, sesame oil, and green onions.

Per Serving

calories: 106 | fat: 6g | protein: 4g | carbs: 8g net carbs: 6g | fiber: 2g

451. Zoodles with Almond-Basil Pesto

Prep time: 10 minutes | Cook time: 10 to 13 minutes | Serves 4

4 medium zucchini (1¼ pounds / 567 g total), spiralized	Parmesan cheese
¾ teaspoon sea salt, divided	⅔ cup extra-virgin olive oil
⅓ cup raw almonds	2 cloves garlic, cut into a few pieces
2 packed cups fresh basil	⅛ teaspoon black pepper
⅓ cup grated	1 tablespoon avocado oil

1. In a colander set in the sink, toss the zucchini noodles with ¼ teaspoon of the sea salt. Let sit for 30 minutes to drain, then squeeze to release more water. You don't have to get every last drop out, just most of it. Pat dry.
2. Meanwhile, preheat the oven to 400ºF (205ºC).
3. Arrange the almonds in a single layer on a baking sheet. Toast in the oven for 6 to 8 minutes, until golden and fragrant. Watch them carefully so they don't burn.
4. Transfer the almonds to a food processor. Pulse a few times until the almonds are broken up into coarse pieces—don't overmix.
5. Add the basil, Parmesan, olive oil, garlic, pepper, and remaining ½ teaspoon sea salt. Pulse on and off, scraping the sides occasionally, until you get a pesto consistency. Adjust sea salt and black pepper to taste—it should be on the salty side, as this will be diluted when you add the zucchini noodles.
6. In a large sauté pan, heat the avocado oil over medium-high heat. Add the zucchini noodles and stir-fry for 3 to 4 minutes, until al dente.
7. Add the pesto and toss to coat. Stir-fry for just 1 more minute, until hot. Serve immediately.

Per Serving

calories: 492 | fat: 48g | protein: 8g | carbs: 10g net carbs: 7g | fiber: 3g

452. Smoked Mackerel and Turnip Patties

Prep time: 5 minutes | Cook time: 14 minutes | Serves 6

1 turnip, diced
1½ cup water
Salt and chili pepper, to taste
3 tablespoons olive oil, plus more for rubbing
4 smoked mackerel steaks, bones removed, flaked
3 eggs, beaten
2 tablespoons mayonnaise
1 tablespoon pork rinds, crushed

1. Bring the turnip to boil in salted water in a saucepan over medium heat for 8 minutes or until tender. Drain the turnip through a colander, transfer to a mixing bowl, and mash the lumps.
2. Add the mackerel, eggs, mayonnaise, pork rinds, salt, and chili pepper; mix and make 6 compact patties. Heat olive oil in a skillet over medium heat and fry the patties for 3 minutes on each side until golden brown. Remove onto a wire rack to cool. Serve with sesame lime dipping sauce.

Per Serving
calories: 348 | fat: 22g | protein: 33g | carbs: 3g net carbs: 2g | fiber: 1g

453. Spicy Onion Rings

Prep time: 15 minutes | Cook time: 20 minutes | Serves 4

1 large onion, sliced into rings
½ cup almond flour
1 egg
½ teaspoon garlic powder
1 teaspoon paprika
1 teaspoon cayenne pepper
1 teaspoon salt

1. Preheat the oven to 400ºF (205ºC), and line a baking sheet with parchment paper.
2. Add the egg to a mixing bowl and then add the almond flour and seasoning to another bowl. Stir the almond flour mixture well.
3. Dip the sliced onions into the egg mixture, followed by the almond flour mix, covering both sides of the sliced onions.
4. Add the onion rings to the baking sheet and bake for about 10 minutes on each side or until crispy.

Per Serving
calories: 51 | fat: 3g | protein: 3g | carbs: 4g net carbs: 3g | fiber: 1g

454. Baked Broccoli Bites

Prep time: 10 minutes | Cook time: 20 minutes | Serves 4

1½ pounds (680 g) broccoli, cut into bite-sized florets
¼ cup extra-virgin olive oil
Juice of ½ lemon
2 cloves garlic, minced
Salt and pepper, to taste
Red pepper flakes (optional)

1. Preheat the oven to 400ºF (205ºC).
2. In a large mixing bowl, combine the broccoli, oil, lemon juice, and garlic and toss until well coated. Season lightly with salt, black pepper, and red pepper flakes, if using.
3. Pour onto a rimmed baking sheet and spread out in a single layer.
4. Bake for 18 to 20 minutes, until lightly golden brown.

Per Serving
calories: 133 | fat: 14g | protein: 1g | carbs: 4g net carbs: 3g | fiber: 1g

455. Herbed Roasted Radishes

Prep time: 5 minutes | Cook time: 16 to 26 minutes | Serves 6

3 tablespoons avocado oil
3 cloves garlic, minced
1 tablespoon fresh thyme, chopped
1 tablespoon fresh rosemary, chopped
1½ teaspoons sea salt
¼ teaspoon black pepper
2 pounds (907 g) radishes, trimmed and halved

1. Preheat the oven to 425ºF (220ºC). Line a baking sheet with foil and grease it.
2. In a large bowl, whisk together the oil, garlic, thyme, rosemary, sea salt, and black pepper. Add the radishes and toss to coat.
3. Arrange the radishes in a single layer on the pan, making sure each one touches the pan. Spread them out as much as possible. Roast for 8 to 13 minutes, until golden on the bottom. Flip and roast for 8 to 13 more minutes.

Per Serving
calories: 98 | fat: 7g | protein: 1g | carbs: 6g net carbs: 4g | fiber: 2g

456. Roasted Brussels Sprouts with Balsamic Glaze

Prep time: 5 minutes | Cook time: 20 to 30 minutes | Serves 8

¼ cup olive oil
2 tablespoons balsamic vinegar
½ teaspoon garlic powder
1 teaspoon sea salt
¼ teaspoon black pepper
1 pound (454 g) Brussels sprouts, trimmed and halved

1. Preheat the oven to 450°F (235°C). Line a large baking sheet with foil.
2. In a large bowl, whisk together the oil, balsamic vinegar, garlic powder, sea salt, and black pepper, until smooth. Add the Brussels sprouts and toss to coat.
3. Spread the Brussels sprouts over the baking sheet in a single layer, so that all the sprouts touch the pan. Roast for 10 to 15 minutes, until browned on the bottom. Flip and repeat for another 10 to 15 minutes.

Per Serving
calories: 88 | fat: 6g | protein: 1g | carbs: 5g net carbs: 3g | fiber: 2g

457. Cheesy Ham Pizza Rolls

Prep time: 15 minutes | Cook time: 30 minutes | Serves 5

Dough:
½ cup Parmesan cheese
1 cup Mozzarella cheese
Filling:
2 cups cooked ham, sliced
1 cup Gouda cheese, sliced
5 tablespoons tomato
3 egg whites
¾ cup coconut flour
1 cup heavy cream

purée
1 teaspoon crushed black pepper, for topping

1. Preheat the oven to 400°F (205°C), and line a baking sheet with parchment paper.
2. In a food processor, combine the ingredients for the crust and process until a smooth dough forms. You may need to add water, a tablespoon at a time, to achieve this result.
3. Flatten the dough into a rectangular shape onto the prepared baking sheet. Bake for about 15 minutes. Remove from the oven and allow to cool slightly.
4. Spread the tomato purée evenly across the dough. Top with the sliced ham and Gouda cheese.
5. Roll the dough carefully into a log. Slice the log into 5 even pieces and place each one back onto the baking sheet. Sprinkle with crushed black pepper.
6. Bake again for about 10 minutes until the dough is golden brown and the cheese is bubbly.

Per Serving
calories: 492 | fat: 35g | protein: 35g | carbs: 6g net carbs: 4g | fiber: 2g

458. Duo-Cheese Lettuce Rolls

Prep time: 5 minutes | Cook time: 5 minutes | Serves 6

½ pound (227 g) gouda cheese, grated
½ pound (227 g) feta cheese, crumbled
1 teaspoon taco
seasoning mix
2 tablespoons olive oil
1½ cups guacamole
1 cup coconut milk
A head lettuce

1. Mix both types of cheese with taco seasoning mix. Set a pan over medium heat and warm the olive oil. Spread the shredded cheese mixture all over the pan. Fry for 5 minutes, turning once. Arrange some of the cheese mixture on each lettuce leaf, top with coconut milk and guacamole, then roll up folding in the ends to secure and serve.

Per Serving
calories: 401 | fat: 30g | protein: 18g | carbs: 10g net carbs: 5g | fiber: 5g

459. Liverwurst and Pistachio Balls

Prep time: 10 minutes | Cook time: 0 minutes | Serves 8

8 bacon slices, cooked and chopped
8 ounces (227 g) Liverwurst
¼ cup chopped
pistachios
1 teaspoon Dijon mustard
6 ounces (170 g) cream cheese

1. Combine the liverwurst and pistachios in the bowl of food the processor. Pulse until smooth. Whisk the cream cheese and mustard in another bowl. Make 12 balls out of the liverwurst mixture.
2. Make a thin cream cheese layer over. Coat with bacon, arrange on a plate and chill for 30 minutes.

Per Serving
calories: 227 | fat: 25g | protein: 9g | carbs: 4g net carbs: 3g | fiber: 1g

460. Spiced Baked Gruyere Crisps

Prep time: 5 minutes | Cook time: 6 minutes | Serves 4

2 cups Gruyere cheese, shredded
½ teaspoon garlic powder
¼ teaspoon onion powder
1 rosemary sprig, minced
½ teaspoon chili powder

1. Set oven to 400°F (205°C). Coat two baking sheets with parchment paper.
2. Mix Gruyere cheese with the seasonings. Take 1 tablespoon of cheese mixture and form small mounds on the baking sheets. Bake for 6 minutes. Leave to cool. Serve.

Per Serving
calories: 276 | fat: 21g | protein: 20g | carbs: 1g net carbs: 1g | fiber: 0g

461. Cauli Rice with Cheddar and Bacon

Prep time: 10 minutes | Cook time: 8 to 10 minutes | Serves 8

1 head cauliflower, cut into florets
2 tablespoons butter
¼ cup sour cream
2 tablespoons heavy cream
3 cloves garlic, minced
1 teaspoon sea salt
1½ cups shredded Cheddar cheese
1/3 cup cooked bacon bits
¼ cup chopped green onions

1. Bring a large pot of water to a boil on the stove top. Add the cauliflower florets and cook for 8 to 10 minutes, until very soft. Drain well and pat dry.
2. Meanwhile, in a microwave-safe bowl or in a saucepan, combine the butter, sour cream, heavy cream, garlic, and sea salt, and heat in the microwave or on the stove until hot and melted.
3. Transfer the cauliflower florets to a food processor. Add the butter-cream mixture and purée until smooth.
4. Transfer the cauliflower to a serving dish. Immediately stir in most of the Cheddar, bacon bits, and green onions, reserving a little of each for the topping. To serve, garnish with the reserved Cheddar, bacon, and green onions.

Per Serving
calories: 180 | fat: 13g | protein: 9g | carbs: 5g net carbs: 3g | fiber: 2g

462. Oven Baked String Beans and Mushrooms

Prep time: 10 minutes | Cook time: 20 to 25 minutes | Serves 4

2 cups string beans, cut in halves
1 pound (454 g) cremini mushrooms, quartered
3 tomatoes, quartered
2 cloves garlic, minced
3 tablespoons olive oil
3 shallots, julienned
½ teaspoon dried thyme
Salt and black pepper, to season

1. Preheat oven to 450°F (235°C). In a bowl, mix the strings beans, mushrooms, tomatoes, garlic, olive oil, shallots, thyme, salt, and pepper. Pour the vegetables in a baking sheet and spread them all around.
2. Place the baking sheet in the oven and bake the veggies for 20 to 25 minutes.

Per Serving
calories: 154 | fat: 11g | protein: 4g | carbs: 13g net carbs: 9g | fiber: 4g

463. Avocado-Bacon Stuffed Eggs

Prep time: 15 minutes | Cook time: 15 minutes | Serves 3

1 ripe avocado
4 large hard-boiled eggs
4 slices bacon, cooked and crumbled
1 red chili pepper, seeded and minced
1 garlic clove, minced
2 tablespoons lemon juice
Salt and black pepper, to taste

1. Peel the eggs, halve them lengthwise and transfer the yolks to a mixing bowl.
2. Add the avocado, chili pepper, garlic and lemon juice to the bowl.
3. Mash with a fork until well combined. Season with salt and black pepper.
4. Scoop the mixture into the egg whites and top with the crumbled bacon.
5. Refrigerate until cold or serve right away.

Per Serving
calories: 455 | fat: 37g | protein: 25g | carbs: 8g net carbs: 3g | fiber: 5g

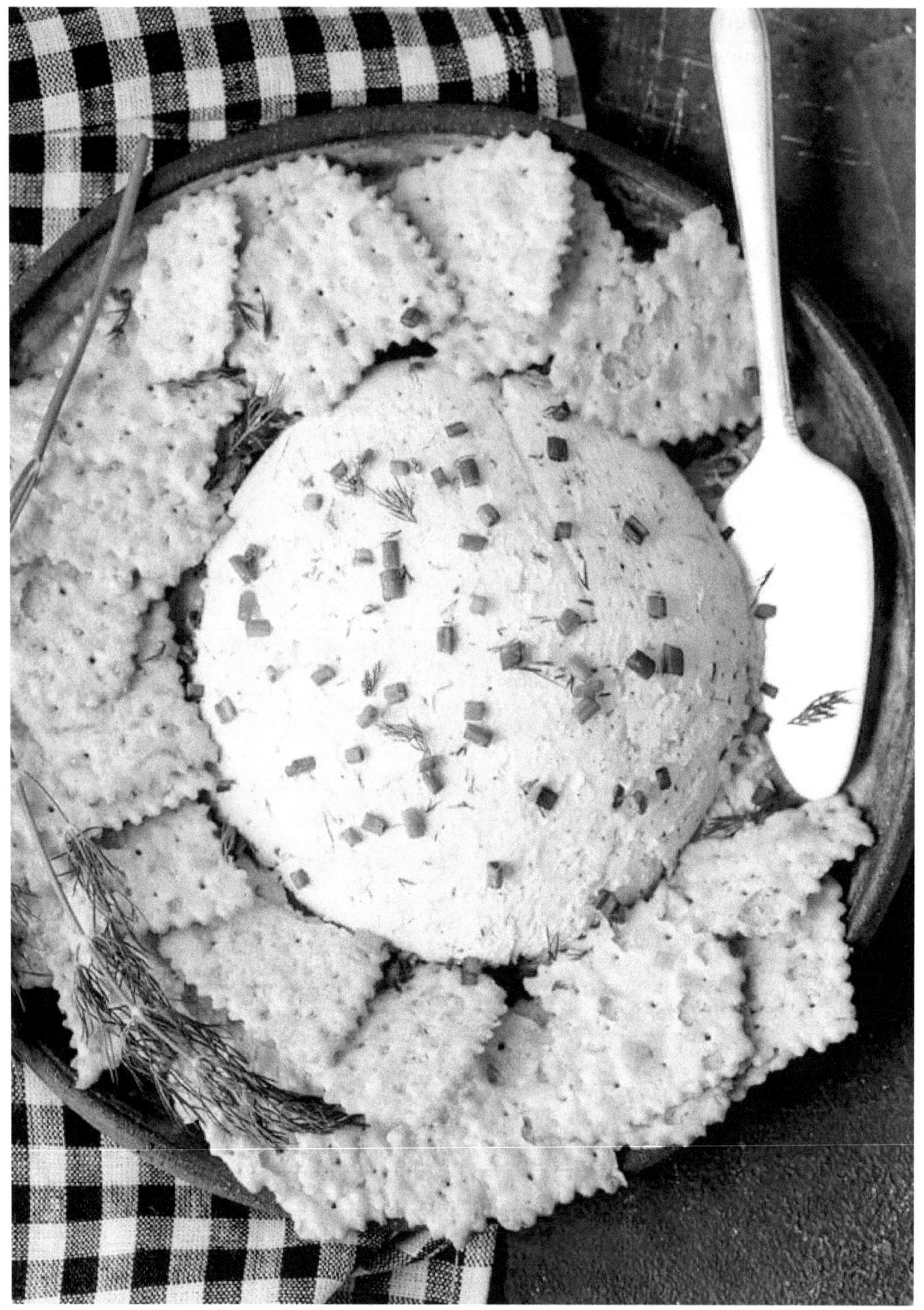

Chapter 12 Appetizers and Snacks

464. Avocado and Ham Stuffed Eggs

Prep time: 5 minutes | Cook time: 12 minutes | Serves 4

4 large eggs
½ avocado, mashed
½ teaspoon yellow mustard
1 garlic clove, minced
2 ounces (57 g) cooked ham, chopped

1. Place the eggs in a saucepan and fill with enough water. Bring the water to a rolling boil; heat off. Cover and allow the eggs to sit for about 12 minutes; let them cool.
2. Slice the eggs into halves; mix the yolks with the avocado, mustard and garlic.
3. Divide the avocado filling among the egg whites. Top with the chopped ham. Bon appétit!

Per Serving
calories: 128 | fat: 9g | protein: 9g | carbs: 3g net carbs: 1g | fiber: 2g

465. Mini Bacon and Kale Muffins

Prep time: 5 minutes | Cook time: 30 minutes | Serves 6

2 slices cooked bacon, chopped
½ cup scallions, chopped
1 garlic clove, minced
1 cup kale, torn into small pieces
4 eggs, well whisked
4 tablespoons Greek yogurt
Kosher salt and ground white pepper, to season

1. Add cupcake liners to a mini muffin tin. Mix the bacon with the scallions, garlic, and kale. Fold in the eggs and yogurt. Mix to combine well.
2. Season with salt and ground white pepper; divide the mixture between the cupcake liners.
3. Bake in the preheated oven at 360ºF (182ºC) for 30 minutes or until your muffins are thoroughly cooked and firm.
4. Let cool for about 5 minutes; lastly, run a butter knife around the edges of each muffin to loosen it. Serve warm or at room temperature. Enjoy!

Per Serving
calories: 88 | fat: 7g | protein: 6g | carbs: 2g net carbs: 1g | fiber: 1g

466. Fajita Spareribs

Prep time: 5 minutes | Cook time: 2 hours 30 minutes | Serves 4

2 pounds (907 g) St. Louis-style spareribs
1 tablespoon Fajita seasoning mix
2 cloves garlic, pressed
½ cup chicken bone broth
1 cup tomato purée

1. Toss the spareribs with the Fajita seasoning mix, garlic, chicken bone broth, and tomato purée until well coated.
2. Arrange the spare ribs on a tinfoil-lined baking sheet.
3. Bake in the preheated oven at 260ºF (127ºC) for 2 hours and 30 minutes.
4. Place under the preheated broiler for about 8 minutes until the sauce is lightly caramelized. Bon appétit!

Per Serving
calories: 344 | fat: 14g | protein: 50g | carbs: 5g net carbs: 4g | fiber: 1g

467. Herbed Provolone Cheese Chips

Prep time: 5 minutes | Cook time: 9 minutes | Serves 5

6 ounces (170 g) (170 g) provolone cheese, grated
½ teaspoon garlic powder
½ teaspoon shallot powder
¼ teaspoon ground black pepper
1 teaspoon dried dill
½ teaspoon dried oregano
1 teaspoon paprika

1. Place the grated provolone cheese in small heaps on a roasting pan lined with Silpat mat. Make sure to leave enough room in between them.
2. Sprinkle the herbs and spices over them.
3. Bake in the preheated oven at 395ºF (202ºC) for about 9 minutes, Transfer to a cooling rack and let it sit for 20 minutes before serving. Serve with a homemade salsa sauce if desired.

Per Serving
calories: 119 | fat: 9g | protein: 9g | carbs: 1g net carbs: 1g | fiber: 0g

468. Crispy Five Seed Crackers

Prep time: 5 minutes | Cook time: 1 hour | Serves 12

¼ cup chia seeds
¼ cup sesame seeds
¼ cup flax seeds
¼ cup sunflower seeds
¼ cup pumpkin seeds
¼ cup almond meal
1 teaspoon psyllium husk powder
Coarse sea salt, to taste
¼ teaspoon ground cumin
¾ cup boiling water
4 tablespoons coconut oil, melted

1. Thoroughly combine the seeds, almond meal, psyllium husk powder, salt, and ground cumin until well mixed.
2. Pour the boiling water over the seed mixture; add in the melted coconut oil.
3. Spread out the batter thinly on a tinfoil-lined baking pan. Bake in the preheated oven at 310ºF (154ºC) for 30 minutes.
4. Rotate the pan and continue to bake an additional 25 to 30 minutes. Heat off. Allow your crackers to dry in the warm oven for 50 to 60 minutes longer. Bon appétit!

Per Serving
calories: 128 | fat: 13g | protein: 4g | carbs: 3g net carbs: 1g | fiber: 2g

469. Traditional Walnut Fat Bombs

Prep time: 5 minutes | Cook time: 1 minute | Serves 10

2 tablespoons keto chocolate protein powder
¼ cup erythritol
5 ounces (142 g) butter
3 ounces (85 g) walnut butter
10 whole walnuts, halved

1. In a sauté pan, melt the butter, protein powder, and Erythritol over a low flame, for 1 minute. Stir until smooth and well mixed.
2. Spoon the mixture into a piping bag and pipe into mini cupcake liners. Add the walnut halves to each mini cupcake.
3. Place in your refrigerator for at least 2 hours. Bon appétit!

Per Serving
calories: 260 | fat: 27g | protein: 5g | carbs: 3g net carbs: 1g | fiber: 2g

470. Avocado-Bacon Sushi

Prep time: 5 minutes | Cook time: 0 minutes | Serves 8

1 teaspoon garlic paste
2 scallions, finely chopped
4 ounces (113 g) cream cheese, softened
1 teaspoon adobo sauce
1 avocado, mashed
2 tablespoons fresh lemon juice
8 bacon slices
1 tablespoon toasted sesame seeds

1. In a mixing bowl, thoroughly combine the garlic paste, scallions, cream cheese, adobo sauce, avocado, and fresh lemon juice.
2. Divide the mixture evenly between the bacon slices. Roll up tightly and garnish with toasted sesame seeds. Enjoy!

Per Serving
calories: 350 | fat: 37g | protein: 2g | carbs: 4g net carbs: 2g | fiber: 2g

471. Bacon-Wrapped Enoki Mushrooms

Prep time: 10 minutes | Cook time: 40 minutes | Serves 5

½ pound (227 g) enoki mushrooms
5 slices bacon, cut into halves
Dipping Sauce:
½ cup water
2 tablespoons sesame oil
2 tablespoons coconut aminos
1 teaspoon monk fruit powder
1 large clove garlic, minced
½ teaspoon ground ginger
1 teaspoon Chinese five-spice powder
Kosher salt and ground black pepper, to taste

1. Wrap the mushrooms with the bacon and secure with toothpicks. Arrange on a parchment-lined baking tray and bake at 380ºF (193ºC) for 40 minutes, flipping once halfway through cooking.
2. In the meantime, make the sauce by whisking all ingredients in a wok or deep saucepan. Cook over medium heat until thickened and reduced.
3. Serve the bacon dippers with the sauce on the side.

Per Serving
calories: 323 | fat: 33g | protein: 2g | carbs: 5g net carbs: 3g | fiber: 2g

472. Paprika Veggie Bites

Prep time: 5 minutes | Cook time: 0 minutes | Serves 3

1 teaspoon Dijon mustard
½ cup cream cheese
¼ cup mayonnaise
1 cucumber, cut into rounds
1 bell pepper, seeded and cut into 4 pieces lengthwise
1 teaspoon paprika

1. Mix the Dijon mustard, cream cheese, and mayonnaise in a bowl; stir to combine.
2. Place the cucumber and bell peppers on a serving platter. Divide the cheese mixture between the vegetables.
3. Sprinkle paprika over the vegetable bites. Serve well chilled.

Per Serving

calories: 164 | fat: 17g | protein: 2g | carbs: 3g | net carbs: 2g | fiber: 1g

473. Herbed Prawn and Veggie Skewers

Prep time: 10 minutes | Cook time: 8 to 9 minutes | Serves 4

2 tablespoons olive oil
1 pound (454 g) king prawns, deveined and cleaned
Sea salt and ground black pepper, to taste
1 teaspoon garlic powder
1 tablespoon fresh sage, minced
1 teaspoon fresh rosemary
2 tablespoons fresh lime juice
2 tablespoons cilantro, chopped
2 bell peppers, diced
1 cup cherry tomatoes

1. Heat the olive oil in a wok over a moderately high heat.
2. Now, cook the prawns for 7 to 8 minutes, until they have turned pink. Stir in the seasonings and cook an additional minute, stirring frequently.
3. Remove from the heat and toss with the lime juice and fresh cilantro. Tread the prawns onto bamboo skewers, alternating them with peppers and cherry tomatoes.
4. Serve on a serving platter. Bon appétit!

Per Serving

calories: 179 | fat: 8g | protein: 20 g | carbs: 5g | net carbs: 4g | fiber: 1g

474. Beef-Stuffed Peppers

Prep time: 5 minutes | Cook time: 30 minutes | Serves 6

¾ pound (340 g) ground beef
½ cup onion, chopped
2 garlic cloves, minced
12 mini peppers, seeded
½ cup Cheddar cheese, shredded

1. Heat up a lightly oiled sauté pan over a moderate flame. Brown the ground beef for 3 to 4 minutes, crumbling with a fork.
2. Stir in the onions and garlic; continue to sauté an additional 2 minutes or until tender and aromatic.
3. Cook the peppers in boiling water until just tender or approximately 7 minutes.
4. Arrange the stuffed peppers on a tinfoil-lined baking pan. Divide the beef mixture among the peppers. Top with the shredded Cheddar cheese.
5. Bake in the preheated oven at 360ºF (182ºC) approximately 17 minutes. Serve at room temperature. Bon appétit!

Per Serving

calories: 207 | fat: 10g | protein: 20g | carbs: 7g | net carbs: 5g | fiber: 2g

475. Spicy Chicken Drumettes

Prep time: 5 minutes | Cook time: 23 minutes | Serves 6

2 pounds (907 g) chicken drumettes
Sea salt and ground black pepper, to taste
½ teaspoon paprika
1 teaspoon cayenne pepper
1 teaspoon dried oregano
⅓ cup hot sauce
1 tablespoon stone-ground mustard
1 teaspoon garlic powder

1. Pat dry the chicken drumettes with paper towels. Season them with salt, black pepper, paprika, cayenne pepper, and oregano.
2. Brush the drumettes with cooking oil and transfer to a roasting pan. Bake at 420ºF (216ºC) for 18 minutes.
3. Toss with the hot sauce, mustard and garlic powder; broil for 5 minutes more or until the chicken drumettes are golden brown and thoroughly cooked. Bon appétit!

Per Serving

calories: 179 | fat: 3g | protein: 34g | carbs: 2g | net carbs: 1g | fiber: 1g

Chapter 12 Appetizers and Snacks

476. Cheesy Ham-Egg Cups

Prep time: 5 minutes | Cook time: 13 minutes | Serves 9

9 slices ham
Coarse salt and ground black pepper, to season
1 teaspoon jalapeño pepper, seeded and minced
½ cup Swiss cheese, shredded
9 eggs

1. Begin by preheating your oven to 390ºF (199ºC). Lightly grease a muffin pan with cooking spray.
2. Line each cup with a slice of ham; add salt, black pepper, jalapeño, and cheese. Crack an egg into each ham cup.
3. Bake in the preheated oven about 13 minutes or until the eggs are cooked through. Bon appétit!

Per Serving

calories: 137 | fat: 9g | protein: 12g | carbs: 2g net carbs: 1g | fiber: 1g

477. Chicken Wings with Ranch Dressing

Prep time: 10 minutes | Cook time: 50 minutes | Serves 6

2 pounds (907 g) chicken wings, pat dry
Nonstick cooking spray
Sea salt and cayenne pepper, to taste
Ranch Dressing:
¼ cup sour cream
¼ cup coconut milk
½ cup mayonnaise
½ teaspoon lemon juice
1 tablespoon fresh parsley, minced
1 clove garlic, minced
2 tablespoons onion, finely chopped
¼ teaspoon dry mustard
Sea salt and ground black pepper, to taste

1. Start by preheating your oven to 420ºF (216ºC).
2. Spritz the chicken wings with a cooking spray. Sprinkle the chicken wings with salt and cayenne pepper. Arrange the chicken wings on a parchment-lined baking pan. Bake in the preheated oven for 50 minutes or until the wings are golden and crispy.
3. In the meantime, make the dressing by mixing all of the above ingredients. Serve with warm wings.

Per Serving

calories: 466 | fat: 37g | protein: 27g | carbs: 2g net carbs: 2g | fiber: 0g

478. Cheesy Ham and Chicken Bites

Prep time: 5 minutes | Cook time: 22 to 24 minutes | Serves 5

5 slices ham
5 chicken fillets, about ¼-inch thin
3 ounces (85 g) Ricotta cheese
⅓ cup Colby cheese, grated
½ cup tomato purée

1. Place a slice of ham on each chicken fillet.
2. Thoroughly combine the Ricotta cheese and Colby cheese until everything is well incorporated.
3. Then, divide the cheese mixture between the chicken fillets. Roll them up and secure with toothpicks.
4. Transfer them to a lightly oiled baking tray. Bake in the preheated oven at 390ºF (199ºC) for 18 minutes, flipping them once or twice.
5. Pour the spicy tomato purée over the chicken roll-ups and bake another 4 to 6 minutes or until everything is thoroughly cooked. Bon appétit!

Per Serving

calories: 289 | fat: 11g | protein: 37 g | carbs: 7g net carbs: 5g | fiber: 2g

479. Baked Romano Zucchini Rounds

Prep time: 5 minutes | Cook time: 15 minutes | Serves 6

2 tablespoons olive oil
2 eggs
½ teaspoon smoked paprika
Sea salt and ground black pepper, to taste
2 pounds (907 g) zucchini, sliced into rounds
½ cup Romano cheese, shredded

1. Begin by preheating an oven to 420ºF (216ºC). Coat a rimmed baking sheet with Silpat mat or parchment paper.
2. In a mixing bowl, whisk the olive oil with eggs. Add in the paprika, salt, and black pepper. Now, dip the zucchini slices into the egg mixture.
3. Top with the shredded Romano cheese.
4. Arrange the zucchini rounds on the baking sheet; bake for 15 minutes until they are golden. Serve at room temperature.

Per Serving

calories: 137 | fat: 10g | protein: 9g | carbs: 6g net carbs: 4g | fiber: 2g

480. Whiskey-Glazed Chicken Wings

Prep time: 5 minutes | Cook time: 50 to 55 minutes | Serves 5

2 tablespoons extra-virgin olive oil
2 pounds (907 g) chicken wings
1 tablespoon whiskey
1 tablespoon Taco seasoning mix
1 cup tomato purée

1. Start by preheating your oven to 410°F (210°C). Toss the chicken wings with the other ingredients until well coated.
2. Place the wings onto a rack in the baking pan. Bake in the preheated oven for 50 to 55 minutes until a meat thermometer reads 165°F (74°C).
3. Serve with dipping sauce, if desired. Enjoy!

Per Serving
calories: 293 | fat: 12g | protein: 41g | carbs: 4g net carbs: 3g | fiber: 1g

481. Deviled Eggs with Roasted Peppers

Prep time: 5 minutes | Cook time: 9 t0 10 minutes | Serves 10

10 eggs
¼ cup sour cream
¼ cup roasted red pepper, chopped
2 tablespoons olive oil
1 teaspoon stone-ground mustard
1 garlic clove, minced
Sea salt, to taste
1 teaspoon red pepper flakes

1. Arrange the eggs in a saucepan. Pour in water (1-inch above the eggs) and bring to a boil. Heat off and let it sit, covered, for 9 to 10 minutes.
2. When the eggs are cool enough to handle, peel away the shells; rinse the eggs under running water. Separate egg whites and yolks.
3. Mix the egg yolks with the sour cream, roasted pepper, olive oil, mustard, garlic, and salt.
4. Stuff the eggs, arrange on a nice serving platter, and garnish with red pepper flakes. Enjoy!

Per Serving
calories: 97 | fat: 8g | protein: 6g | carbs: 1g net carbs: 1g | fiber:0 g

482. Cheesy Prosciutto Balls

Prep time: 5 minutes | Cook time: 0 minutes | Serves 4

2 ounces (57 g) goat cheese, crumbled
2 ounces (57 g) feta cheese crumbled
3 ounces (85 g) prosciutto, chopped
1 red bell pepper, seeded and finely chopped
2 tablespoons sesame seeds, toasted

1. Thoroughly combine the cheese, prosciutto and pepper until everything is well incorporated. Shape the mixture into balls.
2. Arrange these keto balls on a platter and place them in the refrigerator until ready to serve.
3. Roll the keto balls in toasted sesame seeds before serving. Bon appétit!

Per Serving
calories: 176 | fat: 13g | protein: 13g | carbs: 2g net carbs: 1g | fiber: 1g

483. Crispy Fried Dill Pickles

Prep time: 5 minutes | Cook time: 5 minutes | Serves 2

¼ cup avocado oil or coconut oil
3 tablespoons mayonnaise
¼ cup finely grated Parmesan cheese
3 tablespoons golden flaxseed meal
⅛ teaspoon garlic powder
12 dill pickle rounds

1. Heat the oil in a small skillet over medium-high heat.
2. Place the mayonnaise in a bowl. In another bowl, mix together the Parmesan cheese, flaxseed meal, and garlic powder.
3. Place the pickle slices on a paper towel and cover with another paper towel to dry the tops.
4. Dip each pickle slice into the mayonnaise and then into the Parmesan and flaxseed "breading," making sure to coat the slices evenly.
5. When the temperature of the oil reaches 400°F (205°C), gently place the breaded pickles in the hot oil and fry until golden and crispy, 1 to 2 minutes per side. Place the fried pickles on a paper towel-lined plate to absorb the excess oil before serving.

Per Serving
calories: 376 | fat: 38g | protein: 8g | carbs: 5g net carbs: 1g | fiber: 4g

484. Parmesan Crab Dip

Prep time: 15 minutes | Cook time: 25 minutes | Serves 4 to 6

4 ounces (113 g) cream cheese, softened
½ cup shredded Parmesan cheese, plus ½ cup extra for topping (optional)
⅓ cup mayonnaise
¼ cup sour cream
1 tablespoon chopped fresh parsley
2 teaspoons fresh lemon juice
1½ teaspoons Sriracha sauce
½ teaspoon garlic powder
8 ounces (227 g) fresh lump crab meat
Salt and pepper, to taste

1. Preheat the oven to 375ºF (190ºC).
2. Combine all the ingredients except for the crabmeat in a mixing bowl and use a hand mixer to blend until smooth.
3. Put the crabmeat in a separate bowl, check for shells, and rinse with cold water, if needed. Pat dry or allow to rest in a strainer until most of the water has drained.
4. Add the crabmeat to the bowl with the cream cheese mixture and gently fold to combine. Taste for seasoning and add salt and pepper to taste, if needed. Pour into an 8-inch round or square baking dish and bake for 25
5. minutes, until the cheese has melted and the dip is warm throughout.
6. If desired, top the dip with another ½ cup of Parmesan cheese and broil for 2 to 3 minutes, until the cheese has melted and browned slightly.

Per Serving
calories: 275 | fat: 23g | protein: 16g | carbs: 1g net carbs: 1g | fiber: 0g

485. Cheddar Anchovies Fat Bombs

Prep time: 5 minutes | Cook time: 0 minutes | Serves 2

2 (2-ounce / 57-g) cans anchovies, drained
⅓ cup cream cheese, chilled
⅓ cup Cheddar cheese, shredded
1 tablespoon Dijon mustard
2 scallions, chopped

1. Mix all of the above ingredients until everything is well incorporated. Shape the mixture into bite-sized balls.
2. Serve well chilled and enjoy!

Per Serving
calories: 391 | fat: 27g | protein: 34g | carbs: 3g net carbs: 2g | fiber: 1g

486. Turkey and Avocado Roll-Ups

Prep time: 5 minutes | Cook time: 0 minutes | Serves 8

½ fresh lemon, juiced
2 avocados, pitted, peeled and diced
16 slices cooked turkey breasts, deli-sliced
Salt and black pepper, to taste
16 slices Swiss cheese

1. Drizzle fresh lemon juice over your avocados. Place 1-2 avocado pieces on the turkey breast slice.
2. Season with salt and black pepper to taste.
3. Add the slice of Swiss cheese; repeat with the remaining ingredients. Roll them up and arrange on a nice serving platter. Bon appétit!

Per Serving
calories: 332 | fat: 24g | protein: 23g | carbs: 7g net carbs: 3g | fiber: 4g

487. Deviled Eggs with Chives

Prep time: 5 minutes | Cook time: 15 minutes | Serves 8

8 eggs
2 tablespoons cream cheese
1 teaspoon Dijon mustard
1 tablespoon mayonnaise
1 tablespoon tomato purée, no sugar added
1 teaspoon balsamic vinegar
Sea salt and freshly ground black pepper, to taste
¼ teaspoon cayenne pepper
2 tablespoons chives, chopped

1. Place the eggs in a single layer in a saucepan. Add water to cover the eggs and bring to a boil.
2. Cover, turn off the heat, and let the eggs stand for 15 minutes. Drain the eggs and peel them under cold running water.
3. Slice the eggs in half lengthwise; remove the yolks and thoroughly combine them with cream cheese, mustard, mayo, tomato purée, vinegar, salt, black, and cayenne pepper.
4. Next, divide the yolk mixture among egg whites. Garnish with fresh chives and enjoy!

Per Serving
calories: 149 | fat: 11g | protein: 10g | carbs: 2g net carbs: 2g | fiber: 0g

488. Romano Cheese Meatballs

Prep time: 5 minutes | Cook time: 20 minutes | Serves 10

½ ground turkey
1 pound (454 g) ground beef
4 ounces (113 g) pork rinds
¼ cup coconut milk
1 shallot, chopped
2 garlic cloves, minced
Sea salt and ground black pepper, to taste
½ cup Romano cheese, grated

1. Thoroughly combine all ingredients in a mixing bowl; shape the mixture into bite-sized meatballs.
2. Place your meatballs on a parchment-lined baking sheet; brush your meatballs with olive oil.
3. Bake for 10 minutes; rotate the pan and bake for a further 10 minutes. Serve with cocktail sticks and enjoy!

Per Serving
calories: 247 | fat: 18g | protein: 19g | carbs: 1g net carbs: 1g | fiber: 0g

489. Chicken Wings in Spicy Tomato Sauce

Prep time: 10 minutes | Cook time: 45 minutes | Serves 6

3 pounds (1.4 kg) chicken wings
Sea salt and ground black pepper, to taste
½ teaspoon paprika
½ teaspoon cayenne pepper
Sauce:
2 vine-ripe tomatoes
1 onion
2 garlic cloves
1 teaspoon chili pepper

1. Start by preheating your oven to 400°F (205°C). Set a wire rack inside a rimmed baking sheet.
2. Season the chicken wings with salt, black pepper, paprika, and cayenne pepper. Bake the wings approximately 45 minutes or until the skin is crispy.
3. To make the sauce, purée all ingredients in your food processor. Bon appétit!

Per Serving
calories: 309 | fat: 8g | protein: 50g | carbs: 5g net carbs: 4g | fiber: 1g

490. Greek-Style Ricotta Olive Dip

Prep time: 5 minutes | Cook time: 0 minutes | Serves 8

10 ounces (284 g) ricotta cheese
4 tablespoons Greek yogurt
½ teaspoon cayenne pepper
4 tablespoons olives, sliced
½ teaspoon shallot powder
½ teaspoon garlic salt
½ teaspoon black pepper
4 tablespoons cilantro, minced

1. Thoroughly combine the ricotta cheese, Greek yogurt, cayenne pepper, olives, shallot powder, garlic salt, and black pepper in a mixing bowl.
2. Transfer to a nice serving bowl.
3. Garnish with cilantro, serve and enjoy your party!

Per Serving
calories: 72 | fat: 6g | protein: 4g | carbs: 2g net carbs: 2g | fiber: 0g

491. Classic Caprese Skewers

Prep time: 15 minutes | Cook time: 0 minutes | Serves 6

8 ounces (227 g) ciliegini Mozzarella balls, drained and halved
9 grape tomatoes, halved
18 fresh basil leaves
Marinade:
¼ cup extra-virgin olive oil
1 clove garlic, pressed or minced
1 tablespoon chopped fresh parsley
1 tablespoon dried ground oregano
1 tablespoon fresh lemon juice
Kosher salt and ground black pepper, to taste

1. In a medium-sized bowl, combine the Mozzarella balls with the marinade ingredients. Stir well and cover; place in the refrigerator to marinate for 1 hour.
2. To assemble, place a Mozzarella ball, a basil leaf (folded in half lengthwise if needed), and a grape tomato half on a toothpick.
3. Serve right away or store in the refrigerator until ready to serve.

Per Serving
calories: 174 | fat: 16g | protein: 8g | carbs: 2g net carbs: 2g | fiber: 0g

492. Baked Cocktail Franks

Prep time: 5 minutes | Cook time: 12 minutes | Serves 10

2 tablespoons olive oil
18 ounces (510 g) cocktail franks
Sea salt and red pepper flakes, to taste
2 tablespoons wholegrain mustard

1. Start by preheating your oven to 360°F (182°C). Then, brush a baking pan with olive oil. Place the cocktail franks on the baking pan.
2. Sprinkle them with the salt and red pepper; add in the mustard and toss to combine.
3. Bake approximately 12 minutes until they are golden brown. Serve warm and enjoy!

Per Serving

calories: 155 | fat: 12g | protein: 9g | carbs: 5g net carbs: 4g | fiber: 1g

493. Bacon-Loaded Deviled Eggs

Prep time: 10 minutes | Cook time: 14 minutes | Serves 4

6 large eggs
5 slices bacon
¼ cup mayonnaise
½ teaspoon prepared yellow mustard
¼ teaspoon garlic powder
Salt and pepper
⅓ cup shredded Cheddar cheese, for topping
2 green onions, chopped, for topping

1. Place the eggs in a medium-sized saucepan and cover with cold water.
2. Bring to a boil, then immediately remove the pan from the heat. Cover with a lid and allow the eggs to sit in the hot water for 12 to 14 minutes for firm yolks.
3. Meanwhile, fry the bacon in a skillet over medium heat. Set aside on a paper towel-lined plate to cool, then finely chop.
4. Carefully remove the eggs from the hot water and place in a bowl filled with ice water to halt the cooking. When the eggs are cool, peel them.
5. Cut the eggs in half lengthwise. Remove the yolks and place them in a medium-sized mixing bowl. Add the mayonnaise, mustard, garlic powder, two-thirds of the bacon, and salt and pepper to taste; mix well.
6. For easy filling, spoon the egg yolk mixture into a small zip-top plastic bag, seal, and cut off one corner of the bag. Gently squeeze the bag to pipe the yolk mixture into the egg white halves.
7. Top the filled egg white halves with the reserved bacon, Cheddar cheese, and green onions. Eat right away or store in the refrigerator for up to 3 days.

Per Serving

calories: 290 | fat: 26g | protein: 14g | carbs: 2g net carbs: 2g | fiber: 0g

494. Lettuce Wraps with Ham and Tomato

Prep time: 10 minutes | Cook time: 0 minutes | Serves 5

10 Boston lettuce leaves, washed and rinsed well
1 tablespoon lemon juice, freshly squeezed
10 tablespoons cream cheese
10 thin ham slices
1 tomato, chopped
1 red chili pepper, chopped

1. Drizzle lemon juice over the lettuce leaves. Spread cream cheese over the lettuce leaves. Add a ham slice on each leaf.
2. Divide chopped tomatoes between the lettuce leaves. Top with chili peppers and arrange on a nice serving platter. Bon appétit!

Per Serving

calories: 148 | fat: 10g | protein: 11g | carbs: 4g net carbs: 3g | fiber: 1g

495. Lime Brussels Sprout Chips

Prep time: 15 minutes | Cook time: 10 minutes | Serves 2

3 cups Brussels sprouts leaves
Juice of ½ lime
2½ tablespoons avocado oil or melted coconut oil
Pink Himalayan salt

1. Preheat the oven to 400°F (205°C). Line a rimmed baking sheet with parchment paper.
2. Trim off the flat stem ends of the Brussels sprouts and separate the leaves. You should end up with 2 to 3 cups of leaves.
3. Place the separated leaves in a large bowl and add the lime juice.
4. Add the oil and season with salt to taste. Toss until the leaves are evenly coated.
5. Spread the leaves evenly on the prepared baking sheet and bake for 7
6. to 10 minutes, until lightly golden brown.

Per Serving

calories: 173 | fat: 18g | protein: 2g | carbs: 4g net carbs: 2g | fiber: 2g

496. Mozzarella Meatballs

Prep time: 10 minutes | Cook time: 18 to 25 minutes | Serves 8

½ pound (227 g) ground pork
1 pound (454 g) ground turkey
1 garlic clove, minced
4 tablespoons pork rinds, crushed
2 tablespoons shallots, chopped
4 ounces (113 g) Mozzarella string cheese, cubed
1 ripe tomato, puréed
Salt and ground black pepper, to taste

1. In a mixing bowl, thoroughly combine all ingredients, except for the cheese. Shape the mixture into bite-sized balls.
2. Press 1 cheese cube into the center of each ball.
3. Place the meatballs on a parchment-lined baking sheet. Bake in the preheated oven at 350°F (180°C) for 18 to 25 minutes. Bon appétit!

Per Serving
calories: 389 | fat: 31g | protein: 24g | carbs: 2g net carbs:1 g | fiber: 1g

497. Hearty Burger Dip

Prep time: 10 minutes | Cook time: 1 hour 30 minutes | Serves 2

¼ pound (113 g) ground pork
¼ pound (113 g) ground turkey
½ red onion, chopped
1 garlic clove, minced
1 serrano pepper, chopped
1 bell pepper, chopped
2 ounces (57 g) sour cream
½ cup Provolone cheese, grated
2 ounces (57 g) tomato purée
½ teaspoon mustard
½ teaspoon dried oregano
½ teaspoon dried basil
¼ teaspoon dried marjoram

1. Place all of the above ingredients, except for the sour cream and Provolone cheese in your slow cooker.
2. Cook for 1 hour 30 minutes at Low setting. Afterwards, fold in sour cream and cheese.
3. Serve warm with celery sticks if desired. Bon appétit!

Per Serving
calories: 423 | fat: 29g | protein: 32g | carbs: 5g net carbs: 4g | fiber: 1g

498. Italian Cheddar Cheese Crisps

Prep time: 5 minutes | Cook time: 8 minutes | Serves 4

1 cup sharp Cheddar cheese, grated
¼ teaspoon ground black pepper
½ teaspoon cayenne pepper
1 teaspoon Italian seasoning

1. Start by preheating an oven to 400°F (205°C). Line a baking sheet with a parchment paper.
2. Mix all of the above ingredients until well combined.
3. Then, place tablespoon-sized heaps of the mixture onto the prepared baking sheet.
4. Bake at the preheated oven for 8 minutes, until the edges start to brown. Allow the cheese crisps to cool slightly; then, place them on paper towels to drain the excess fat. Enjoy!

Per Serving
calories: 134 | fat: 11g | protein: 5g | carbs: 1g net carbs: 1g | fiber: 0g

499. Ranch Chicken-Bacon Dip

Prep time: 10 minutes | Cook time: 20 minutes | Serves 6

3 slices bacon
1½ cups shredded cooked chicken
1 (8-ounce / 227-g) package cream cheese, softened
½ cup Buffalo sauce
½ cup ranch dressing
Chopped green onions, for garnish (optional)

1. Preheat the oven to 375°F (190°C).
2. In a skillet over medium heat, fry the bacon until crispy. Set aside on a paper towel-lined plate to cool, then chop.
3. In a large bowl, combine the shredded chicken, cream cheese, Buffalo sauce, ranch dressing, and bacon; mix well. (If desired, reserve some of the bacon to sprinkle on top, as pictured.)
4. Transfer the chicken mixture to a shallow 1-quart baking dish and bake for 20 minutes, until warm throughout.
5. Garnish with chopped green onions, if desired.

Per Serving
calories: 286 | fat: 25g | protein: 11g | carbs: 3g net carbs: 3g | fiber: 0g

500. Cheesy Charcuterie Board

Prep time: 15 minutes | Cook time: 0 minutes | Serves 6 to 8

4 ounces (113 g) prosciutto, sliced
4 ounces (113 g) Calabrese salami, sliced
4 ounces (113 g) capicola, sliced
7 ounces (198 g) Parrano Gouda cheese
7 ounces (198 g) aged Manchego cheese
7 ounces (198 g) Brie cheese
½ cup roasted almonds
½ cup mixed olives
12 cornichons (small, tart pickles)
1 sprig fresh rosemary or other herbs of choice, for garnish

1. Arrange the meats, cheeses, and almonds on a large wooden cutting board.
2. Place the olives and pickles in separate bowls and set them on or alongside the cutting board. Garnish with a spring of rosemary or other fresh herbs of your choice.

Per Serving

calories: 445 | fat: 35g | protein: 31g | carbs: 3g net carbs: 2g | fiber: 1g

501. Cheese Crisps with Basil

Prep time: 5 minutes | Cook time: 8 minutes | Serves 2

½ cup shredded Cheddar cheese
½ cup shredded Parmesan cheese
½ teaspoon dried basil
¼ teaspoon garlic powder

1. Preheat the oven to 400°F (205°C). Line a baking sheet with parchment paper.
2. In a medium-sized bowl, mix together all the ingredients.
3. 3 Scoop up a heaping tablespoon of the mixture and place it on the parchment paper. Repeat, making a total of 8 small piles, spacing them 2 inches apart to prevent the cheese from running together.
4. Bake for 8 minutes, until golden brown. Let cool for 5 minutes before removing from the parchment paper.

Per Serving

calories: 195 | fat: 13g | protein: 15g | carbs: 3g net carbs: 3g | fiber: 0g

502. Creamy Herb Dip

Prep time: 15 minutes | Cook time: 5 minutes | Serves 7

1 (8-ounce / 227-g) package cream cheese
½ cup heavy whipping cream
¼ cup sour cream
3 tablespoons finely chopped fresh chives
2 tablespoons finely chopped onions
2 tablespoons finely chopped fresh parsley
½ teaspoon garlic powder

1. Place the cream cheese and heavy whipping cream in a microwave-safe bowl and microwave on high for 1 minute; stir and repeat until the texture is smooth.
2. Add the remaining ingredients and stir to combine.
3. Place in the refrigerator to chill for at least 30 minutes before serving.

Per Serving

calories: 156 | fat: 14g | protein: 3g | carbs: 2g net carbs: 2g | fiber: 1g

503. Fresh Homemade Guacamole

Prep time: 15 minutes | Cook time: 0 minutes | Serves 4

2 ripe avocados
½ tomato, chopped
¼ cup minced red onions
2 tablespoons finely chopped fresh cilantro
1 tablespoon fresh lime juice
½ teaspoon minced garlic
½ teaspoon salt
1 tablespoon sour cream (optional)

1. Slice the avocados in half lengthwise, remove the pits, and scoop the flesh into a medium-sized serving bowl. Mash the avocado flesh.
2. Stir in the tomato, onions, cilantro, lime juice, garlic, and salt. Fold in the sour cream, if using.
3. Serve right away or place in the refrigerator to chill until ready to serve.

Per Serving

calories: 133 | fat: 12g | protein: 2g | carbs: 8g net carbs: 3g | fiber: 5g

504. Lemony Bacon Chips

Prep time: 5 minutes | Cook time: 10 minutes | Serves 12

1½ pounds (680 g) bacon, cut into 1-inch squares
¼ cup lemon juice
1 teaspoon Ranch seasoning mix
1 tablespoon hot sauce

1. Toss the bacon squares with the lemon juice, Ranch seasoning mix, and hot sauce. Arrange the bacon squares on a parchment-lined baking sheet.
2. Roast in the preheated oven at 375°F (190°C) approximately 10 minutes or until crisp.
3. Let it cool completely before storing. Bon appétit!

Per Serving
calories: 232 | fat: 23g | protein: 7g | carbs: 1g net carbs: 1g | fiber: 0g

505. Mexican Shrimp-Stuffed Avocados

Prep time: 10 minutes | Cook time: 15 minutes | Serves 4

2 avocados, halved and pitted
12 large cooked shrimp, peeled and deveined
3 tablespoons salsa
¼ cup shredded Mexican cheese blend
Finely chopped fresh cilantro, for garnish (optional)
Sour cream, for garnish (optional)

1. Preheat the oven to 350°F (180°C). Line a rimmed baking sheet with parchment paper.
2. Rinse the shrimp and halve lengthwise. Place in a bowl and top with the salsa. Stir to coat the shrimp evenly with the salsa.
3. Place the avocado halves cut side up on the lined baking sheet. Fill each half with salsa-coated shrimp and top with the cheese.
4. Bake for 15 minutes, until the cheese is melted.
5. Serve garnished with cilantro and/or topped with sour cream, if desired.

Per Serving
calories: 185 | fat: 13g | protein: 11g | carbs: 7g net carbs: 6g | fiber: 1g

506. Blue Cheese and Ranch Dip

Prep time: 5 minutes | Cook time: 0 minutes | Serves 10

½ cup Greek-style yogurt
1 cup blue cheese, crumbled
½ cup mayonnaise
1 tablespoon lime juice
Freshly ground black pepper, to taste
2 tablespoons ranch seasoning

1. In a mixing bowl, thoroughly combine all ingredients until well incorporated.
2. Serve well chilled with your favorite keto dippers. Bon appétit!

Per Serving
calories: 94 | fat: 8g | protein: 4g | carbs: 1g net carbs: 1g | fiber: 0g

507. Italian Fried Mozzarella Sticks

Prep time: 10 minutes | Cook time: 4 minutes | Serves 5

1 large egg
¼ cup grated Parmesan cheese
¼ cup golden flaxseed meal
½ teaspoon Italian seasoning
¼ teaspoon garlic powder
Pinch salt
5 Mozzarella cheese sticks, cut in half crosswise to make 10 pieces
1 tablespoon avocado oil or coconut oil, for frying
Ranch dressing, warm, for serving

1. In a small bowl, beat the egg.
2. In another bowl, combine the Parmesan cheese, flaxseed meal, Italian seasoning, garlic powder, and salt; mix with a fork.
3. Dip each cheese stick into the beaten egg and then into the Parmesan cheese mixture. Press the Parmesan mixture into the cheese sticks to coat them evenly on all sides.
4. Place the breaded cheese sticks on a plate and place in the freezer for 30 to 45 minutes, until the Parmesan crust is firm and fully frozen.
5. In a small skillet, heat the oil over medium-high heat. When the temperature of the oil reaches 400°F (205°C), add the cheese sticks and fry for 1 to 2 minutes, then flip and fry for 1 to 2 more minutes, until golden brown on both sides.
6. Serve with ranch dressing or marinara for dipping.

Per Serving
calories: 185 | fat: 14g | protein: 11g | carbs: 3g net carbs: 2g | fiber: 1g

508. Margherita Pizza with Mushrooms

Prep time: 5 minutes | Cook time: 18 minutes | Serves 4

4 medium portobello mushroom caps, stemmed
Dash of salt
¼ cup no-sugar-added marinara sauce
4 tomato slices
4 ounces (113 g) fresh Mozzarella, cut into 4 slices
4 teaspoons extra-virgin olive oil or avocado oil
2 small cloves or 1 large clove garlic, minced
1 tablespoon chopped fresh basil, for garnish

1. Preheat the oven to 375°F (190°C). Place a wire rack in a rimmed baking sheet.
2. Set the mushroom caps on top of the wire rack. Place 1 tablespoon of marinara and a slice of tomato in each cap, then a Mozzarella slice. Drizzle with olive oil, then top with the minced garlic.
3. Bake for 15 to 18 minutes, until the cheese is melted and the mushrooms are tender.
4. Remove from the oven and top with the basil before serving.

Per Serving
calories: 141 | fat: 10g | protein: 8g | carbs: 6g net carbs: 4g | fiber: 2g

509. Oven-Baked Prosciutto-Wrapped Asparagus

Prep time: 5 minutes | Cook time: 12 minutes | Serves 6

18 asparagus spears, ends trimmed
2 tablespoons coconut oil, melted
6 slices prosciutto
1 teaspoon garlic powder

1. Preheat the oven to 400°F (205°C). Line a rimmed baking sheet with parchment paper.
2. Place the asparagus and coconut oil in a large zip-top plastic bag. Seal and toss until the asparagus is evenly coated.
3. Wrap a slice of prosciutto around 3 grouped asparagus spears. Repeat with the remaining prosciutto and asparagus, making a total of 6 bundles.
4. Arrange the bundles in a single layer on the lined baking sheet. Sprinkle the garlic powder over the bundles.
5. Bake for 8 to 12 minutes, until the asparagus is tender.

Per Serving
calories: 122 | fat: 10g | protein: 8g | carbs: 3g net carbs: 2g | fiber: 1g

510. Cheesy Bacon-Stuffed Jalapeño Poppers

Prep time: 15 minutes | Cook time: 20 minutes | Serves 3

5 slices bacon
6 jalapeño peppers
3 ounces (85 g) cream cheese, softened
¼ cup shredded Cheddar cheese
¼ teaspoon garlic powder

1. In a skillet over medium heat, fry the bacon until crispy. Set aside on a paper towel–lined plate to cool. When cool enough to handle, chop the bacon into bits.
2. Preheat the oven to 400°F (205°C). Line a rimmed baking sheet with parchment paper.
3. Slice the jalapeño peppers in half lengthwise. Use a spoon to scrape out the seeds and membranes. (If you prefer spicy food, feel free to incorporate the jalapeño seeds and membranes into the cheese sauce instead of discarding them.)
4. In a medium-sized bowl, use a fork to combine the cream cheese, Cheddar cheese, garlic powder, and bacon bits. Spoon some of the mixture into each jalapeño half and set the peppers cheese side up on the lined baking sheet. Bake for 18 to 20 minutes, until the cheese is melted and slightly crisp on top.

Per Serving
calories: 203 | fat: 16g | protein: 9g | carbs: 3g net carbs: 2g | fiber: 1g

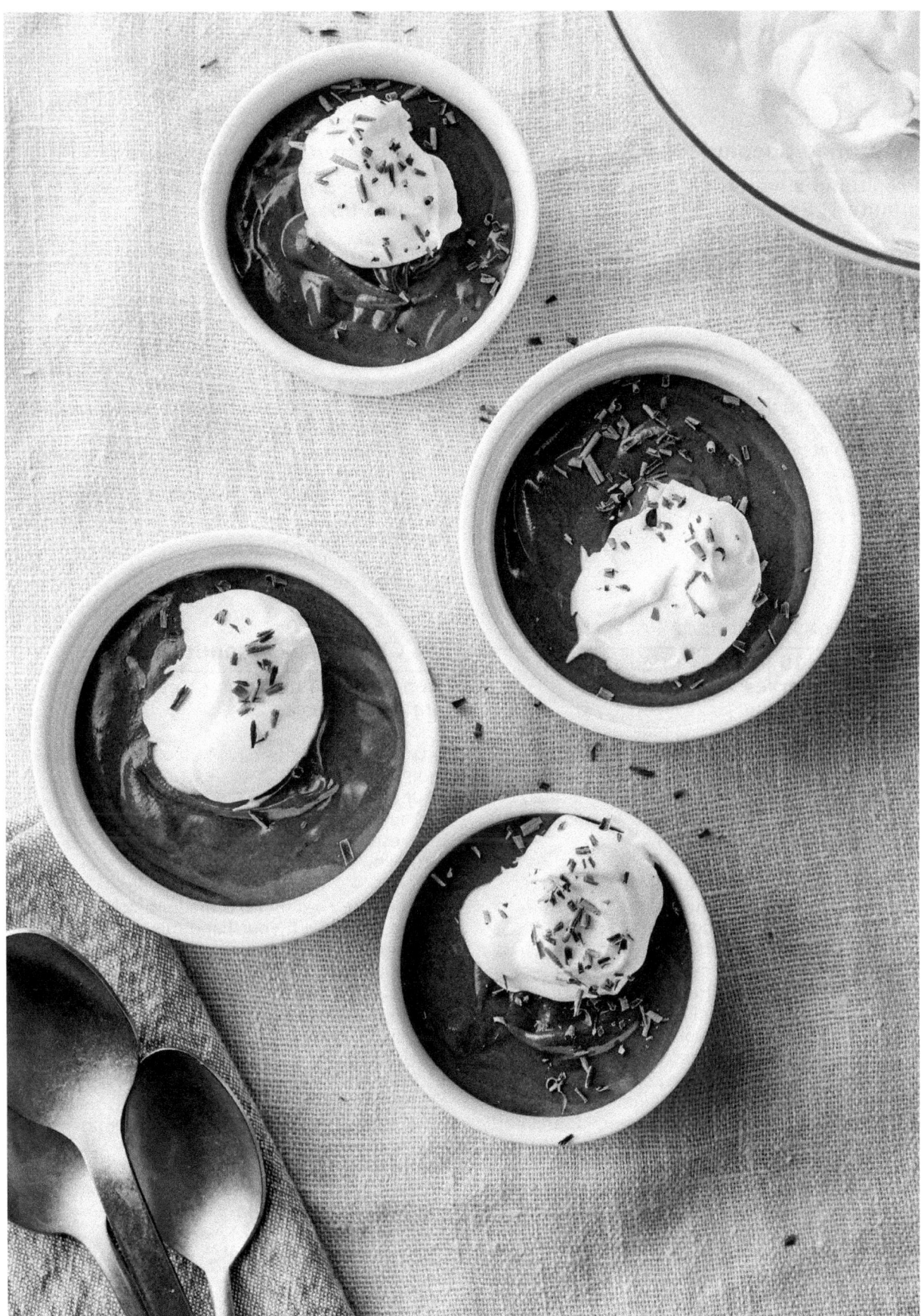

Chapter 13 Desserts

511. Coffee-Coconut Ice Pops

Prep time: 5 minutes | Cook time: 0 minutes | Serves 4

2 cups brewed coffee, cold
¾ cup coconut cream
2 teaspoons Swerve natural sweetener or 2 drops liquid stevia
2 tablespoons sugar-free chocolate chips

1. In a food processor (or blender), mix together the coffee, coconut cream, and sweetener until thoroughly blended.
2. Pour into ice pop molds, and drop a few chocolate chips into each mold.
3. Freeze for at least 2 hours before serving.

Per Serving
calories: 105 | fat: 10g | protein: 1g | carbs: 7g net carbs: 2g | fiber: 5g

512. Cheesy Lemonade Fat Bomb

Prep time: 10 minutes | Cook time: 0 minutes | Serves 2

½ lemon
4 ounces (113 g) cream cheese, at room temperature
2 ounces (57 g) butter, at room temperature
2 teaspoons Swerve natural sweetener or 2 drops liquid stevia
Pinch pink Himalayan salt

1. Zest the lemon half with a very fine grater into a small bowl. Squeeze the juice from the lemon half into the bowl with the zest.
2. In a medium bowl, combine the cream cheese and butter. Add the sweetener, lemon zest and juice, and pink Himalayan salt. Using a hand mixer, beat until fully combined.
3. Spoon the mixture into the fat bomb molds. (I use small silicone cupcake molds. If you don't have molds, you can use cupcake paper liners that fit into the cups of a muffin tin.)
4. Freeze for at least 2 hours, unmold, and eat! Keep extras in your freezer in a zip-top bag so you and your loved ones can have them anytime you are craving a sweet treat. They will keep in the freezer for up to 3 months.

Per Serving
calories: 404 | fat: 43g | protein: 4g | carbs: 8g net carbs: 4g | fiber: 4g

513. Coconut-Fudge Ice Pops

Prep time: 5 minutes | Cook time: 0 minutes | Serves 4

½ (13.5-ounce / 383-g) can coconut cream
2 teaspoons Swerve natural sweetener
2 tablespoons unsweetened cocoa powder
2 tablespoons sugar-free chocolate chips

1. In a food processor (or blender), mix together the coconut cream, sweetener, and unsweetened cocoa powder.
2. Pour into ice pop molds, and drop chocolate chips into each mold.
3. Freeze for at least 2 hours before serving.

Per Serving
calories: 193 | fat: 20g | protein: 2g | carbs: 9g net carbs: 3g | fiber: 6g

514. Chocolate-Coconut Shake

Prep time: 10 minutes | Cook time: 0 minutes | Serves 2

¾ cup heavy (whipping) cream
4 ounces (113 g) coconut milk
1 tablespoon Swerve natural sweetener
¼ teaspoon vanilla extract
2 tablespoons unsweetened cocoa powder

1. Pour the cream into a medium cold metal bowl, and with your hand mixer and cold beaters, beat the cream just until it forms peaks.
2. Slowly pour in the coconut milk, and gently stir it into the cream. Add the sweetener, vanilla, and cocoa powder, and beat until fully combined.
3. Pour into two tall glasses, and chill in the freezer for 1 hour before serving. I usually stir the shakes twice during this time.

Per Serving
calories: 444 | fat: 47g | protein: 4g | carbs: 15g net carbs: 7g | fiber: 8g

515. Crispy Strawberry Chocolate Bark

Prep time: 10 minutes | Cook time: 1 minute | Serves 2

½ (2.8-ounce / 79-g) keto-friendly chocolate bar
1 tablespoon heavy (whipping) cream
2 tablespoons salted almonds
1 fresh strawberry, sliced

1. Line a baking sheet with parchment paper.
2. Break up the chocolate bar half into small pieces, and put them in a microwave-safe bowl with the cream.
3. Heat in the microwave for 45 seconds at 50 percent power. Stir the chocolate, and cook for 20 seconds more at 50 percent power. Stir again, making sure the mixture is fully melted and combined. If not, microwave for another 20 seconds.
4. Pour the chocolate mixture onto the parchment paper and spread it in a thin, uniform layer.
5. Sprinkle on the almonds, then add the strawberry slices.
6. Refrigerate until hardened, about 2 hours.
7. Once the bark is nice and hard, break it up into smaller pieces to nibble on. Yum!
8. The bark will keep for up to 4 days in a sealed container in the refrigerator.

Per Serving

calories: 111 | fat: 10g | protein: 3g | carbs: 9g net carbs: 4g | fiber: 5g

516. Creamy Strawberry Shake

Prep time: 10 minutes | Cook time: 0 minutes | Serves 2

¾ cup heavy (whipping) cream
2 ounces (57 g) cream cheese, at room temperature
1 tablespoon Swerve
natural sweetener
¼ teaspoon vanilla extract
6 strawberries, sliced
6 ice cubes

1. In a food processor (or blender), combine the heavy cream, cream cheese, sweetener, and vanilla. Mix on high to fully combine.
2. Add the strawberries and ice, and blend until smooth.
3. Pour into two tall glasses and serve.

Per Serving

calories: 407 | fat: 42g | protein: 4g | carbs: 13g net carbs: 6g | fiber: 7g

517. Fresh Strawberry Cheesecake Mousse

Prep time: 10 minutes | Cook time: 0 minutes | Serves 2

4 ounces (113 g) cream cheese, at room temperature
1 tablespoon heavy (whipping) cream
1 teaspoon Swerve
natural sweetener or 1 drop liquid stevia
1 teaspoon vanilla extract
4 fresh strawberries, sliced

1. Break up the cream cheese block into smaller pieces and distribute evenly in a food processor (or blender). Add the cream, sweetener, and vanilla.
2. Mix together on high. I usually stop and stir twice and scrape down the sides of the bowl with a small rubber scraper to make sure everything is mixed well.
3. Add the strawberries to the food processor, and mix until combined.
4. Divide the strawberry cheesecake mixture between two small dishes, and chill for 1 hour before serving.

Per Serving

calories: 221 | fat: 21g | protein: 4g | carbs: 11g net carbs: 4g | fiber: 7g

518. Cheesecake Fat Bomb with Berries

Prep time: 10 minutes | Cook time: 0 minutes | Serves 2

4 ounces (113 g) cream cheese, at room temperature
4 tablespoons butter, at room temperature
2 teaspoons Swerve
natural sweetener or 2 drops liquid stevia
1 teaspoon vanilla extract
¼ cup berries, fresh or frozen

1. In a medium bowl, use a hand mixer to beat the cream cheese, butter, sweetener, and vanilla.
2. In a small bowl, mash the berries thoroughly. Fold the berries into the cream-cheese mixture using a rubber scraper.
3. Spoon the cream-cheese mixture into fat bomb molds.
4. Freeze for at least 2 hours, unmold them, and eat! Leftover fat bombs can be stored in the freezer in a zip-top bag for up to 3 months. It's nice to have some in your freezer for when you are craving a sweet treat.

Per Serving

calories: 414 | fat: 43g | protein: 4g | carbs: 9g net carbs: 4g | fiber: 5g

519. Simple Peanut Butter Fat Bomb

Prep time: 10 minutes | Cook time: 1 minute | Serves 2

1 tablespoon butter, at room temperature
1 tablespoon coconut oil
2 tablespoons all-natural peanut butter or almond butter
2 teaspoons Swerve natural sweetener or 2 drops liquid stevia

1. In a microwave-safe medium bowl, melt the butter, coconut oil, and peanut butter in the microwave for 1 minute on 50 percent power. Mix in the sweetener.
2. Pour the mixture into fat bomb molds.
3. Freeze for 30 minutes, unmold them, and eat! Keep some extras in your freezer so you can eat them anytime you are craving a sweet treat.

Per Serving
calories: 196 | fat: 20g | protein: 3g | carbs: 8g | net carbs: 3g | fiber: 5g

520. Keto Peanut Butter Cookies

Prep time: 5 minutes | Cook time: 10 minutes | Makes 15 cookies

1 cup natural crunchy peanut butter
½ cup Swerve natural sweetener
1 egg

1. Preheat the oven to 350°F (180°C). Line a baking sheet with a silicone baking mat or parchment paper.
2. In a medium bowl, use a hand mixer to mix together the peanut butter, sweetener, and egg.
3. Roll up the batter into small balls about 1 inch in diameter.
4. Spread out the cookie-dough balls on the prepared pan. Press each dough ball down with the tines of a fork, then repeat to make a crisscross pattern.
5. Bake for about 12 minutes, or until golden.
6. Let the cookies cool for 10 minutes on the lined pan before serving. If you try to move them too soon, they will crumble.
7. Store leftover cookies covered in the refrigerator for up to 5 days.

Per Serving (1 cookie)
calories: 98 | fat: 8g | protein: 4g | carbs: 10g | net carbs: 3g | fiber: 7g

521. Baked Cheesecake Bites

Prep time: 10 minutes | Cook time: 30 minutes | Serves 4

4 ounces (113 g) cream cheese, at room temperature
¼ cup sour cream
2 large eggs
⅓ cup Swerve natural sweetener
¼ teaspoon vanilla extract

1. Preheat the oven to 350°F (180°C).
2. In a medium mixing bowl, use a hand mixer to beat the cream cheese, sour cream, eggs, sweetener, and vanilla until well mixed.
3. Place silicone liners (or cupcake paper liners) in the cups of a muffin tin.
4. Pour the cheesecake batter into the liners, and bake for 30 minutes.
5. Refrigerate until completely cooled before serving, about 3 hours. Store extra cheesecake bites in a zip-top bag in the freezer for up to 3 months.

Per Serving
calories: 169 | fat: 15g | protein: 5g | carbs: 18g | net carbs: 2g | fiber: 16g

522. Pumpkin Cheesecake Bites

Prep time: 10 minutes | Cook time: 30 minutes | Serves 4

4 ounces (113 g) pumpkin purée
4 ounces (113 g) cream cheese, at room temperature
2 large eggs
⅓ cup Swerve natural sweetener
2 teaspoons pumpkin pie spice

1. Preheat the oven to 350°F (180°C).
2. In a medium mixing bowl, use a hand mixer to mix the pumpkin purée, cream cheese, eggs, sweetener, and pumpkin pie spice until thoroughly combined.
3. Place silicone liners (or cupcake paper liners) into the cups of a muffin tin.
4. Pour the batter into the liners, and bake for 30 minutes.
5. Refrigerate until completely cooled before serving, about 3 hours. Put leftover cheesecake bites in a zip-top plastic bag and store in the freezer for up to 3 months.

Per Serving
calories: 156 | fat: 12g | protein: 5g | carbs: 21g | net carbs: 4g | fiber: 17g

523. Chocolate Pecan-Berry Mascarpone Bowl

Prep time: 5 minutes | Cook time: 0 minutes | Serves 2

1 cup chopped pecans
1 teaspoon Swerve natural sweetener or 1 drop liquid stevia
¼ cup mascarpone
30 Lily's dark-chocolate chips
6 strawberries, sliced

1. Divide the pecans between two dessert bowls.
2. In a small bowl, mix the sweetener into the mascarpone cheese. Top the nuts with a dollop of the sweetened mascarpone.
3. Sprinkle in the chocolate chips, top each dish with the strawberries, and serve.

Per Serving
calories: 462 | fat: 47g | protein: 6g | carbs: 15g net carbs: 6g | fiber: 9g

524. Chocolate Chip Ice Cream with Mint

Prep time: 10 minutes | Cook time: 30 minutes | Serves 2

½ tablespoon butter
1 tablespoon Swerve natural sweetener
10 tablespoons heavy (whipping) cream, divided
¼ teaspoon peppermint extract
2 tablespoons sugar-free chocolate chips

1. Put a medium metal bowl and your hand-mixer beaters in the freezer to chill.
2. In a small, heavy saucepan over medium heat, melt the butter. Whisk in the sweetener and 5 tablespoons of cream.
3. Turn the heat up to medium-high and bring the mixture to a boil, stirring constantly. Turn the heat down to low and simmer, stirring occasionally, for about 30 minutes. You want the mixture to be thick, so it sticks to the back of a spoon.
4. Stir in the peppermint extract.
5. Pour the thickened mixture into a medium bowl and refrigerate to cool.
6. Remove the metal bowl and the mixer beaters from the freezer. Pour the remaining 5 tablespoons of cream into the bowl. With the electric beater, whip the cream until it is thick and fluffy and forms peaks. Don't overbeat, or the cream will turn to butter. Take the cream mixture out of the refrigerator.
7. Using a rubber scraper, gently fold the whipped cream into the cooled mixture.
8. Transfer the mixture to a small metal container that can go in the freezer.
9. Mix in the chocolate chips, and cover the container with foil or plastic wrap.
10. Freeze the ice cream for 4 to 5 hours before serving, stirring it twice during that time.

Per Serving
calories: 325 | fat: 33g | protein: 3g | carbs: 17g net carbs: 4g | fiber: 13g

525. Creamsicle Float

Prep time: 5 minutes | Cook time: 0 minutes | Serves 2

1 can diet lemon lime soda
4 tablespoons heavy (whipping) cream
1 teaspoon vanilla extract
6 ice cubes

1. In a food processor (or blender), combine the lemon lime soda, cream, vanilla, and ice.
2. Blend well, pour into two tall glasses, and serve.

Per Serving
calories: 56 | fat: 6g | protein: 1g | carbs: 3g net carbs: 1g | fiber: 2g

526. Creamy Chocolate Mousse

Prep time: 10 minutes | Cook time: 0 minutes | Serves 2

1½ tablespoons heavy (whipping) cream
4 tablespoons butter, at room temperature
1 tablespoon unsweetened cocoa powder
4 tablespoons cream cheese, at room temperature
1 tablespoon Swerve natural sweetener

1. In a medium chilled bowl, use a whisk or fork to whip the cream. Refrigerate to keep cold.
2. In a separate medium bowl, use a hand mixer to beat the butter, cocoa powder, cream cheese, and sweetener until thoroughly combined.
3. Take the whipped cream out of the refrigerator. Gently fold the whipped cream into the chocolate mixture with a rubber scraper.
4. Divide the pudding between two dessert bowls.
5. Cover and chill for 1 hour before serving.

Per Serving
calories: 460 | fat: 50g | protein: 4g | carbs: 10g net carbs: 4g | fiber: 6g

527. Avocado-Chocolate Pudding

Prep time: 5 minutes | Cook time: 0 minutes | Serves 2

1 ripe medium avocado, cut into chunks
2 ounces (57 g) cream cheese, at room temperature
1 tablespoon Swerve natural sweetener
4 tablespoons unsweetened cocoa powder
¼ teaspoon vanilla extract
Pinch pink Himalayan salt

1. In a food processor (or blender), combine the avocado with the cream cheese, sweetener, cocoa powder, vanilla, and pink Himalayan salt. Blend until completely smooth.
2. Pour into two small dessert bowls, and chill for 30 minutes before serving.

Per Serving

calories: 281 | fat: 27g | protein: 8g | carbs: 27g net carbs: 12g | fiber: 15g

528. Slow Cooker Chocolate Pot De Crème

Prep time: 10 minutes | Cook time: 3 hours | Serves 6

6 egg yolks
2 cups heavy (whipping) cream
⅓ cup cocoa powder
1 tablespoon pure vanilla extract
½ teaspoon liquid stevia
Whipped coconut cream, for garnish (optional)
Shaved dark chocolate, for garnish (optional)

1. In a medium bowl, whisk together the yolks, heavy cream, cocoa powder, vanilla, and stevia.
2. Pour the mixture into a 1½-quart baking dish and place the dish in the insert of the slow cooker.
3. Pour in enough water to reach halfway up the sides of the baking dish.
4. Cover and cook on low for 3 hours.
5. Remove the baking dish from the insert and cool to room temperature on a wire rack.
6. Chill the dessert completely in the refrigerator and serve, garnished with the whipped coconut cream and shaved dark chocolate (if desired).

Per Serving

calories: 198 | fat: 18g | protein: 5g | carbs: 4g net carbs: 3g | fiber: 1g

529. Lemon Custard

Prep time: 10 minutes | Cook time: 3 hours | Serves 4

5 egg yolks
¼ cup freshly squeezed lemon juice
1 tablespoon lemon zest
1 teaspoon pure vanilla extract
⅓ teaspoon liquid stevia
2 cups heavy (whipping) cream
1 cup whipped coconut cream

1. In a medium bowl, whisk together the yolks, lemon juice and zest, vanilla, and liquid stevia.
2. Whisk in the heavy cream and divide the mixture between 4 ramekins.
3. Place a rack at the bottom of the insert of the slow cooker and place the ramekins on it.
4. Pour in enough water to reach halfway up the sides of the ramekins.
5. Cover and cook on low for 3 hours.
6. Remove the ramekins from the insert and cool to room temperature.
7. Chill the ramekins completely in the refrigerator and serve topped with whipped coconut cream.

Per Serving

calories: 319 | fat: 30g | protein: 7g | carbs: 3g net carbs: 3g | fiber: 0g

530. Ginger-Pumpkin Pudding

Prep time: 5 minutes | Cook time: 3 to 4 hours | Serves 8

1 tablespoon coconut oil
2 cups pumpkin purée
1½ cups coconut milk
2 eggs
½ cup almond flour
1 ounce (28 g) protein powder
1 tablespoon grated fresh ginger
¾ teaspoon liquid stevia
Pinch ground cloves
1 cup whipped coconut cream

1. Lightly grease the insert of the slow cooker with coconut oil.
2. In a large bowl, stir together pumpkin, coconut milk, eggs, almond flour, protein powder, ginger, liquid stevia, and cloves.
3. Transfer the mixture to the insert.
4. Cover and cook on low 3 to 4 hours.
5. Serve warm with whipped coconut cream.

Per Serving

calories: 217 | fat: 19g | protein: 8g | carbs: 7g net carbs: 3g | fiber: 4g

531. Pumpkin Compote with Mix Berries

Prep time: 10 minutes | Cook time: 3 to 4 hours | Serves 10

1 tablespoon coconut oil
2 cups diced pumpkin
1 cup cranberries
1 cup blueberries
½ cup granulated erythritol
Juice and zest of 1 lemon
½ cup coconut milk
1 teaspoon ground cinnamon
½ teaspoon ground allspice
¼ teaspoon ground nutmeg
1 cup whipped cream

1. Lightly grease the insert of the slow cooker with the coconut oil.
2. Place the pumpkin, cranberries, blueberries, erythritol, lemon juice and zest, coconut milk, cinnamon, allspice, and nutmeg in the insert.
3. Cover and cook on low for 3 to 4 hours.
4. Let the compote cool for 1 hour and serve warm with a generous scoop of whipped cream.

Per Serving
calories: 113 | fat: 9g | protein: 4g | carbs: 7g net carbs: 4g | fiber: 3g

532. Almond-Sour Cream Cheesecake

Prep time: 15 minutes | Cook time: 5 to 6 hours | Serves 10

¼ cup butter, melted, divided
1 cup ground almonds
¾ cup plus 1 tablespoon granulated erythritol, divided
¼ teaspoon ground cinnamon
12 ounces (340 g) cream cheese, at room temperature
2 eggs
2 teaspoons pure vanilla extract
1 cup sour cream

1. Lightly grease a 7-inch springform pan with 1 tablespoon of the butter.
2. In a small bowl, stir together the almonds, 1 tablespoon of the erythritol, and cinnamon until blended.
3. Add the remaining 3 tablespoons of the butter and stir until coarse crumbs form.
4. Press the crust mixture into the springform pan along the bottom and about 2 inches up the sides.
5. In a large bowl, using a handheld mixer, beat together the cream cheese, eggs, vanilla, and remaining ¾ cup of the erythritol. Beat the sour cream into the cream-cheese mixture until smooth.
6. Spoon the batter into the springform pan and smooth out the top.
7. Place a wire rack in the insert of the slow cooker and place the springform pan on top.
8. Cover and cook on low for 5 to 6 hours, or until the cheesecake doesn't jiggle when shaken.
9. Cool completely before removing from pan.
10. Chill the cheesecake completely before serving, and store leftovers in the refrigerator.

Per Serving
calories: 279 | fat: 25g | protein: 8g | carbs: 4g net carbs: 3g | fiber: 1g

533. Almond-Peanut Butter Cheesecake

Prep time: 15 minutes | Cook time: 5 to 6 hours | Serves 10

¼ cup butter, melted, divided
1 cup ground almonds
2 tablespoons cocoa powder
1 cup granulated erythritol, divided
12 ounces (340 g) cream cheese, room temperature
½ cup natural peanut butter
2 eggs, room temperature
1 teaspoon pure vanilla extract

1. Lightly grease a 7-inch springform pan with 1 tablespoon butter.
2. In a small bowl, stir together the almonds, cocoa powder, and ¼ cup erythritol until blended. Add the remaining 3 tablespoons of the butter and stir until coarse crumbs form.
3. Press the crust mixture into the springform pan along the bottom and about 2 inches up the sides.
4. In a large bowl, using a handheld mixer, beat together the cream cheese and peanut butter until smooth. Beat in the remaining ¾ cup of the erythritol, eggs, and vanilla.
5. Spoon the batter into the springform pan and smooth out the top.
6. Place a wire rack in the insert of slow cooker and place the springform pan on the wire rack.
7. Cover and cook on low for 5 to 6 hours, or until the cheesecake doesn't jiggle when shaken.
8. Cool completely before removing from pan.
9. Chill the cheesecake completely before serving, and store leftovers in the refrigerator.

Per Serving
calories: 311 | fat: 28g | protein: 11g | carbs: 5g net carbs: 3g | fiber: 2g

534. Blackberry Cobbler with Almonds

Prep time: 15 minutes | Cook time: 3 to 4 hours | Serves 10

For the Filling:
1 tablespoon coconut oil
6 cups blackberries
½ cup granulated erythritol
1 teaspoon ground cinnamon

For the Topping:
2 cups ground almonds
½ cup granulated erythritol
1 tablespoon baking powder
½ teaspoon salt
1 cup heavy (whipping) cream
½ cup butter, melted

1. Lightly grease the insert of a 4-quart slow cooker with the coconut oil.
2. Add the blackberries, erythritol, and cinnamon to the insert. Mix to combine.
3. In a large bowl, stir together the almonds, erythritol, baking powder, and salt. Add the heavy cream and butter and stir until a thick batter forms.
4. Drop the batter by the tablespoon on top of the blackberries.
5. Cover and cook on low for 3 to 4 hours.
6. Serve warm.

Per Serving
calories: 281 | fat: 31g | protein: 8g | carbs: 10g net carbs: 4g | fiber: 6g

535. Almond Chocolate Cookies

Prep time: 15 minutes | Cook time: 10 minutes | Makes 20 cookies

1 cup grass-fed butter, at room temperature
¾ cup monk fruit sweetener, granulated form
2 eggs
1 tablespoon vanilla extract
3½ cups almond flour
1 teaspoon baking soda
½ teaspoon sea salt
1½ cups dark chocolate chips

1. Preheat the oven. Set the oven temperature to 350ºF (180ºC). Line a baking sheet with parchment paper and set it aside.
2. Mix the wet ingredients. In a large bowl, cream the butter and sweetener until the mixture is very fluffy, either by hand or with a hand mixer. Add the eggs and vanilla and beat until everything is well blended.
3. Mix the dry ingredients. In a medium bowl, stir together the almond flour, baking soda, and salt until they're well mixed together.
4. Add the dry to the wet ingredients. Stir the dry ingredients into the wet ingredients and mix until everything is well combined. Stir in the chocolate chips.
5. Bake. Drop the batter by tablespoons onto the baking sheet about 2 inches apart and flatten them down slightly. Bake the cookies for 10 minutes, or until they're golden. Repeat with any remaining dough. Transfer the cookies to a wire rack and let them cool.
6. Store. Store the cookies in a sealed container in the refrigerator for up to five days, or in the freezer for up to one month.

Per Serving (2 cookies)
calories: 226 | fat: 27g | protein: 3g | carbs: 1g net carbs: 0g | fiber: 1g

536. Citrus Raspberry Custard Cake

Prep time: 15 minutes | Cook time: 3 hours | Serves 8

1 teaspoon coconut oil
6 eggs, separated
2 cups heavy (whipping) cream
¾ cup granulated erythritol
½ cup coconut flour
¼ teaspoon salt
Juice and zest of 2 limes
½ cup raspberries

1. Lightly grease a 7-inch springform pan with the coconut oil.
2. In a large bowl, using a handheld mixer, beat the egg whites until stiff peaks form, about 5 minutes.
3. In a large bowl, whisk together the yolks, heavy cream, erythritol, coconut flour, salt, and lime juice and zest.
4. Fold the egg whites into the mixture.
5. Transfer the batter to the springform pan and sprinkle the raspberries over the top.
6. Place a wire rack in the insert of the slow cooker and place the springform pan on the wire rack.
7. Cover and cook on low for 3 hours, or until a toothpick inserted in the center comes out clean.
8. Remove the cover and allow the cake to cool to room temperature.
9. Place the springform pan in the refrigerator for at least 2 hours, until the cake is firm.
10. Carefully remove the sides of the springform pan. Slice and serve.

Per Serving
calories: 165 | fat: 15g | protein: 6g | carbs: 4g net carbs: 3g | fiber: 1g

537. Peanut Butter Cupcake

Prep time: 15 minutes | Cook time: 3 to 4 hours | Serves 8

2 tablespoons coconut oil, divided
1 cup almond flour
1 cup granulated erythritol, divided
1 teaspoon baking powder
¼ teaspoon salt
¾ cup natural peanut butter
½ cup heavy (whipping) cream
1 teaspoon pure vanilla extract
1 cup boiling water
¼ cup cocoa powder

1. Lightly grease the insert of a 4-quart slow cooker with 1 tablespoon of the coconut oil.
2. In a large bowl, stir together the almond flour, ½ cup of the erythritol, baking powder, and salt.
3. In a medium bowl, whisk together the peanut butter, heavy cream, and vanilla until smooth.
4. Add the peanut butter mixture to the dry ingredients and stir to combine.
5. Transfer the batter to the insert and spread it out evenly.
6. In a small bowl, stir together the remaining ½ cup of the erythritol, boiling water, and cocoa powder.
7. Pour the chocolate mixture over the batter.
8. Cover and cook on low for 3 to 4 hours.
9. Let the cake stand for 30 minutes and serve warm.

Per Serving

calories: 244 | fat: 20g | protein: 11g | carbs: 6g net carbs: 3g | fiber: 3g

538. Blueberry-Pecan Crisp

Prep time: 10 minutes | Cook time: 3 to 4 hours | Serves 8

5 tablespoons coconut oil, melted, divided
4 cups blueberries
¾ cup plus 2 tablespoons granulated erythritol
1 cup ground pecans
1 teaspoon baking soda
½ teaspoon ground cinnamon
2 tablespoons coconut milk
1 egg

1. Lightly grease a 4-quart slow cooker with 1 tablespoon of the coconut oil.
2. Add the blueberries and 2 tablespoons of erythritol to the insert.
3. In a large bowl, stir together the remaining ¾ cup of the erythritol, ground pecans, baking soda, and cinnamon until well mixed.
4. Add the coconut milk, egg, and remaining coconut oil, and stir until coarse crumbs form.
5. Top the contents in the insert with the pecan mixture.
6. Cover and cook on low for 3 to 4 hours.
7. Serve warm.

Per Serving

calories: 222 | fat: 19g | protein: 9g | carbs: 9g net carbs: 5g | fiber: 4g

539. Vanilla-Flavored Hazelnut Ice Cream

Prep time: 5 minutes | Cook time: 20 minutes | Serves 5

1⅓ cups blanched hazelnuts, divided into 1 cup whole and ⅓ cup coarsely chopped
1½ cups unsweetened vanilla almond milk
½ cup powdered erythritol
4 large egg yolks
1½ cups heavy cream

1. In a food processor or high-powered blender, pulse 1 cup of the whole hazelnuts, scraping down the sides frequently, until it reaches a nut flour consistency.
2. Transfer the hazelnut flour to a large saucepan. Stir in the almond milk and powdered erythritol, and bring to a boil over medium heat. Remove from the heat.
3. In a medium bowl, whisk the egg yolks until smooth. Slowly pour the mixture from the saucepan into the yolks while whisking constantly. This is called tempering and needs to be done slowly to avoid cooking the eggs in the process.
4. Return the mixture to the saucepan and cook over low heat for about 10 minutes, stirring frequently, until the mixture coats the back of a spoon. Keep the heat very low and watch closely to avoid curdling.
5. Pour the mixture into a cheesecloth-lined strainer set over a large bowl and squeeze all the liquid into the bowl (about 1 cup). Cool for about 10 minutes, until warm but no longer hot.
6. Stir the heavy cream into the bowl.
7. Transfer the mixture to an ice cream maker and process according to the manufacturer's instructions. (For most ice cream makers, you'll turn the ice cream maker on, pour the mixture into the frozen freezer bowl, and let it mix until thickened, 15 to 20 minutes.)
8. Five minutes before the churning is completed, add the ⅓ cup chopped hazelnuts and let them mix in completely. Transfer to a container and freeze for at least 4 hours, until firm.

Per Serving

calories: 349 | fat: 35g | protein: 5g | carbs: 18g net carbs: 3g | fiber: 15g

540. Tender Almond Pound Cake

Prep time: 10 minutes | Cook time: 5 to 6 hours | Serves 8

1 tablespoon coconut oil	tartar
2 cups almond flour	Pinch salt
1 cup granulated erythritol	1 cup butter, melted
½ teaspoon cream of	5 eggs
	2 teaspoons pure vanilla extract

1. Lightly grease an 8-by-4-inch loaf pan with the coconut oil.
2. In a large bowl, stir together the almond flour, erythritol, cream of tartar, and salt, until well mixed.
3. In a small bowl, whisk together the butter, eggs, and vanilla.
4. Add the wet ingredients to the dry ingredients and stir to combine.
5. Transfer the batter to the loaf pan.
6. Place the loaf pan in the insert of the slow cooker.
7. Cover and cook until a toothpick inserted in the center comes out clean, about 5 to 6 hours on low.
8. Serve warm.

Per Serving

calories: 281 | fat: 29g | protein: 5g | carbs: 1g net carbs: 1g | fiber: 0g

541. Old-fashioned Gingerbread Cake

Prep time: 10 minutes | Cook time: 3 hours | Serves 8

1 tablespoon coconut oil	cinnamon
2 cups almond flour	½ teaspoon ground nutmeg
¾ cup granulated erythritol	¼ teaspoon ground cloves
2 tablespoons coconut flour	Pinch salt
2 tablespoons ground ginger	¾ cup heavy (whipping) cream
2 teaspoons baking powder	½ cup butter, melted
2 teaspoons ground	4 eggs
	1 teaspoon pure vanilla extract

1. Lightly grease the insert of the slow cooker with coconut oil.
2. In a large bowl, stir together the almond flour, erythritol, coconut flour, ginger, baking powder, cinnamon, nutmeg, cloves, and salt.
3. In a medium bowl, whisk together the heavy cream, butter, eggs, and vanilla.
4. Add the wet ingredients to the dry ingredients and stir to combine.
5. Spoon the batter into the insert.
6. Cover and cook on low for 3 hours, or until a toothpick inserted in the center comes out clean.
7. Serve warm.

Per Serving

calories: 259 | fat: 23g | protein: 7g | carbs: 6g net carbs: 3g | fiber: 3g

542. Pecan-Carrot Muffins

Prep time: 10 minutes | Cook time: 25 to 35 minutes | Makes 10 muffins

4 tablespoons butter	almond flour
½ cup erythritol	2 teaspoons baking powder
2 teaspoons ground cinnamon	¼ teaspoon sea salt
1 teaspoon vanilla extract	1 loosely packed cup grated carrots
3 large eggs	1½ cups chopped pecans, divided
3 cups blanched	

1. Preheat the oven to 350ºF (180ºC). Line 10 cups of a muffin tin with parchment paper liners.
2. In a large bowl, with an electric hand mixer, beat the butter and erythritol at medium speed, until fluffy and light yellow in color.
3. Beat in the cinnamon and vanilla. Beat in the eggs, one at a time.
4. Beat in the almond flour, baking powder, and sea salt until well mixed. (The batter will be very thick, which is normal.)
5. Stir in the grated carrots and 1 cup of the chopped pecans.
6. Divide the batter among the lined muffin cups, filling almost to the top. Sprinkle remaining ½ cup chopped pecans over the muffins. Press gently into the top so that they won't fall off.
7. Bake for 25 to 35 minutes, until the top is golden brown and an inserted toothpick comes out clean. If the top browns before the inside is done, tent with foil and continue to bake until done inside.
8. Cool to firm up the texture before enjoying.

Per Serving (1 muffin)

calories: 368 | fat: 33g | protein: 10g | carbs: 14g net carbs: 6g | fiber: 8g

543. Chocolate Brownie Cake

Prep time: 10 minutes | Cook time: 3 hours | Serves 12

½ cup plus 1 tablespoon unsalted butter, melted, divided
1½ cups almond flour
¾ cup cocoa powder
¾ cup granulated erythritol
1 teaspoon baking powder
¼ teaspoon fine salt
1 cup heavy (whipping) cream
3 eggs, beaten
2 teaspoons pure vanilla extract
1 cup whipped cream

1. Generously grease the insert of the slow cooker with 1 tablespoon of the melted butter.
2. In a large bowl, stir together the almond flour, cocoa powder, erythritol, baking powder, and salt.
3. In a medium bowl, whisk together the remaining ½ cup of the melted butter, heavy cream, eggs, and vanilla until well blended.
4. Whisk the wet ingredients into the dry ingredients and spoon the batter into the insert.
5. Cover and cook on low for 3 hours, and then remove the insert from the slow cooker and let the cake sit for 1 hour.
6. Serve warm with the whipped cream.

Per Serving
calories: 185 | fat: 16g | protein: 5g | carbs: 7g net carbs: 6g | fiber: 1g

544. Coconut Lemon Truffles with Pecans

Prep time: 30 minutes | Cook time: 0 minutes | Makes 16 truffles

3 cups shredded unsweetened coconut, divided
½ cup pecans
2 tablespoons coconut oil
Zest and juice of 1 lemon
½ cup monk fruit sweetener, granulated form
Pinch sea salt

1. Make the truffle base. Put 2 cups of the coconut and the pecans in a food processor and pulse until the mixture looks like a paste, about 5 minutes.
2. Add the remaining ingredients. Add the coconut oil, lemon zest, lemon juice, sweetener, and salt to the processor and pulse until the mixture forms a big ball, about 2 minutes.
3. Form the truffles. Scoop the mixture out with a tablespoon and roll it into 16 balls. Roll the truffles in the remaining 1 cup of coconut.
4. Store. Store the truffles in a sealed container in the refrigerator for up to one week or in the freezer for up to one month.

Per Serving (1 truffle)
calories: 160 | fat:16 g | protein: 2g | carbs: 5g net carbs: 2g | fiber: 3g

545. Keto Almond Butter Fudge

Prep time: 10 minutes | Cook time: 0 minutes | Makes 36 pieces

1 cup coconut oil, at room temperature
1 cup almond butter
¼ cup heavy (whipping) cream
10 drops liquid stevia
Pinch sea salt

1. Line a 6-by-6-inch baking dish with parchment paper and set aside.
2. In a medium bowl, whisk together the coconut oil, almond butter, heavy cream, stevia, and salt until very smooth.
3. Spoon the mixture into the baking dish and smooth the top with a spatula.
4. Place the dish in the refrigerator until the fudge is firm, about 2 hours.
5. Cut into 36 pieces and store the fudge in an airtight container in the freezer for up to 2 weeks.

Per Serving (2 pieces)
calories: 204 | fat: 22g | protein: 3g | carbs: 3g net carbs: 2g | fiber: 1g

546. Super Easy Peanut Butter Mousse

Prep time: 10 minutes | Cook time: 0 minutes | Serves 4

1 cup heavy (whipping) cream
¼ cup natural peanut butter
1 teaspoon alcohol-free pure vanilla extract
4 drops liquid stevia

1. In a medium bowl, beat together the heavy cream, peanut butter, vanilla, and stevia until firm peaks form, about 5 minutes.
2. Spoon the mousse into 4 bowls and place in the refrigerator to chill for 30 minutes.
3. Serve.

Per Serving
calories: 280 | fat: 28g | protein: 6g | carbs: 4g net carbs: 3g | fiber: 1g

547. Classic Almond Golden Cake

Prep time: 15 minutes | Cook time: 3 hours | Serves 8

½ cup coconut oil, divided
1½ cups almond flour
½ cup coconut flour
½ cup granulated erythritol
2 teaspoons baking powder
3 eggs
½ cup coconut milk
2 teaspoons pure vanilla extract
½ teaspoon almond extract

1. Line the insert of a 4-quart slow cooker with aluminum foil and grease the aluminum foil with 1 tablespoon of the coconut oil.
2. In a medium bowl, mix the almond flour, coconut flour, erythritol, and baking powder.
3. In a large bowl, whisk together the remaining coconut oil, eggs, coconut milk, vanilla, and almond extract.
4. Add the dry ingredients to the wet ingredients and stir until well blended.
5. Transfer the batter to the insert and use a spatula to even the top.
6. Cover and cook on low for 3 hours, or until a toothpick inserted in the center comes out clean.
7. Remove the cake from the insert and cool completely before serving.

Per Serving
calories: 234 | fat: 22g | protein: 6g | carbs: 3g | net carbs: 2g | fiber: 1g

548. Almond Butter Fat Bombs

Prep time: 10 minutes | Cook time: 4 minutes | Makes 12 fat bombs

¾ cup coconut oil
¼ cup cocoa powder
¼ cup almond butter
⅛ teaspoon chili powder
3 drops liquid stevia

1. Line a mini muffin tin with paper liners and set aside.
2. Put a small saucepan over low heat and add the coconut oil, cocoa powder, almond butter, chili powder, and stevia.
3. Heat for 4 minutes until the coconut oil is melted, then whisk to blend.
4. Spoon the mixture into the muffin cups and place the tin in the refrigerator until the bombs are firm, about 15 minutes.
5. Transfer the cups to an airtight container and store the fat bombs in the freezer until you want to serve them.

Per Serving (1 fat bomb)
calories: 117 | fat: 12g | protein: 2g | carbs: 2g | net carbs: 2g | fiber: 0g

549. Banana Fat Bombs

Prep time: 10 minutes | Cook time: 0 minutes | Makes 12 fat bombs

1¼ cups cream cheese, at room temperature
¾ cup heavy (whipping) cream
1 tablespoon pure banana extract
6 drops liquid stevia

1. Line a baking sheet with parchment paper and set aside.
2. In a medium bowl, beat together the cream cheese, heavy cream, banana extract, and stevia until smooth and very thick, about 5 minutes.
3. Gently spoon the mixture onto the baking sheet in mounds, leaving some space between each mound, and place the baking sheet in the refrigerator until firm, about 1 hour.
4. Store the fat bombs in an airtight container in the refrigerator for up to 1 week.

Per Serving (1 fat bomb)
calories: 134 | fat: 12g | protein: 3g | carbs: 1g | net carbs: 1g | fiber: 0g

550. Easy Dark Chocolate Fudge

Prep time: 15 minutes | Cook time: 0 minutes | Makes 30 pieces

1 cup coconut oil, melted
1 cup cocoa powder
1 teaspoon vanilla extract
½ cup monk fruit sweetener, granulated form
Pinch sea salt

1. Prepare a baking dish. Line a 9-by-9-inch glass baking dish with plastic wrap and set it aside.
2. Make the fudge. Place the coconut oil, cocoa powder, vanilla, sweetener, and salt in a blender and process until the mixture is smooth and blended. Pour the mixture into the baking dish and place more plastic wrap over it.
3. Refrigerate. Place the fudge in the refrigerator for at least 4 hours, until it is set up and firm.
4. Cut and store. Remove the fudge from the baking dish, cut it into roughly 1½-inch squares and store in the freezer in a sealed container for up to one month.

Per Serving (2 pieces)
calories: 139 | fat: 15g | protein: 1g | carbs: 3g | net carbs: 1g | fiber: 2g

551. Simple Blueberry Fat Bombs

Prep time: 10 minutes | Cook time: 0 minutes | Makes 12 fat bombs

½ cup coconut oil, at room temperature
½ cup cream cheese, at room temperature
½ cup blueberries, mashed with a fork
6 drops liquid stevia
Pinch ground nutmeg

1. Line a mini muffin tin with paper liners and set aside.
2. In a medium bowl, stir together the coconut oil and cream cheese until well blended.
3. Stir in the blueberries, stevia, and nutmeg until combined.
4. Divide the blueberry mixture into the muffin cups and place the tray in the freezer until set, about 3 hours.
5. Place the fat bombs in an airtight container and store in the freezer until you wish to eat them.

Per Serving (1 fat bomb)
calories: 115 | fat: 12g | protein: 1g | carbs: 1g net carbs: 1g | fiber: 0g

552. Almond Flour Crusted Cheesecake

Prep time: 5 minutes | Cook time: 1 hour | Serves 16

Almond Flour Crust:
2 cups blanched almond flour
5 tablespoons plus 1 teaspoon butter, melted
3 tablespoons erythritol
1 teaspoon vanilla extract
Cheesecake Filling:
32 ounces (907 g) cream cheese, softened at room temperature
1¼ cups powdered erythritol
3 large eggs, at room temperature
1 tablespoon lemon juice
1 teaspoon vanilla extract

1. Position a rack in the center of the oven and preheat the oven to 350°F (180°C). Grease the sides of a 9-inch springform pan and line the bottom with a circle of parchment paper.
2. Make the almond flour crust: In a medium bowl, stir the almond flour, melted butter, erythritol, and vanilla until well combined. The dough will be slightly crumbly. Press the dough into the bottom of the prepared pan. Bake for 10 to 12 minutes, until barely golden. Let cool at least 10 minutes. Leave the oven on.
3. Meanwhile, make the cheesecake filling: In a bowl, with an electric hand mixer, beat the cream cheese and powdered erythritol together at low to medium speed for about 2 minutes, until fluffy. Keeping the mixer at low to medium the whole time (too high a speed will introduce too many air bubbles, which we don't want), beat in the eggs, one at a time. Finally, beat in the lemon juice and vanilla, scraping down the sides of the bowl periodically.
4. Pour the filling into the pan over the crust. Smooth the top with a spatula (use an icing spatula for a smoother top if you have one). Tap the pan on the counter to release any air bubbles.
5. Bake for 40 to 55 minutes, until the center is almost set, but still jiggly.
6. Remove the cheesecake from the oven. If the edges are stuck to the pan, run a knife around the edge (don't remove the springform edge yet). Cool in the pan on the counter to room temperature, then refrigerate for at least 4 hours, preferably overnight, until completely set. (Do not try to remove the cake from the pan before chilling.)

Per Serving
calories: 328 | fat: 31g | protein: 7g | carbs: 18g net carbs: 5g | fiber: 13g

553. Coconut-Vanilla Ice Pops

Prep time: 10 minutes | Cook time: 5 minutes | Makes 8 ice pops

2 cups almond milk
1 cup heavy (whipping) cream
1 vanilla bean, halved lengthwise
1 cup shredded unsweetened coconut

1. Place a medium saucepan over medium heat and add the almond milk, heavy cream, and vanilla bean.
2. Bring the liquid to a simmer and reduce the heat to low. Continue to simmer for 5 minutes.
3. Remove the saucepan from the heat and let the liquid cool.
4. Take the vanilla bean out of the liquid and use a knife to scrape the seeds out of the bean into the liquid.
5. Stir in the coconut and divide the liquid between the ice pop molds.
6. Freeze until solid, about 4 hours, and enjoy.

Per Serving (1 ice pop)
calories: 166 | fat: 15g | protein: 3g | carbs: 4g net carbs: 2g | fiber: 2g

554. Blueberry-Almond Muffins

Prep time: 5 minutes | Cook time: 25 minutes | Makes 10 muffins

2½ cups blanched almond flour
½ cup erythritol
1½ teaspoons baking powder
¼ teaspoon sea salt
⅓ cup coconut oil, melted
⅓ cup unsweetened almond milk
3 large eggs
½ teaspoon vanilla extract
¾ cup blueberries

1. Preheat the oven to 350ºF (180ºC). Line 10 cups of a muffin tin with silicone or parchment paper liners.
2. In a large bowl, stir together the almond flour, erythritol, baking powder, and sea salt.
3. Stir in the melted coconut oil, almond milk, eggs, and vanilla. Fold in the blueberries.
4. Distribute the batter evenly among the muffin cups. Bake for about 25 minutes, until the tops are golden and an inserted toothpick comes out clean.

Per Serving (1 muffin)
calories: 254 | fat: 23g | protein: 8g | carbs: 11g net carbs: 5g | fiber: 6g

555. Pumpkin-Almond Fat Bombs

Prep time: 10 minutes | Cook time: 0 minutes | Makes 16 fat bombs

½ cup butter, at room temperature
½ cup cream cheese, at room temperature
⅓ cup pure pumpkin purée
3 tablespoons chopped almonds
4 drops liquid stevia
½ teaspoon ground cinnamon
¼ teaspoon ground nutmeg

1. Line an 8-by-8-inch pan with parchment paper and set aside.
2. In a small bowl, whisk together the butter and cream cheese until very smooth.
3. Add the pumpkin purée and whisk until blended.
4. Stir in the almonds, stevia, cinnamon, and nutmeg.
5. Spoon the pumpkin mixture into the pan. Use a spatula or the back of a spoon to spread it evenly in the pan, then place it in the freezer for about 1 hour.
6. Cut into 16 pieces and store the fat bombs in a tightly sealed container in the freezer until ready to serve.

Per Serving (1 fat bomb)
calories: 87 | fat: 9g | protein: 1g | carbs: 1g net carbs: 1g | fiber: 0g

556. Hazelnut Shortbread Cookies

Prep time: 10 minutes | Cook time: 10 minutes | Makes 18 cookies

½ cup butter, at room temperature, plus more for greasing
½ cup granulated sweetener
1 teaspoon alcohol-free pure vanilla extract
1½ cups almond flour
½ cup ground hazelnuts
Pinch sea salt

1. In a medium bowl, cream together the butter, sweetener, and vanilla until well blended.
2. Stir in the almond four, ground hazelnuts, and salt until a firm dough is formed.
3. Roll the dough into a 2-inch cylinder and wrap it in plastic wrap. Place the dough in the refrigerator for at least 30 minutes until firm.
4. Preheat the oven to 350ºF (180ºC). Line a baking sheet with parchment paper and lightly grease the paper with butter; set aside.
5. Unwrap the chilled cylinder, slice the dough into 18 cookies, and place the cookies on the baking sheet.
6. Bake the cookies until firm and lightly browned, about 10 minutes.
7. Allow the cookies to cool on the baking sheet for 5 minutes and then transfer them to a wire rack to cool completely.

Per Serving (1 cookie)
calories: 105 | fat: 10g | protein: 3g | carbs: 2g net carbs: 1g | fiber: 1g

557. Coconut-Chocolate Treats

Prep time: 10 minutes | Cook time: 3 minutes | Makes 16 treats

⅓ cup coconut oil
¼ cup unsweetened cocoa powder
4 drops liquid stevia
Pinch sea salt
¼ cup shredded unsweetened coconut

1. Line a 6-by-6-inch baking dish with parchment paper and set aside.
2. In a small saucepan over low heat, stir together the coconut oil, cocoa, stevia, and salt for about 3 minutes.
3. Stir in the coconut and press the mixture into the baking dish.
4. Place the baking dish in the refrigerator until the mixture is hard, about 30 minutes.
5. Cut into 16 pieces and store the treats in an airtight container in a cool place.

Per Serving (1 treat)
calories: 43 | fat: 5g | protein: 1g | carbs: 1g net carbs: 1g | fiber: 0g

558. Vanilla-Raspberry Cheesecake

Prep time: 10 minutes | Cook time: 25 to 30 minutes | Serves 12

⅔ cup coconut oil, melted	granulated sweetener
½ cup cream cheese, at room temperature	1 teaspoon alcohol-free pure vanilla extract
6 eggs	½ teaspoon baking powder
3 tablespoons	¾ cup raspberries

1. Preheat the oven to 350°F (180°C). Line an 8-by-8-inch baking dish with parchment paper and set aside.
2. In a large bowl, beat together the coconut oil and cream cheese until smooth.
3. Beat in the eggs, scraping down the sides of the bowl at least once.
4. Beat in the sweetener, vanilla, and baking powder until smooth.
5. Spoon the batter into the baking dish and use a spatula to smooth out the top. Scatter the raspberries on top.
6. Bake until the center is firm, about 25 to 30 minutes.
7. Allow the cheesecake to cool completely before cutting into 12 squares.

Per Serving (1 square)
calories: 176 | fat: 18g | protein: 6g | carbs: 3g net carbs: 2g | fiber: 1g

559. Blueberry-Vanilla Pudding

Prep time: 10 minutes | Cook time: 10 minutes | Serves 6

3 cups coconut milk	1 tablespoon coconut oil
⅓ cup monk fruit sweetener, granulated form	1 tablespoon pure vanilla extract
¼ cup arrowroot flour	1 cup fresh blueberries
1 egg	

1. Cook the base. In a large saucepan, whisk together the coconut milk, sweetener, and arrowroot. Bring the mixture to a boil then reduce the heat to low, whisking constantly, until the pudding is thick, about 5 minutes. Whisk the egg into the pudding and cook, while still whisking, for about 30 seconds.
2. Add the remaining ingredients. Whisk the coconut oil and vanilla into the pudding until it's smooth.
3. Cool. Transfer the pudding to a medium bowl and cover it with plastic wrap, pressing the wrap down to the surface of the pudding, then place it in the refrigerator to cool completely, about 2 hours.
4. Serve. Spoon the pudding into bowls and top with the blueberries.

Per Serving
calories: 286 | fat: 27g | protein: 3g | carbs: 9g net carbs: 7g | fiber: 2g

560. Cream Cheese Chocolate Mousse

Prep time: 10 minutes | Cook time: 0 minutes | Serves 2

3 ounces (85 g) cream cheese, softened	¼ cup Swerve
½ cup heavy cream	2 tablespoons cocoa powder
1 teaspoon vanilla extract	1 pinch salt

1. Beat the cream cheese in a large mixing bowl with an electric beater until it makes fluffy mixture.
2. Switch the beater to low speed, and add the vanilla extract, heavy cream, salt, Swerve, and cocoa powder to beat for 2 minutes until it is completely smooth.
3. Chill in the refrigerator until ready to serve.

Per Serving
calories: 270 | fat: 26.4g | total carbs: 6.0g fiber: 2.0g | protein: 4.2g

561. Keto Vanilla Ice Cream

Prep time: 10 minutes | Cook time: 0 minutes | Serves 3

1 cup heavy whipping cream	1 teaspoon vanilla extract
2 tablespoons Swerve confectioners' style sweetener	¼ teaspoon xanthan gum
1 tablespoon vodka	1 pinch salt

1. Add the cream, vodka, xanthan gum, Swerve, vanilla extract, and salt in a large jar.
2. Beat the cream mixture with a hand blender until the cream has thickened, and it makes soft peaks, after 60 to 75 seconds.
3. Cover this cream jar and place in your freezer for 3 to 4 hours, stirring occasionally.
4. Serve the vanilla ice cream in scoops and enjoy.

Per Serving
calories: 143 | fat: 14.8g | total carbs: 1.6g fiber: 0g | protein: 0.8g

562. Spicy Almond Fat Bombs

Prep time: 10 minutes | Cook time: 4 minutes | Serves 12

¾ cup coconut oil
¼ cup almond butter
¼ cup cocoa powder
3 drops liquid stevia
⅛ teaspoon chili powder

SPECIAL EQUIPMENT:
A 12-cup muffin pan

1. Line a muffin pan with 12 paper liners. Keep aside.
2. Heat the oil in a small saucepan over low heat, then add the almond butter, cocoa powder, stevia, and chili powder. Stir to combine well.
3. Divide the mixture evenly among the muffin cups and keep the muffin pan in the refrigerator for 15 minutes, or until the bombs are set and firm.
4. Serve immediately or refrigerate to chill until ready to serve.

Per Serving
calories: 160 | fat: 16.8g | total carbs: 2.0g fiber: 1.2g | protein: 1.5g

563. Microwaved Rhubarb Cakes

Prep time: 5 minutes | Cook time: 2 minutes | Serves 2

¼ teaspoon vanilla extract or powder
1 tablespoon plus 1 teaspoon erythritol
3 tablespoons refined macadamia nut oil or avocado oil
1 large egg
¼ teaspoon baking powder
¼ teaspoon ground nutmeg
1 teaspoon ground cinnamon
¼ cup roughly ground flaxseeds
1 (2½-inch) piece rhubarb, diced
1 to 2 fresh strawberries, hulled and sliced, for garnish

1. In a small bowl, whisk together the vanilla, erythritol, oil, and egg.
2. In another bowl, combine the baking powder, nutmeg, cinnamon and flaxseeds. Pour into the egg mixture. Stir in the rhubarb.
3. Divide evenly among 2 microwave-safe containers and microwave for about 2 minutes. You can check the doneness by inserting a toothpick in the center of the cake. If it comes out clean, then it is ready to serve.
4. Top with strawberries and serve.

Per Serving
calories: 335 | fat: 32.7g | total carbs: 9.5g fiber: 7.1g | protein: 7.7g

564. Chia Pudding with Blueberries

Prep time: 10 minutes | Cook time: 0 minutes | Serves 2

1 cup unsweetened vanilla almond milk
1½ tablespoons stevia
¼ cup chia seeds
4 to 6 fresh blueberries

1. Put the milk and stevia in a blender and process for 1 minute to combine well.
2. Pour the chia seeds in a glass and add the mixture.
3. Make the pudding: Stir the mixture well and then cover the glass with plastic wrap and refrigerate for 6 to 8 hours.
4. Transfer the pudding into a glass and add the blueberries on top before serving

Per Serving
calories: 125 | fat: 10.2g | total carbs: 12.9g fiber: 9.8g | protein: 5.2g

565. Almond and Cinnamon Truffles

Prep time: 20 minutes | Cook time: 0 minutes | Makes 10 truffles

½ cup unsweetened almond butter
¼ cup plus 2 tablespoons melted cacao butter
1 tablespoon plus 1 teaspoon ground cinnamon
1 tablespoon erythritol
½ teaspoon vanilla extract
1 pinch of gray sea salt
3 tablespoons roasted almonds, smashed to ⅛-inch thick

1. Line a rimmed baking sheet with parchment paper.
2. Make the truffle: Pour almond butter, cacao butter, cinnamon, erythritol, vanilla extract, and salt in a bowl and stir until it's smooth. Refrigerate for about 45 minutes.
3. Remove the truffle mixture from the fridge, shape 1 tablespoon of the mixture into 10 eraser sized bricks. Pour the smashed almonds in a separate bowl.
4. Pick up the little bricks, coat it with almond pieces and then set it on the baking sheet already prepared. Repeat the process until you have 10 coated truffle pieces.
5. Serve the truffle in the baking sheet under room temperature.

Per Serving
calories: 186 | fat: 18.1g | total carbs: 3.6g fiber: 0.7g | protein: 2.8g

566. Macadamia Nut and Chocolate Fat Bombs

Prep time: 5 minutes | Cook time: 1 minute | Makes 8 fat bombs

¼ cup sugar-free dark chocolate chips
Sea salt, to taste
1 tablespoon coconut oil
24 raw macadamia nut halves

SPECIAL EQUIPMENT:
8 baking cups or truffle molds

1. Melt the chocolate chips in a microwave for 50 seconds and mix it with sea salt and oil. Stir it until well mixed.
2. Arrange 3 macadamia nut halves inside each small baking cup and completely cover the nuts in chocolate by spooning the melted chocolate over each nut. Sprinkle a pinch of sea salt over the chocolate.
3. Place the cups inside the freezer for 30 to 40 minutes or until solid.

Per Serving
calories: 161 | fat: 14.8g | total carbs: 7.5g fiber: 2.2g | protein: 1.7g

567. Strawberry Popsicles

Prep time: 5 minutes | Cook time: 0 minutes | Makes 6 popsicles

8 fresh strawberries, hulled and quartered
1 cup heavy whipping cream
½ cup unsweetened almond milk
2 ounces (57 g) softened cream cheese
2½ tablespoons stevia
½ teaspoon vanilla extract

SPECIAL EQUIPMENT:
6 ice pop molds

1. Blend the strawberries and cream in a blender until they form soft peaks
2. Add almond milk, cream cheese, sweetener and vanilla extract, and pulse the blender until smooth.
3. Make the Popsicles: Pour the mixture in the blender into the ice pop molds and freeze them for at least three hours.
4. To separate the ice molds and Popsicles before serving, run the molds through lukewarm or hot water.

Per Serving
calories: 120 | fat: 11.3g | total carbs: 3.2g fiber: 0.3g | protein: 1.7g

568. No-Bake Hemp Seeds and Chocolate Cookies

Prep time: 20 minutes | Cook time: 0 minutes | Serves 14

½ teaspoon ground cinnamon
½ teaspoon vanilla extract or powder
¼ cup melted coconut oil or cacao butter
1¼ cups hulled hemp seeds
2 drops liquid stevia
¼ cup sugar-free dark chocolate chips

1. Line parchment paper on a baking sheet.
2. In a medium bowl, combine cinnamon, vanilla, coconut oil, hemp seeds and stevia.
3. Blend the mixture in a food processor until the dough is ready. To check if it's ready, pinch it with your fingers; it is ready if it sticks together.
4. Add the chocolate chips and mix.
5. Scoop the dough with a round spoon into the baking sheet to make 14 cookies.
6. Refrigerate for at least 30 minutes and then serve.

Per Serving
calories: 127 | fat: 11.6g | total carbs: 1.3g fiber: 0g | protein: 4.3g

569. Cardamom Orange Bark

Prep time: 15 minutes | Cook time: 0 minutes | Serves 6

⅛ teaspoon finely ground gray sea salt
½ teaspoon orange extract
½ teaspoon vanilla extract
¾ cup melted coconut oil
1¾ teaspoons ground cardamom
2 teaspoons ginger powder
2 tablespoons erythritol
⅔ cup raw walnut pieces, roasted

1. Pour all the ingredients except for the walnuts in a food processor and pulse for 20 seconds or until smooth and creamy.
2. Add the crushed walnuts. Pulse the food processor until each walnut is about ¼ inch in size.
3. Pour the mixture into a parchment-lined square baking pan, and leave it in the freezer for about an hour.
4. Remove the frozen mixture from the pan and break it into six pieces to serve.

Per Serving
calories: 336 | fat: 35.8g | total carbs: 2.4g fiber: 1.1g | protein: 2.1g

570. Gingersnap Nutmeg Cookies

Prep time: 13 minutes | Cook time: 12 minutes | Serves 8

1 teaspoon vanilla essence
1 large egg
¼ cup butter, unsalted
1 cup erythritol
2 cups almond flour
½ teaspoon ground cinnamon
2 teaspoons ground ginger
¼ teaspoon ground nutmeg
¼ teaspoon ground cloves
¼ teaspoon salt

1. Start by preheating the oven to 350°F (180°C) and line a baking sheet with parchment paper.
2. With an electric mixer, add vanilla essence, egg, butter, erythritol, and mix.
3. Add almond flour, cinnamon, ginger, nutmeg, cloves and salt and stir until smooth.
4. Spoon the dough into cookies with a cookie scoop and arrange them on the baking sheet.
5. Bake for 12 minutes in the preheated oven.
6. Remove from oven and cool for 3 minutes and serve.

Per Serving
calories: 238 | fat: 20.5g | total carbs: 6.5g fiber: 0.2g | protein: 7.0g

571. Lemony Poppy Seed Cookies

Prep time: 10 minutes | Cook time: 13 to 18 minutes | Makes 14 cookies

Cookies:
½ cup butter, softened at room temperature
1/3 cup erythritol
½ teaspoon vanilla extract
2 cups blanched almond flour
1 tablespoon lemon zest, plus more for garnish (optional)
2 teaspoons poppy seeds

Glaze:
¼ cup powdered erythritol
1 tablespoon lemon juice

1. Preheat the oven to 350°F (180°C). Line a cookie sheet with parchment paper.
2. Make the cookies: In a bowl, with an electric hand mixer, beat the butter and erythritol together at medium speed for about 2 minutes, until fluffy. Beat in the gelatin (if using) and vanilla.
3. Beat in the almond flour, ½ cup at a time.
4. Mix in lemon zest and poppy seeds with a spoon or spatula, pressing with the back of the spoon or spatula to incorporate. You can also use your hands to bring it together.
5. Use a medium cookie scoop to scoop the dough onto the lined cookie sheet, at least 1½ inches apart. Flatten using your palm.
6. Bake for 13 to 18 minutes, until golden on top. The cookies will still be very soft to the touch. Set aside to cool without moving from the pan.
7. Meanwhile, make the glaze: In a small bowl, whisk together the powdered erythritol and lemon juice. If it's too thick for drizzling, thin out with a bit more lemon juice.
8. When the cookies have cooled to warm and are no longer hot, drizzle the glaze over them. Immediately garnish with more lemon zest on top (if using) and poppy seeds. Cool completely to crisp up and set the glaze.

Per Serving (1 cookie)
calories: 154 | fat: 14g | protein: 4g | carbs: 10g net carbs: 2g | fiber: 8g

572. Keto Matcha Brownies with Pistachios

Prep time: 10 minutes | Cook time: 18 minutes | Serves 4

¼ cup butter, unsalted and melted
4 tablespoons Swerve
A pinch of salt
1 egg
1 tablespoon matcha powder
¼ cup coconut flour
½ teaspoon baking powder
½ cup pistachios, chopped

1. Preheat your oven to 350°F (180°C) and line a baking pan with parchment paper.
2. Add butter, Swerve, and a pinch of salt to a mixing bowl, and whisk until well combined.
3. Break the egg into the butter mixture and beat the mixture until well mixed.
4. Sift matcha powder coconut flour and baking powder through a fine-mesh sieve into the bowl of the egg mixture. Stir until well mixed.
5. Add the chopped pistachios and stir well to combine. Pour the mixture into the prepared baking pan and bake in the preheated oven for 18 minutes.
6. Remove from the oven and let rest for 5 minutes. Cut into brownie cubes to serve.

Per Serving
calories: 239 | fat: 21.9g | total carbs: 8.5g | fiber: 1.6g | protein: 6.5g

573. Easy Peanut Butter Cookies

Prep time: 1 hour | Cook time: 15 minutes | Serves 6

1 egg
½ cup peanut butter
½ cup Swerve

1. Start by preheating the oven to 350°F (180°C). Line a parchment paper on a baking pan.
2. Put egg, peanut butter and Swerve in a bowl to make the dough and mix until bubbly.
3. Using a cookie spoon to scoop the dough into balls, then arrange them in the baking pan. Press the balls with a fork.
4. Put the baking pan in the preheated oven and bake for 15 minutes.
5. Cool for 10 minutes and serve.

Per Serving
calories: 155 | fat: 12.7g | total carbs: 5.0g fiber: 1.1g | protein: 6.3g

574. Raspberry and Chocolate Fat Bombs

e: 1 hour 5 minutes | Cook time: 0 minutes | Serves 12

½ cup coconut oil, melted
2 ounces (57 g) cacao butter
½ cup dried raspberries
¼ cup Swerve

SPECIAL EQUIPMENT:
A 12-cup muffin pan

1. Line a muffin pan with 12 paper liners and set it aside.
2. Combine the melted coconut oil and cocoa butter in a bowl.
3. Blend the raspberries in a blender until smooth and pour into the bowl of coconut oil mixture. Drizzle with the Swerve.
4. Divide the mixture equally among the muffin cups.
5. Refrigerate for at least 1 hour, or until steady and then serve.

Per Serving
calories: 127 | fat: 13.9g | total carbs: 0.7g fiber: 0.4g | protein: 0.1g

575. Strawberries in Chocolate

Prep time: 5 minutes | Cook time: 1 minute | Serves 2

¼ cup sugar-free dark chocolate chips
1½ teaspoons coconut oil
10 medium-sized fresh strawberries, rinsed and drained

1. Melt the chocolate chips by placing it in a small microwave-safe bowl and microwaving it for 1 minute or until it's completely melted.
2. Remove the bowl from the microwave, add chocolate chips into the bowl and mix until it completely dissolves.
3. Add the oil to the melted chocolate and mix thoroughly.
4. Line the parchment paper on a baking sheet. Dip ⅔ of each strawberry inside the melted chocolate and set it on the parchment paper.
5. Place the baking sheet inside a refrigerator for 15 minutes to allow the chocolate to set.
6. Remove them from the refrigerator and serve chill.

Per Serving
calories: 133 | fat 12.6g | total carbs 5.6g | fiber: 1.2g | protein 0.4g

576. Healthy Blueberry Fat Bombs

Prep time: 10 minutes | Cook time: 0 minutes | Serves 12

½ cup cream cheese, at room temperature
½ cup coconut oil, at room temperature
½ cup blueberries, mashed with a fork
Pinch ground nutmeg
6 drops liquid stevia

1. Use the silicone mold or line a mini-sized muffin tin with paper liners. Keep it aside.
2. Combine the cream cheese with coconut oil in a medium mixing bowl and stir to blend well.
3. Fold in the blueberries, nutmeg, and stevia, and mix well.
4. Spoon the mixture into the muffin cups evenly and keep the muffin tin or mold in the refrigerator for 3 hours or until firm.

Per Serving
calories: 119 | fat: 12.5g | total carbs: 1.3g fiber: 0.2g | protein: 0.6g

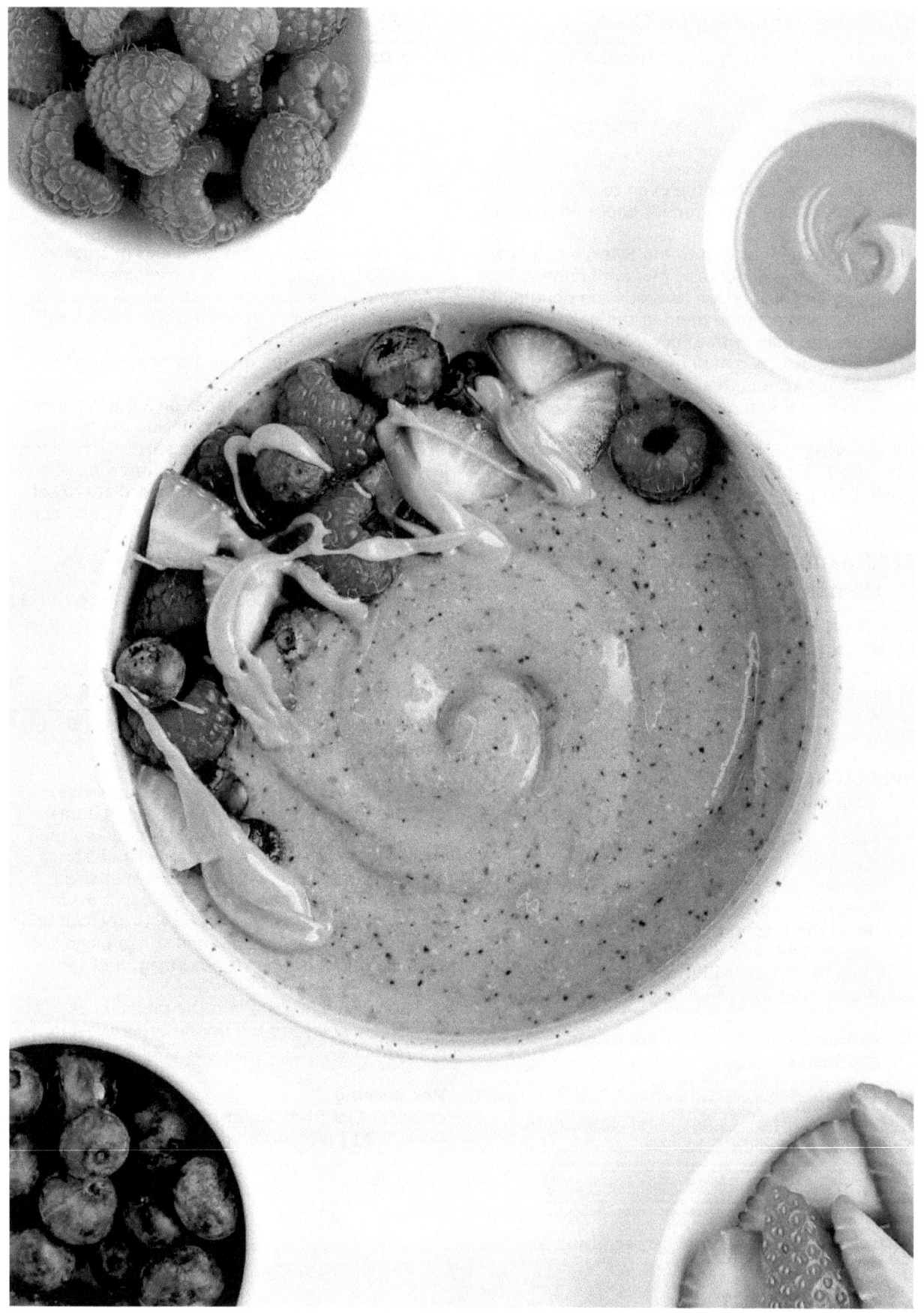

Chapter 14 Smoothies

577. Avocado and Berry Smoothie

Prep time: 5 minutes | Cook time: 0 minutes | Serves 2

1 cup unsweetened full-fat coconut milk
1 scoop Perfect Keto Exogenous Ketone Powder in chocolate sea salt
½ avocado
2 tablespoons almond butter
½ cup berries, fresh or frozen (no sugar added if frozen)
½ cup ice cubes
¼ teaspoon liquid stevia (optional)

1. In a blender, combine the coconut milk, protein powder, avocado, almond butter, berries, ice, and stevia (if using).
2. Blend until thoroughly mixed and frothy.
3. Pour into two glasses and enjoy.

Per Serving
calories: 446 | fat: 43g | protein: 7g | carbs: 16g net carbs: 9g | fiber: 7g

578. Blueberry-Almond Butter Smoothie

Prep time: 5 minutes | Cook time: 0 minutes | Serves 1

1 cup unsweetened almond milk, plus more as needed
¼ cup frozen blueberries
2 tablespoons unsweetened almond butter
1 tablespoon ground flaxseed or chia seeds
1 tablespoon extra-virgin olive oil or avocado oil
1 to 2 teaspoons stevia or monk fruit extract (optional)
½ teaspoon vanilla extract
¼ teaspoon ground cinnamon

1. In a blender or a large wide-mouth jar, if using an immersion blender, combine the almond milk, blueberries, almond butter, flaxseed, olive oil, stevia (if using), vanilla, and cinnamon and blend until smooth and creamy, adding more almond milk to achieve your desired consistency.

Per Serving
calories: 460 | fat: 40g | protein: 9g | carbs: 20g net carbs: 10g | fiber: 10g

579. Morning Five Greens Smoothie

Prep time: 5 minutes | Cook time: 0 minutes | Serves 4

6 kale leaves, chopped
3 stalks celery, chopped
1 ripe avocado, skinned, pitted, sliced
1 cup ice cubes
2 cups spinach, chopped
1 large cucumber, peeled and chopped
Chia seeds, for garnish

1. In a blender, add the kale, celery, avocado, and ice cubes, and blend for 45 seconds. Add the spinach and cucumber, and process for another 45 seconds until smooth.
2. Pour the smoothie into glasses, garnish with chia seeds and serve the drink immediately.

Per Serving
calories: 133 | fat: 9g | protein: 5g | carbs: 13g net carbs: 6g | fiber: 7g

580. Spiced Pistachio-Lemon Smoothie

Prep time: 5 minutes | Cook time: 0 minutes | Serves 1

½ cup plain whole-milk Greek yogurt
½ cup unsweetened almond milk, plus more as needed
Zest and juice of 1 lemon
1 tablespoon extra-virgin olive oil
1 tablespoon shelled pistachios, coarsely chopped
1 to 2 teaspoons monk fruit extract or stevia (optional)
¼ to ½ teaspoon ground allspice or unsweetened pumpkin pie spice
¼ teaspoon ground cinnamon
¼ teaspoon vanilla extract

1. In a blender or a large wide-mouth jar, if using an immersion blender, combine the yogurt, ½ cup almond milk, lemon zest and juice, olive oil, pistachios, monk fruit extract (if using), allspice, cinnamon, and vanilla and blend until smooth and creamy, adding more almond milk to achieve your desired consistency.

Per Serving
calories: 264 | fat: 22g | protein: 6g | carbs: 12g net carbs: 10g | fiber: 2g

581. Easy Peanut Butter Smoothie

Prep time: 5 minutes | Cook time: 0 minutes | Serves 2

1 cup water
¾ cup coconut cream
1 scoop chocolate protein powder
2 tablespoons natural peanut butter
3 ice cubes

1. Put the water, coconut cream, protein powder, peanut butter, and ice in a blender and blend until smooth.
2. Pour into 2 glasses and serve immediately.

Per Serving
calories: 486 | fat: 40g | protein: 30g | carbs: 11g net carbs: 6g | fiber: 5g

582. Classic PB and J Smoothie

Prep time: 5 minutes | Cook time: 0 minutes | Serves 2

¾ cup frozen mixed berries (blueberries, raspberries, and blackberries)
¼ cup full-fat sour cream
½ cup full-fat coconut milk
¼ cup water
1½ tablespoons all-natural peanut butter (no added sugar)
½ tablespoon granulated erythritol/monk fruit blend (optional)

1. In a blender, blend the frozen mixed berries, sour cream, coconut milk, water, peanut butter, and erythritol/monk fruit blend (if using). Pulse a few times to get the ingredients to fall to the bottom, and blend for about 1 minute, or until smooth. If the blender struggles, add a few tablespoons of water and try again. Serve and enjoy immediately.

Per Serving
calories: 266 | fat: 23g | protein: 5g | carbs: 11g net carbs: 9g | fiber: 2g

583. Raspberry and Kale Smoothie

Prep time: 10 minutes | Cook time: 0 minutes | Serves 2

1 cup water
½ cup raspberries
½ cup shredded kale
¾ cup cream cheese
1 tablespoon coconut oil
1 scoop vanilla protein powder

1. Put the water, raspberries, kale, cream cheese, coconut oil, and protein powder in a blender and blend until smooth.
2. Pour into 2 glasses and serve immediately.

Per Serving
calories: 436 | fat: 36g | protein: 28g | carbs: 11g net carbs: 6g | fiber: 5g

584. Creamy Cashew Lemon Smoothie

Prep time: 5 minutes | Cook time: 0 minutes | Serves 1

1 cup unsweetened cashew milk
¼ cup heavy (whipping) cream
¼ cup freshly squeezed lemon juice
1 scoop plain protein powder
1 tablespoon coconut oil
1 teaspoon Swerve

1. Put the cashew milk, heavy cream, lemon juice, protein powder, coconut oil, and sweetener in a blender and blend until smooth.
2. Pour into a glass and serve immediately.

Per Serving
calories: 503 | fat: 45g | protein: 29g | carbs: 15g net carbs: 11g | fiber: 4g

585. Spinach and Cucumber Smoothie

Prep time: 5 minutes | Cook time: 0 minutes | Serves 1

1 small very ripe avocado, peeled and pitted
1 cup almond milk or water, plus more as needed
1 cup tender baby spinach leaves, stems removed
½ medium cucumber, peeled and seeded
1 tablespoon extra-virgin olive oil or avocado oil
8 to 10 fresh mint leaves, stems removed
Juice of 1 lime (about 1 to 2 tablespoons)

1. In a blender or a large wide-mouth jar, if using an immersion blender, combine the avocado, almond milk, spinach, cucumber, olive oil, mint, and lime juice and blend until smooth and creamy, adding more almond milk or water to achieve your desired consistency.

Per Serving
calories: 330 | fat: 30g | protein: 4g | carbs: 19g net carbs:10 g | fiber: 9g

586. Spinach-Cucumber Smoothie

Prep time: 5 minutes | Cook time: 0 minutes | Serves 2

1 cup coconut milk
1 cup spinach
½ English cucumber, chopped
½ cup blueberries
1 scoop plain protein powder
2 tablespoons coconut oil
4 ice cubes
Mint sprigs, for garnish

1. Put the coconut milk, spinach, cucumber, blueberries, protein powder, coconut oil, and ice in a blender and blend until smooth.
2. Pour into 2 glasses, garnish each with the mint, and serve immediately.

Per Serving
calories: 353 | fat: 32g | protein: 15g | carbs: 9g net carbs: 6g | fiber: 3g

587. Creamy Vanilla Smoothie

Prep time: 5 minutes | Cook time: 0 minutes | Serves 2

2 cups coconut milk
1 scoop vanilla protein powder
5 drops liquid stevia
1 teaspoon ground cinnamon
½ teaspoon alcohol-free vanilla extract

1. Put the coconut milk, protein powder, stevia, cinnamon, and vanilla in a blender and blend until smooth.
2. Pour into 2 glasses and serve immediately.

Per Serving
calories: 492 | fat: 47g | protein: 18g | carbs: 8g net carbs: 6g | fiber: 2g

588. Vanilla Coconut Smoothie

Prep time: 5 minutes | Cook time: 0 minutes | Serves 1

1 cup full-fat coconut milk
½ teaspoon vanilla extract
1 scoop vanilla bone broth protein
½ cup water
1 cup ice
Pinch of sea salt
2 to 3 drops liquid stevia (optional)

1. Place all the ingredients in a high-speed blender and blend until smooth.

Per Serving
calories: 549 | fat: 49g | protein: 25g | carbs: 9g net carbs: 9g | fiber: 0g

589. Double-Berry Coconut Smoothie

Prep time: 5 minutes | Cook time: 0 minutes | Serves 4

½ cup water
1½ cups coconut milk
1 cup frozen strawberries
2 cups fresh blueberries
¼ teaspoon vanilla extract
1 tablespoon protein powder

1. Using a blender, combine all the ingredients and blend well until you attain a uniform and creamy consistency. Divide in glasses and serve!

Per Serving
calories: 281 | fat: 22g | protein: 4g | carbs: 21g net carbs: 16g | fiber: 5g

590. Apple-Almond Butter Smoothie

Prep time: 5 minutes | Cook time: 0 minutes | Serves 1

½ Granny Smith apple, cored
¼ cup almond butter
½ cup coconut cream
½ cup unsweetened almond milk
½ tablespoon cinnamon
¼ teaspoon powdered ginger
5 to 10 drops liquid stevia
1 cup ice

1. Place all the ingredients in a high-speed blender and blend until smooth.

Per Serving
calories: 388 | fat: 33g | protein: 5g | carbs: 26g net carbs: 18g | fiber: 8g

591. Blueberry-Spinach Smoothie

Prep time: 5 minutes | Cook time: 0 minutes | Serves 1

½ cup full-fat coconut milk
½ cup fresh baby spinach
½ cup frozen wild blueberries
1 scoop keto collagen powder
1 tablespoon almond butter

1. Place all the ingredients in a high-speed blender and blend until smooth.

Per Serving
calories: 454 | fat: 36g | protein: 20g | carbs: 16g net carbs: 12g | fiber: 4g

592. Refreshing Green Smoothie

Prep time: 5 minutes | Cook time: 0 minutes | Serves 1

1 cup unsweetened almond, cashew, or coconut milk
½ medium cucumber, peeled and halved lengthwise
1 tablespoon vanilla protein powder
½ lime, peeled and seeded
1 tablespoon hemp seeds
1 avocado, sliced
1 cup frozen kale, stems removed
1 tablespoon coconut oil, melted
5 to 6 stevia drops
1 cup ice cubes

1. In a high-powered blender, combine the milk, cucumber, protein powder, lime, hemp seeds, avocado, kale, and coconut oil. Blend for 30 seconds.
2. Add the stevia and ice cubes, and then blend on high for 1 minute.
3. Pour into a glass and serve.

Per Serving
calories: 634 | fat: 46g | protein: 21g | carbs: 32g net carbs: 14g | fiber: 18g

593. Avocado Smoothie with Mixed Berries

Prep time: 5 minutes | Cook time: 0 minutes | Serves 4

1 avocado, pitted and sliced
3 cups mixed blueberries and strawberries
2 cups unsweetened almond milk
6 tablespoons heavy cream
2 teaspoons erythritol
1 cup ice cubes
⅓ cup nuts and seeds mix

1. Combine the avocado slices, blueberries, strawberries, almond milk, heavy cream, erythritol, ice cubes, nuts and seeds in a smoothie maker; blend in high-speed until smooth and uniform.
2. Pour the smoothie into drinking glasses, and serve immediately.

Per Serving
calories: 336 | fat: 25g | protein: 8g | carbs: 18g net carbs: 12g | fiber: 6g

594. Lemony Berry Smoothie

Prep time: 5 minutes | Cook time: 0 minutes | Serves 5

2 cups unsweetened vanilla almond milk
2 cups raspberries, fresh or frozen
1 cup blueberries, fresh or frozen
½ cup monk fruit/erythritol sweetener blend (1:1 sugar replacement)
½ cup almond butter, no sugar added
½ cup lemon juice
¼ cup chia seeds

1. In a blender, combine all the ingredients and blend until smooth. If using fresh berries, chill the smoothie for 30 minutes.

Per Serving
calories: 256 | fat: 18g | protein: 8g | carbs: 39g net carbs: 11g | fiber: 28g

595. Creamy Flaxseed-Ginger Smoothie

Prep time: 5 minutes | Cook time: 0 minutes | Serves 1

1 cup full-fat coconut milk
1 tablespoon coconut cream
1 teaspoon finely diced fresh ginger
½ teaspoon spirulina powder
¼ teaspoon ground cardamom
¼ teaspoon ground cinnamon
1 tablespoon vanilla protein powder
1 cup ice cubes
1 teaspoon flaxseed

1. In a high-powered blender, combine the coconut milk, coconut cream, ginger, spirulina, cardamom, and cinnamon. Blend for 30 seconds.
2. Add the protein powder and ice cubes, and blend on high for 1 minute.
3. Pour the smoothie into a glass, sprinkle the flaxseed on top, and enjoy.

Per Serving
calories: 708 | fat: 60g | protein: 15g | carbs: 27g net carbs: 19g | fiber: 8g

596. Coconut Strawberry Smoothie

Prep time: 5 minutes | Cook time: 0 minutes | Serves 1

¾ cup fresh strawberries, hulled, plus extra for garnish (optional)
1 cup coconut milk, chilled
2 tablespoons heavy whipping cream
2 tablespoons unsweetened coconut flakes
1 scoop unflavored collagen peptides
¼ teaspoon liquid stevia
¼ teaspoon pink Himalayan salt

1. Put all the ingredients in a blender and blend until smooth, 30 to 45 seconds. Pour into a glass and serve immediately, garnished with strawberries, if desired.

Per Serving
calories: 294 | fat: 23g | protein: 12g | carbs: 13g net carbs: 9g | fiber: 4g

597. Spinach and Hemp Heart Smoothie

Prep time: 5 minutes | Cook time: 0 minutes | Serves 1

1 cup frozen spinach
1 cup unsweetened almond milk
2 tablespoons hemp hearts
1 tablespoon MCT oil
1 scoop chocolate-flavored protein powder

1. Put all the ingredients in a blender and blend until smooth, 30 to 45 seconds. Pour into a glass and serve immediately.

Per Serving
calories: 416 | fat: 27g | protein: 35g | carbs: 7g net carbs: 4g | fiber: 3g

598. Avocado and Almond Smoothie

Prep time: 5 minutes | Cook time: 0 minutes | Serves 2

⅓ ripe avocado, peeled and pitted
3 teaspoons cacao powder, unsweetened
¼ teaspoon grated nutmeg
2 teaspoons granulated erythritol
1 cup almond milk
½ cup water

1. Purée all ingredients in a blender until smooth and uniform.
2. Spoon into two glasses and enjoy!

Per Serving
calories: 140 | fat: 9g | protein: 4g | carbs: 7g net carbs: 4g | fiber: 3g

599. Avocado and Seed Smoothie Bowl

Prep time: 5 minutes | Cook time: 0 minutes | Serves 2

½ ripe avocado, peeled and pitted
½ cup canned coconut milk
½ cup water
2 teaspoons sunflower seeds
2 tablespoons sesame seeds
2 teaspoons granulated erythritol
1 teaspoon ground cinnamon

1. Purée all the ingredients in your blender or food processor.
2. Divide the mixture between two serving bowls and serve well-chilled.

Per Serving
calories: 286 | fat: 28g | protein: 5g | carbs: 8g net carbs: 5g | fiber: 3g

600. Turmeric Avocado Smoothie

Prep time: 5 minutes | Cook time: 0 minutes | Serves 1

¾ cup full-fat coconut milk
¼ cup unsweetened almond milk
1 teaspoon ground turmeric
½ teaspoon ground ginger
¼ teaspoon cinnamon
¼ teaspoon freshly ground black pepper
1 scoop collagen protein
5 drops liquid stevia
5 to 6 ice cubes
½ avocado

1. Place all the ingredients, except the ice cubes and avocado, in a high-speed blender. Pulse several times.
2. Add the ice cubes and avocado and blend at high speed until smooth.

Per Serving
calories: 536 | fat: 51g | protein: 11g | carbs: 17g net carbs: 10g | fiber: 7g

Appendix 1: Measurement Conversion Chart

VOLUME EQUIVALENTS(DRY)

US STANDARD	METRIC (APPROXIMATE)
1/8 teaspoon	0.5 mL
1/4 teaspoon	1 mL
1/2 teaspoon	2 mL
3/4 teaspoon	4 mL
1 teaspoon	5 mL
1 tablespoon	15 mL
1/4 cup	59 mL
1/2 cup	118 mL
3/4 cup	177 mL
1 cup	235 mL
2 cups	475 mL
3 cups	700 mL
4 cups	1 L

VOLUME EQUIVALENTS(LIQUID)

US STANDARD	US STANDARD (OUNCES)	METRIC (APPROXIMATE)
2 tablespoons	1 fl.oz.	30 mL
1/4 cup	2 fl.oz.	60 mL
1/2 cup	4 fl.oz.	120 mL
1 cup	8 fl.oz.	240 mL
1 1/2 cup	12 fl.oz.	355 mL
2 cups or 1 pint	16 fl.oz.	475 mL
4 cups or 1 quart	32 fl.oz.	1 L
1 gallon	128 fl.oz.	4 L

WEIGHT EQUIVALENTS

US STANDARD	METRIC (APPROXIMATE)
1 ounce	28 g
2 ounces	57 g
5 ounces	142 g
10 ounces	284 g
15 ounces	425 g
16 ounces (1 pound)	455 g
1.5 pounds	680 g
2 pounds	907 g

TEMPERATURES EQUIVALENTS

FAHRENHEIT(F)	CELSIUS(C) (APPROXIMATE)
225 °F	107 °C
250 °F	120 °C
275 °F	135 °C
300 °F	150 °C
325 °F	160 °C
350 °F	180 °C
375 °F	190 °C
400 °F	205 °C
425 °F	220 °C
450 °F	235 °C
475 °F	245 °C
500 °F	260 °C

Appendix 2: Recipe Index

A

Alaskan Cod Fillet	71
Almond and Cinnamon Truffles	184
Almond Butter Fat Bombs	180
Almond Chocolate Cookies	176
Almond Flour Crusted Cheesecake	181
Almond Soup with Sour Cream and Cilantro	124
Almond-Peanut Butter Cheesecake	175
Almond-Sour Cream Cheesecake	175
Anchovies and Veggies Wraps	67
Anchovies with Caesar Dressing	67
Apple-Almond Butter Smoothie	191
Asian Peanut Sauce	23
Asian Salmon and Veggies Salad	69
Asian Scallop and Vegetable	82
Asian-Flavored Beef and Broccoli	55
Asparagus Parmesan Soup	131
Avocado and Almond Smoothie	193
Avocado and Berry Smoothie	189
Avocado and Ham Stuffed Eggs	157
Avocado and Seed Smoothie Bowl	193
Avocado Crostini Nori with Walnuts	148
Avocado Mayonnaise	18
Avocado Smoothie with Mixed Berries	192
Avocado-Bacon Stuffed Eggs	155
Avocado-Bacon Sushi	158
Avocado-Chocolate Pudding	174

B

Baby Arugula and Walnuts Salad	139
Bacon and Pork Omelet	34
Bacon Fat Browned Chicken	100
Bacon Frittata with Olives and Herbs	31
Bacon on Cheesy Chicken Breast	99
Bacon-Loaded Deviled Eggs	164
Bacon-Wrapped Chicken with Asparagus	92
Bacon-Wrapped Enoki Mushrooms	158
Bacon, Avocado, and Veggies Salad	137
Baked Broccoli Bites	153
Baked Cheesecake Bites	172
Baked Cheesy Chicken and Spinach	93
Baked Cheesy Chicken and Zucchini	96
Baked Cheesy Pork and Veggies	34
Baked Chicken and Chorizo Sausages	96
Baked Chicken in Tomato Purée	100
Baked Chicken Skewers and Celery Fries	97
Baked Cocktail Franks	164
Baked Halibut Steaks	76
Baked Pork Sausage and Bell Pepper	43
Baked Romano Zucchini Rounds	160
Baked Spinach Cheese Balls	148
Baked Stuffed Peppers with Olives	116
Baked Zucchini Sticks with Garlic Aioli	147
Balsamic Broccoli Salad	113
Balsamic Brussels Sprouts Cheese Salad	136
Balsamic Glazed Meatloaf	59
Balsamic Glazed Meatloaf	61
Balsamic Pork Loin Chops	36
Balsamic Pork Loin Chops	46
Balsamic Zucchini Salad	112
Banana Fat Bombs	180
Basil Dressing	20
Basil Feta Flank Steak Pinwheels	52
Basil Kale Pesto	22
Basil Lamb Shoulder with Pine Nuts	53
Basil Turkey Meatballs	90
BBQ Grilled Pork Spare Ribs	39
Beef and Cauliflower Curry with Cilantro	64
Beef and cauliflower rice Casserole	52
Beef and Egg cauliflower rice Bowls	65
Beef and Mushroom Cheeseburgers	54
Beef and Mushrooms in Red Wine	64
Beef and Onion Stuffed Zucchinis	54
Beef Brisket with Red Wine	53
Beef Casserole with Cauliflower	62
Beef Chuck Roast with Veggies	62
Beef Lasagna with Zucchinis	58
Beef Meatball Salad with Dilled Yogurt	61
Beef Meatloaf with Balsamic Glaze	60
Beef Ragout with Green Beans	56
Beef Sausage Casserole with Okra	57
Beef Steaks with Mushrooms and Bacon	59
Beef Stew with Black Olives	57
Beef-Cabbage Casserole	65
Beef-Stuffed Peppers	159
Beef-Stuffed Zucchini Boats	58
Blackberry Cobbler with Almonds	176
Blue Cheese and Ranch Dip	167
Blueberry-Almond Butter Smoothie	189
Blueberry-Almond Muffins	182
Blueberry-Pecan Crisp	177
Blueberry-Spinach Smoothie	191
Blueberry-Vanilla Pudding	183
Boiled Eggs with Lemony Avocado	29
Bolognese Sauce	19
Bolognese Sauce	20
Braised Chicken and Veggies	91
Braised Mushrooms and Cabbage	111
Braised Mushrooms with Parsley	110
Broccoli and Cauliflower Omelet	29
Broccoli Salad with Tahini Dressing	117
Broccoli-Cabbage Soup	107
Browned Chicken and Mushrooms	92
Buffalo Cheese Chicken Soup	130
Buttered Mushrooms with Sage	151
Buttered Pork Chops	37
Butternut Squash Soup	129
Buttery Habanero and Beef Balls	59
Button Mushroom Stroganoff	118

C

Caesar Salad with Chicken and Cheese	140
Caesar Salad with Salmon and Egg	134
Cajun Tilapia Fish Burgers	72
Cardamom Orange Bark	185
Catfish Flakes and Cauliflower Casserole	80
Cauli Rice with Cheddar and Bacon	155
Cauliflower and Celery Soup	104
Cauliflower Chowder with Fresh Dill	108

Cheddar Anchovies Fat Bombs	162	Classic PB and J Smoothie	190
Cheddar Buffalo Chicken Bake	145	Coconut Cheesy Cauliflower Soup	125
Cheese Crisps with Basil	166	Coconut Lemon Truffles with Pecans	179
Cheesecake Fat Bomb with Berries	171	Coconut Strawberry Smoothie	193
Cheesy Bacon Salad with Walnuts	142	Coconut-Chicken Breasts	97
Cheesy Bacon-Stuffed Jalapeño Poppers	168	Coconut-Chocolate Treats	182
Cheesy Beef Gratin	62	Coconut-Fudge Ice Pops	170
Cheesy Broccoli and Bacon Soup	131	Coconut-Vanilla Ice Pops	181
Cheesy Broccoli and Spinach Soup	129	Cod Fillet and Mustard Greens	77
Cheesy Broccoli Bake	107	Cod Fillet with Lemony Sesame Sauce	78
Cheesy Broccoli Soup	127	Cod Fillet with Parsley Pistou	81
Cheesy Cauli Bake with Mayo	146	Cod Fillet with Summer Salad	75
Cheesy Cauliflower Soup	124	Cod Patties with Creamed Horseradish	74
Cheesy Charcuterie Board	166	Coffee-Coconut Ice Pops	170
Cheesy Chicken and Tomato Packets	88	Colby Bacon-Wrapped Jalapeño Peppers	149
Cheesy Cod Fillet	76	Colby Broccoli Bake	111
Cheesy Egg-Stuffed Avocados	106	Colden Gazpacho Soup	123
Cheesy Green Salad with Bacon	138	Cooked Chicken in Creamy Spinach Sauce	91
Cheesy Ham and Chicken Bites	160	Cranberry Pork Roast	48
Cheesy Ham Pizza Rolls	154	Cream Cheese Chocolate Mousse	183
Cheesy Ham-Egg Cups	160	Creamsicle Float	173
Cheesy Hot Crab Sauce	19	Creamy Broccoli and Zucchini Soup	108
Cheesy Lemonade Fat Bomb	170	Creamy Broccoli-Spinach Soup	114
Cheesy Omelet and Vegetables	26	Creamy Cabbage and Cauliflower	112
Cheesy Pork Nachos	35	Creamy Caesar Dressing	18
Cheesy Pork Patties Salad	137	Creamy Cashew Lemon Smoothie	190
Cheesy Prosciutto Balls	161	Creamy Cauliflower and Leek Soup	129
Cheesy Shrimp Stuffed Mushrooms	70	Creamy Cauliflower Soup with Sausage	128
Cheesy Spinach Basil Pesto	21	Creamy Chicken Soup	127
Cheesy Spinach Stuffed Chicken	94	Creamy Chocolate Mousse	173
Cheesy Spinach Stuffed Chicken	99	Creamy Flaxseed-Ginger Smoothie	192
Cheesy Tilapia Omelet	81	Creamy Herb Dip	166
Cheesy Tomato and Onion Soup	130	Creamy Pork Chops and Canadian Ham	38
Cheesy Tomato Frittata	31	Creamy Reuben Soup with Sauerkraut	52
Cheesy Veggie Fritters	109	Creamy Strawberry Shake	171
Chepala Vepudu	83	Creamy Summer Stew with Chives	109
Chia Pudding with Blueberries	184	Creamy Tomato Soup	124
Chicken Breast Fritters with Dill Dip	146	Creamy Tomato Soup	131
Chicken Breast with Anchovy Tapenade	99	Creamy Tomato Soup with Basil	130
Chicken Fingers	95	Creamy Turkey and Celery Soup	121
Chicken Garam Masala	97	Creamy Vanilla Smoothie	191
Chicken in Creamy Mushroom Sauce	102	Creamy Vegetable Chowder	116
Chicken Paella and Chorizo	93	Creamy-Cheesy Cauliflower Soup	123
Chicken Wings in Spicy Tomato Sauce	163	Creamy-Lemony Chicken Soup	125
Chicken Wings with Ranch Dressing	160	Creamy-Lemony Chicken Thighs	92
Chicken with Mayo-Avocado Sauce	96	Creole Beef Tripe Stew with Onions	51
Chicken-Stuffed Cucumber Bites	145	Crispy Chorizo with Parsley	147
Chili Chicken Breast	98	Crispy Five Seed Crackers	158
Chinese Cabbage Stir-Fry	113	Crispy Fried Dill Pickles	161
Chocolate Brownie Cake	179	Crispy Strawberry Chocolate Bark	171
Chocolate Chip Ice Cream with Mint	173	Crustless Cheesy Quiche Lorraine	30
Chocolate Pecan-Berry Mascarpone Bowl	173	Curry Green Beans and Shrimp Soup	126
Chocolate-Coconut Shake	170	Curry Tilapia	80
Chunky Lemony Blue Cheese	19	Curry White Fish Fillet	68
Cioppino	123	Crispy Keto Creamy Fish Casserole	69
Citrus Asparagus and Cherry Tomato Salad	105		
Citrus Raspberry Custard Cake	176	**D**	
Classic Almond Golden Cake	180	Deviled Eggs with Chives	162
Classic Caprese Salad	142	Deviled Eggs with Roasted Peppers	161
Classic Caprese Skewers	163	Dijon Broccoli Slaw Salad	141
Classic Carnitas	48	Dijon Cauliflower Salad	142
Classic Devilled Eggs with Sriracha Mayo	146	Dijon Chicken Thighs	92
Classic Greek Salad	134	Dijon Egg Salad	143
Classic Jerk Chicken	89	Dijon Sea Bass Fillet	77

Dilled Egg Salad with Dijon Mayo	32
Double Cheese Braised Vegetables	116
Double Cheese Kale Bake	104
Double Cheese Stuffed Bell Peppers	25
Double-Berry Coconut Smoothie	191
Duo-Cheese Lettuce Rolls	154

E

Easy Dark Chocolate Fudge	180
Easy Peanut Butter Cookies	187
Easy Peanut Butter Smoothie	190
Easy Roasted Asparagus with Mayo Sauce	110
Egg and Bacon Muffins with Kale	30
Egg and Chicken Salad in Lettuce Cups	135
Egg Muffins	25
Egg, Scallion, Jalapeño Pepper Salad	27

F

Fajita Spareribs	157
Feta Zucchini and Pepper Gratin	149
Fettuccine Alfredo	20
Flank Steak and Kale Roll	62
French Scrambled Eggs	26
Fresh Homemade Guacamole	166
Fresh Strawberry Cheesecake Mousse	171
Fried Cauliflower Rice with Peppers	152
Fried Eggs with Canadian Bacon	31
Fried Veggies with Eggs	113

G

Gambas al Ajillo	68
Garlic Aioli Sauce	23
Garlicky Cauliflower-Pecan Casserole	117
Garlicky Chicken Salad	136
Garlicky Chicken Thighs	101
Garlicky Creamed Swiss Chard	107
Garlicky Lamb Chops in White Wine	54
Garlicky Lamb Chops with Sage	64
Garlicky Mackerel Fillet	68
Garlicky Mayonnaise	22
Garlicky Pork and Bell Peppers	48
Garlicky Roasted Broccoli	150
Garlicky Roasted Vegetable Mix	148
Garlicky Sweet Chicken Skewers	98
Garlicky Voodles with Avocado Sauce	117
Ginger-Pumpkin Pudding	174
Gingersnap Nutmeg Cookies	186
Goan Sole Fillet Stew	75
Goat Cheese Omelet	31
Goat Cheese Stuffed Squid	83
Golden Pork Burgers	37
Gouda Cauli-Broccoli Casserole	119
Greek Roasted Cauliflower with Feta Cheese	116
Greek Scrambled Eggs	28
Greek-Style Aubergine-Egg Casserole	106
Greek-Style Ricotta Olive Dip	163
Green Minestrone Soup	126
Grilled Beef Skewers with Fresh Salad	61
Grilled Lamb Kebabs	54
Grilled Lemony Chicken Wings	89
Grilled Prosciutto-Chicken Wraps	151
Grilled Ribeye Steaks with Green Beans	53
Grilled Salmon Steak	73
Ground Beef and Cauliflower Curry	52

H

Haddock and Turkey Smoked Sausage	82
Haddock with Mediterranean Sauce	67
Halászlé with Paprikash	83
Halloumi Asparagus Frittata	106
Ham, Cheese and Egg Cups	27
Hazelnut Shortbread Cookies	182
Healthy Blueberry Fat Bombs	187
Hearty Burger Dip	165
Hearty Pork Stew Meat	43
Hearty Stuffed Chicken	94
Hearty Veggie Stir-Fry	111
Heavy Cream-Cheese Broccoli Soup	130
Herbed Cheese Balls	25
Herbed Cheese Balls with Walnuts	113
Herbed Monkfish Fillet	79
Herbed Pork Chops with Cranberry Sauce	42
Herbed Pork Chops with Raspberry Sauce	47
Herbed Prawn and Veggie Skewers	159
Herbed Provolone Cheese Chips	157
Herbed Roasted Radishes	153
Herbed Turkey Breast	88
Herbed Turkey with Cucumber Salsa	87
Hollandaise Sauce	21
Homemade Albacore Tuna Salad	143
Homemade Coleslaw with Cauliflower	115
Homemade Dijon Vinaigrette	18
Homemade Pork Osso Bucco	45
Homemade Poulet en Papillote	101
Hungarian Chicken Thighs	91

I

Indian Tomato Soup with Raita	114
Italian Bacon Omelet	27
Italian Beef Roast with Jalapeño	63
Italian Broccoli and Spinach Soup	110
Italian Cheddar Cheese Crisps	165
Italian Fried Mozzarella Sticks	167
Italian Haddock Fillet	74
Italian Pepper and Mushrooms Stew	115
Itanlian Chicken Cacciatore	90

J

Jalapeño Pepper Cream Cheese Omelet	28
Juicy Beef Meatballs with Parsley	64
Juicy Beef with Thyme and Rosemary	55

K

Keto Almond Butter Fudge	179
Keto Matcha Brownies with Pistachios	186
Keto Peanut Butter Cookies	172
Keto Vanilla Ice Cream	183
King Size Beef Burgers	51

L

Lebanese Tabbouleh Salad	119
Lemon Custard	174
Lemon-Mint Grilled Lamb Chops	53
Lemon-Mustard Beef Rump Steak	63
Lemony Bacon Chips	167
Lemony Berry Smoothie	192
Lemony Chicken Skewers	94
Lemony Chicken Wings	91
Lemony Cucumber-Avocado Salad	105
Lemony Peanuts Pork Chops	36
Lemony Poppy Seed Cookies	186
Lemony Pork Chops and Brussel Sprouts	40
Lemony Pork Chops and Brussels Sprouts	46

Recipe	Page
Lemony Pork Chops with Veggies	39
Lemony Pork Loin and Brussels Sprouts	38
Lemony Pork Loin Roast	49
Lemony Prawn and Arugula Salad	134
Lemony Rosemary Chicken Thighs	87
Lemony Shrimp and Veggie Bowl	75
Lettuce Wraps with Ham and Tomato	164
Lime Brussels Sprout Chips	164
Liverwurst and Pistachio Balls	154
Lush Greek Salad	141
Lush Vegetable Soup	127

M

Recipe	Page
Macadamia Nut and Chocolate Fat Bombs	185
Mackerel and Green Bean Salad	137
Mackerel Fillet and Clam	84
Mahi Mahi Ceviche	77
Mangalore-Style Egg Curry	32
Margherita Pizza with Mushrooms	168
Marinara Sauce	21
Marinated Chicken with Peanut Sauce	95
Mascarpone Beef Balls with Cilantro	56
Mascarpone Turkey Pastrami Pinwheels	150
Mashed Cauliflower with Bacon and Chives	147
Mediterranean Aïoli	25
Mediterranean Cauliflower Quiche	114
Mediterranean Halibut Fillet	74
Mediterranean Pork	36
Mediterranean Shakshuka	30
Mediterranean Tomato and Avocado Salad	135
Mexican Chicken Mole	98
Mexican Shrimp-Stuffed Avocados	167
Mexican-Flavored Stuffed Peppers	106
Microwaved Rhubarb Cakes	184
Mini Bacon and Kale Muffins	157
Monkfish Mayonnaise Salad	77
Morning Five Greens Smoothie	189
Mozzarella Bacon and Tomato Salad	138
Mozzarella Creamed Salad with Basil	118
Mozzarella Meatballs	165
Mozzarella Prosciutto Wraps with Basil	152
Mushroom and Bell Pepper Omelet	104
Mushroom and Zucchini Stew	104
Mustard Eggs Salad	140
Mustard Pork Meatballs	34

N

Recipe	Page
Nacho Soup	122
New Orleans Halibut and Crabmeat	79
No-Bake Hemp Seeds and Chocolate Cookies	185

O

Recipe	Page
Oasted Chicken	102
Old Bay Prawns	79
Old Bay Sea Bass Fillet	73
Old-fashioned Gingerbread Cake	178
Old-Fashioned Greek Tirokroketes	29
Oregano Balsamic Vinegar	23
Oven Baked String Beans and Mushrooms	155
Oven-Baked Prosciutto-Wrapped Asparagus	168

P

Recipe	Page
Paprika Chicken with Steamed Broccoli	99
Paprika Egg Salad with Mayo	29
Paprika Roast Beef Brisket	63
Paprika Veggie Bites	159
Parma Ham-Wrapped Stuffed Chicken	101
Parmesan Bacon-Stuffed Pork Roll	44
Parmesan Cauliflower Fritters	150
Parmesan Chicken Wings with Yogurt Sauce	102
Parmesan Crab Dip	162
Parmesan Creamed Spinach	151
Parmesan Zoodles with Avocado Sauce	112
Peanut Butter Crêpes with Coconut	105
Peanut Butter Cupcake	177
Pecan-Carrot Muffins	178
Pecorino Mushroom Burgers	148
Peppery Omelet with Cheddar Cheese	112
Pesto Turkey with Zucchini Spaghetti	90
Pork and Beef Meatballs	34
Pork and Butternut Squash Stew	42
Pork and Mashed Cauliflower Crust	35
Pork and Vegetable Soup	126
Pork and Veggies Burgers	37
Pork and Yellow Squash Traybake	42
Pork Chops and Bacon	35
Pork Chops with Blackberry Gravy	38
Pork Chops with Broccoli	37
Pork Chops with Greek Salsa	41
Pork Kofte with Cauliflower Mash	45
Pork Lettuce Wraps	40
Pork Loin Chops	40
Pork Meatballs in Pasta Sauce	43
Pork Medallions with Rosemary	39
Pork Patties with Caramelized Onion Rings	49
Pork Pie	45
Pork Shoulder and Sauerkraut Casserole	36
Pork Steaks with Broccoli	40
Pork Steaks with Chimichurri Sauce	35
Pork Tenderloin with Lemon Chimichurri	47
Pork with Cranberry Sauce	47
Pork with Raspberry Sauce	39
Pork Wraps with Veggies	44
Power Green Soup	124
Prosciutto and Egg Muffins	28
Prosciutto-Wrapped Piquillo Peppers	149
Provençal Lemony Fish Stew	71
Provençal Ratatouille Casserole	119
Provolone Zucchini Lasagna	108
Pumpkin Cheesecake Bites	172
Pumpkin Compote with Mix Berries	175
Pumpkin-Almond Fat Bombs	182

R

Recipe	Page
Rack of Lamb with Pepper Butter Sauce	57
Ranch Chicken-Bacon Dip	165
Raspberry and Chocolate Fat Bombs	187
Raspberry and Kale Smoothie	190
Red Curry Shrimp and Bean Soup	128
Red Snapper Fillet and Salad	75
Refreshing Green Smoothie	192
Reuben Beef Soup	126
Rich Cheesy Bacon-Cauliflower Soup	121
Rich Taco Soup	121
Ricotta Spinach Gnocchi	149
Ritzy Baked Chicken with Vegetable	93
Ritzy Chicken Salad with Tzatziki Sauce	139
Roast Herbs Stuffed Chicken	90
Roasted Brussels Sprouts with Balsamic Glaze	145
Roasted Brussels Sprouts with Balsamic Glaze	154

Roasted Cauliflower with Serrano Ham	145
Roasted Chicken Breasts with Capers	86
Roasted Stuffed Pork Loin Steak	44
Romano Cheese Meatballs	163
Rosemary Lamb Chops	46
Rosemary-Lemon Snapper Fillet	82
Rump Steak Salad	60

S

Saffron Coconut Shrimp Soup	122
Salmon Fillet	78
Salmon Fillet and Spinach Cobb Salad	135
Salmon Tacos with Guajillo Sauce	76
Salsa Verde Chicken Soup	127
Sardine Burgers	69
Sausage Frittatas with Goat Cheese	32
Scallops and Calamari	81
Scrambled Eggs and Baby Spinach	26
Scrambled Eggs with Swiss Chard Pesto	150
Seafood Chowder	68
Seared Ribeye Steak with Shitake Mushrooms	63
Shirataki Mushroom Ramen	105
Shrimp and Sea Scallop	78
Shrimp Jambalaya	72
Shrimp Salad with Lemony Mayonnaise	136
Shrimp, Cauliflower and Avocado Salad	138
Simple Blueberry Fat Bombs	181
Simple Boiled Stuffed Eggs	147
Simple Buttery Broccoli	146
Simple Peanut Butter Fat Bomb	172
Sirloin Steak Skewers with Ranch Dressing	55
Sirloin Steak with Sauce Diane	58
Skirt Steak and Pickled Peppers Salad	141
Skirt Steak with Green Beans	51
Skirt Steak, Veggies, and Pecan Salad	138
Slow Cooked Chicken Cacciatore	87
Slow Cooked Faux Lasagna Soup	125
Slow Cooked Spaghetti Squash	115
Slow Cooker Chocolate Pot De Crème	174
Smoked Haddock Burgers	72
Smoked Mackerel and Turnip Patties	153
Smoked Paprika Beef Ragout	60
Sole Fish Jambalaya	71
Spanish Cod à La Nage	73
Spanish Queso Sauce	22
Spiced Baked Gruyere Crisps	155
Spiced Chicken Breast	87
Spiced Chicken Wings	88
Spiced Cucumber Soup	132
Spiced Mashed Cauliflower	110
Spiced Pistachio-Lemon Smoothie	189
Spiced Pumpkin Soup	132
Spiced-Pumpkin Soup	122
Spicy Almond Fat Bombs	184
Spicy Brown Mushroom Omelet	26
Spicy Chicken Drumettes	159
Spicy Chicken Skewers	89
Spicy Chicken Soup	128
Spicy Enchilada Sauce	19
Spicy Onion Rings	153
Spicy Pork and Capers with Olives	44
Spicy Roasted Eggplant with Avocado	118
Spicy Tiger Prawns	76
Spinach and Cucumber Smoothie	190
Spinach and Egg Salad	117
Spinach and Hemp Heart Smoothie	193
Spinach and Zucchini Chowder	109
Spinach Mozzarella Soup	132
Spinach-Cucumber Smoothie	191
Spring Vegetable Salad with Cheese Balls	139
Sriracha Mayonnaise	20
Stewed Pork and Veggies	38
Stir-Fried Chicken, Broccoli and Cashew	95
Stir-Fried Scallops with Cauliflower	84
Strawberries in Chocolate	187
Strawberry and Spinach Salad	137
Strawberry Popsicles	185
Super Easy Peanut Butter Mousse	179
Swedish Herring and Spinach Salad	73
Swiss Zucchini Gratin	107
Swordfish with Greek Yogurt Sauce	84

T-V

Tangy Avocado Crema	18
Tangy Cucumber and Avocado Soup	121
Tangy Pork Rib Roast	41
Tangy Shrimp Ceviche Salad	141
Tangy Squid and Veggies Salad	140
Tangy-Garlicky Pork Chops	41
Tender Almond Pound Cake	178
Thai Tuna Fillet	74
Three-Cheese Beef Sausage Casserole	65
Tilapia and Shrimp Soup	80
Tilapia Fillet	78
Tomato purée Pork Chops	45
Traditional Chicken Stroganoff	100
Traditional Italian Bolognese Sauce	55
Traditional Thai Tom Kha Soup	115
Traditional Walnut Fat Bombs	158
Tuna Cheese Caprese Salad	136
Tuna Fillet Salade Niçoise	67
Tuna Niçoise Salad	70
Tuna Salad with Olives and Lettuce	134
Tuna-Mayo Topped Dill Pickles	151
Tuna, Ham and Avocado Wraps	72
Turkey and Avocado Roll-Ups	162
Turkey and Pumpkin Ragout	89
Turkey and Veggies Soup	131
Turkey and Walnuts Salad	143
Turmeric Avocado Smoothie	193
Turnip and Soup with Pork Sausage	129
Tuscan Chicken Breast Sauté	86
Tuscan Kale Salad with Lemony Anchovies	140
Two-Cheese Sausage Balls	32
Tzatziki Sauce	22
Vanilla Coconut Smoothie	191
Vanilla-Flavored Hazelnut Ice Cream	177
Vanilla-Raspberry Cheesecake	183
Vegetable Stir-Fry with Seeds	109
Veggie cauliflower rice with Beef Steak	56
Vinegary Cucumber Salad	143

W-Z

Whiskey-Glazed Chicken Wings	161
White Chowder	70
White Mushroom Cream Soup with Herbs	128
Yogurt and Swiss Cheese Soup	27
Zoodles with Almond-Basil Pesto	152
Zoodles with Beef Bolognese Sauce	51

CPSIA information can be obtained
at www.ICGtesting.com
Printed in the USA
BVHW062116300721
613251BV00004B/586